VOLUME **1**

Neurostimulation for the Treatment of Chronic Pain

Interventional and Neuromodulatory Techniques for Pain Management

VOLUME

1 Neurostimulation for the Treatment of Chronic Pain

Volume Editors

Salim M. Hayek, MD, PhD

Associate Professor
Department of Anesthesiology
Case Western Reserve University
Chief
Division of Pain Medicine
University Hospitals, Case Medical Center
Cleveland, Ohio

Robert Levy, MD, PhD

Professor of Neurological Surgery, Physiology, and Radiation Oncology
Feinberg School of Medicine
Northwestern University
Chicago, Illinois

Series Editor

Timothy R. Deer, MD, DABPM, FIPP

President and CEO
The Center for Pain Relief
Clinical Professor of Anesthesiology
West Virginia University School of Medicine
Charleston, West Virginia

ELSEVIER
SAUNDERS

1600 John F. Kennedy Blvd.
Ste 1800
Philadelphia, PA 19103-2899

NEUROSTIMULATION FOR THE TREATMENT OF CHRONIC PAIN
(Volume 1: A Volume in the Interventional and Neuromodulatory
Techniques for Pain Management Series by Timothy Deer)   ISBN: 978-1-4377-2216-1

Library of Congress Cataloging-in-Publication Data
Interventional and neuromodulatory techniques for pain management.
    p. ; cm.
  Includes bibliographical references and indexes.
    ISBN 978-1-4377-3791-2 (series package : alk. paper)—ISBN 978-1-4377-2216-1 (hardcover, v. 1 : alk. paper)—
ISBN 978-1-4377-2217-8 (hardcover, v. 2 : alk. paper)—ISBN 978-1-4377-2218-5 (hardcover, v. 3 : alk. paper)—
ISBN 978-1-4377-2219-2 (hardcover, v. 4 : alk. paper)—ISBN 978-1-4377-2220-8 (hardcover, v. 5 : alk. paper)
    1. Pain—Treatment.   2. Nerve block.   3. Spinal anesthesia.   4. Neural stimulation.   5. Analgesia.
  I. Deer, Timothy R.
    [DNLM: 1. Pain—drug therapy.   2. Pain—surgery.   WL 704]
    RB127.I587 2012
    616′.0472—dc23

                                                                        2011018904

Acquisitions Editor: Pamela Hetherington
Developmental Editor: Lora Sickora
Publishing Services Manager: Jeff Patterson
Project Manager: Megan Isenberg
Design Direction: Lou Forgione

Printed in China

Last digit is the print number: 9   8   7   6   5   4   3   2   1

For Missy for all your love and support.

For Morgan, Taylor, Reed, and Bailie for your inspiration.

To those who have taught me a great deal:
John Rowlingson, Richard North, Giancarlo Barolat, Sam Hassenbusch,
Elliot Krames, K. Dean Willis, Peter Staats, Nagy Mekhail, Robert Levy, David Caraway,
Kris Kumar, Joshua Prager, and Jim Rathmell.

To my team:
Christopher Kim, Richard Bowman, Matthew Ranson, Doug Stewart,
Wilfredo Tolentino, Jeff Peterson, and Michelle Miller.

Timothy R. Deer

To my parents who raised me to be who I am today.
To Timothy Deer for his confidence in me and for his friendship.
To my mentors and teachers who generously taught me invaluable skills.
Most importantly, to my wife Addie—mother of our beautiful children Elena, Zoe, and
Michael—for her endless love, support, and understanding.

Salim M. Hayek

To our patients.

Robert Levy

Contributors

Marina V. Abramova, MD
Department of Neurosurgery, LSU Health Sciences Center, New Orleans, Louisiana
Chapter 13, Nerve Root, Sacral, and Pelvic Stimulation

Kenneth M. Alò, MD
Clinical Member, The Methodist Hospital Research Institute; President, Houston Texas Pain Management, Houston, Texas
Houston Texas Pain Management, Houston, Texas
Chapter 13, Nerve Root, Sacral, and Pelvic Stimulation

Tipu Z. Aziz, MD, DMEDSC, FRCS(SN)
Consultant Neurosurgeon and Professor of Neurosurgery, Oxford Functional Neurosurgery, Department of Neurological Surgery, The West Wing, Nuffield Department of Surgery, Oxford University, The John Radcliffe Hospital, Oxford, United Kingdom
Chapter 22, Deep Brain Stimulation

Diaa Bahgat, MD
Lecturer, Fayoum University, Al Fayyum, Egypt; Fellow, Stereotactic and Functional Neurosurgery, Department of Neurological Surgery, Oregon Health & Science University, Portland, Oregon
Chapter 16, Peripheral Nerve Stimulation

Giancarlo Barolat, MD
Director, Barolat Neuroscience; Presbyterian/St. Luke's Medical Center, Denver, Colorado
Chapter 20, Peripheral Subcutaneous Stimulation for Intractable Pain

David Barrows, MD
Assistant Professor, Department of Anesthesia, Uniformed Services University of the Health Sciences, Bethesda, Maryland; Staff Anesthesiologist, Department of Anesthesia, Walter Reed National Military Medical Center, Bethesda, Maryland
Chapter 11, Spinal Cord Stimulation for Refractory Angina and Peripheral Vascular Disease

Marshall D. Bedder, MD, FRCP (C)
Director, Department of Interventional Pain, Pacific Medical Centers, Seattle, Washington
Chapter 15, Complications of Spinal Cord Stimulation

Kim J. Burchiel, MD
John Raaf Professor and Chairman, Department of Neurological Surgery, Oregon Health & Science University, Portland, Oregon
Chapter 16, Peripheral Nerve Stimulation

Timothy R. Deer, MD, DABPM, FIPP
President and CEO, The Center for Pain Relief, Clinical Professor of Anesthesiology, West Virginia University School of Medicine, Charleston, West Virginia
Chapter 19, Occipital Neurostimulation;
Chapter 23, Coding and Billing for Neurostimulation

Daniel M. Doleys, PhD
Director, Pain and Rehabilitation Institute, Birmingham, Alabama
Chapter 4, Patient Selection: Psychological Considerations

Steven M. Falowksi, MD
Physician, Department of Neurological Surgery, Thomas Jefferson University Hospitals, Philadelphia, Pennsylvania
Chapter 5, Spinal Cord Stimulation: General Indications

Claudio Andres Feler, MD, FACS
Associate Professor, Department of Neurosurgery, University of Tennessee Health Sciences, Memphis, Tennessee
Chapter 7, Spinal Cord Stimulation: Parameter Selection and Equipment Choices;
Chapter 21, Motor Cortex Stimulation for Relief of Chronic Pain

Robert D. Foreman, PhD, FAHA
George Lynn Cross Research Professor, Department of Physiology, University of Oklahoma Health Sciences Center, Oklahoma City, Oklahoma
Chapter 2, Mechanisms of Spinal Neuromodulation

Salim M. Hayek, MD, PhD
Associate Professor, Department of Anesthesiology, Case Western Reserve University; Chief, Division of Pain Medicine, University Hospitals, Case Medical Center, Cleveland, Ohio
Chapter 3, Medical Considerations in Spinal Cord Stimulation;
Chapter 9, Neurostimulation in Complex Regional Pain Syndrome;
Chapter 19, Occipital Neurostimulation

Marc A. Huntoon, MD
Professor of Anesthesiology, Department of Anesthesiology, College of Medicine, Mayo Clinic, Rochester, Minnesota
Chapter 18, Peripheral Nerve Stimulation: Percutaneous Technique

Leonardo Kapural, MD, PhD
Professor of Anesthesiology, Wake Forest University, School of Medicine; Director, Pain Medicine Center, Wake Forest Baptist Health, Winston-Salem, North Carolina
Chapter 12, Spinal Cord Stimulation for Visceral Abdominal Pain

Al-Amin A. Khalil, MD
Associate Professor, Department of Anesthesiology, Case Western Reserve University, University Hospitals, Cleveland, Ohio
Chapter 3, Medical Considerations in Spinal Cord Stimulation

Krishna Kumar, MB, MS, FRCS (C), FACS
Department of Neurosurgery, Regina General Hospital, Regina, Saskatchewan, Canada
Chapter 10, Spinal Cord Stimulation for Peripheral Vascular Disease

Bengt Linderoth, MD, PhD
Professor and Head, Functional Neurosurgery and Applied Neuroscience Research Program, Department of Neurosurgery, Karolinska Institutet and Karolinska University Hospital, Stockholm, Sweden; Adjunct Professor, Department of Physiology, University of Oklahoma Health Sciences Center, Oklahoma City, Oklahoma
Chapter 2, Mechanisms of Spinal Neuromodulation

Andre G. Machado, MD, PhD
Director, Center for Neurological Restoration, Department of Neurosurgery, Neurological Institute, Cleveland Clinic, Cleveland, Ohio
Chapter 6, Spinal Cord Stimulation: Implantation Techniques

Sean Mackey, MD, PhD
Chief, Division of Pain Management, Associate Professor, Department of Anesthesiology, Stanford University, Palo Alto, California
Chapter 11, Spinal Cord Stimulation for Refractory Angina and Peripheral Vascular Disease

Patrick J. McIntyre, MD, JD
Assistant Professor, Department of Anesthesiology, University Hospitals Case Medical Center, Cleveland, Ohio
Chapter 15, Complications of Spinal Cord Stimulation

Jonathan Miller, MD
Director, Functional and Restorative Neurosurgery; Assistant Professor of Neurosurgery, University Hospitals, Case Medical Center, Case Western Reserve University, Cleveland, Ohio
Chapter 16, Peripheral Nerve Stimulation

Sean Nagel, MD
Clinical Fellow, Center for Neurological Restoration, Department of Neurosurgery, Neurological Institute, Cleveland Clinic, Cleveland, Ohio
Chapter 6, Spinal Cord Stimulation: Implantation Techniques

Samer Narouze, MD, MSc, DABPM, FIPP
Clinical Professor of Anesthesiology and Pain Medicine, OUCOM; Clinical Professor of Neurological Surgery, OSU; Associate Professor of Surgery, NEOUCOM; Chairman, Center for Pain Medicine, Summa Western Reserve Hospital, Cuyahoga Falls, Ohio
Chapter 19, Occipital Neurostimulation

Rita Nguyen, MD
College of Medicine, Regina General Hospital, Regina, Saskatchewan, Canada
Chapter 10, Spinal Cord Stimulation for Peripheral Vascular Disease

James L. North, MD
Clinical Assistant Professor, Department of Anesthesiology and Pain Medicine, Wake Forest University Health Sciences; Chief of Pain Medicine, Department of Pain Medicine, Forsyth Medical Center; Attending Physician, Carolinas Pain Institute, Winston-Salem, North Carolina
Chapter 6, Spinal Cord Stimulation: Implantation Techniques

Richard B. North, MD
Professor (retired), Departments of Neurosurgery, Anesthesiology, and Critical Care Medicine, Johns Hopkins University School of Medicine, Baltimore, Maryland; Sinai Hospital, Baltimore, Maryland
Chapter 8, Spinal Cord Stimulation as a Treatment of Failed Back Surgery Syndrome

Erlick A.C. Pereira, MA, BM, BCH, MRCS(ENG)
Specialty Registrar in Neurosurgery, Department of Neurological Surgery, The West Wing, Nuffield Department of Surgery, Oxford University, The John Radcliffe Hospital, Oxford, United Kingdom
Chapter 22, Deep Brain Stimulation

Jeffrey T.B. Peterson
Chief Operating Officer, The Center for Pain Relief, Charleston, West Virginia
Chapter 1, History of Neurostimulation; Chapter 23, Coding and Billing for Neurostimulation

Joshua P. Prager, MD, MS
Clinical Assistant Professor of Medicine, Clinical Assistant Professor of Anesthesiology, David Geffen School of Medicine at UCLA; Director, California Pain Medicine Centers, Center for Rehabilitation of Pain Syndromes (CRPS), Los Angeles, California
Chapter 9, Neurostimulation in Complex Regional Pain Syndrome

Matthew T. Ranson, MD
Assistant Director, Staff Physician, Center for Pain Relief, St. Francis Hospital, Charleston, West Virginia
Chapter 25, The Future of Neurostimulation

Richard L. Rauck, MD
Medical Director, Carolinas Pain Institute, Center for Clinical Research, Winston-Salem, North Carolina
Chapter 6, Spinal Cord Stimulation: Implantation Techniques

Erich O. Richter, MD
Department of Neurosurgery, LSU Health Sciences Center, New Orleans, Louisiana
Chapter 13, Nerve Root, Sacral, and Pelvic Stimulation

Binit J. Shah, MD
Senior Instructor, Department of Psychiatry, Case Western Reserve University, University Hospitals, Cleveland, Ohio
Chapter 3, Medical Considerations in Spinal Cord Stimulation

Ashwini Sharan, MD
Associate Professor, Program Director, Department of Neurosurgery, Jefferson Medical College, Philadelphia, Pennsylvania
Chapter 5, Spinal Cord Stimulation: General Indications

Konstantin V. Slavin, MD
Professor of Stereotactic and Functional Neurosurgery, Department of Neurosurgery, University of Illinois at Chicago, Chicago, Illinois
Chapter 14, Emerging Indications and Other Applications of Spinal Cord Stimulation

Michael Stanton-Hicks, MB, BS, MD, FRCA, ABPM, FIPP
Professor, Department of Anesthesia, Case Western Reserve University, Lerner School of Medicine; Staff Physician, Department of Pain Management, Cleveland Clinic; Consulting Staff, Department of Pediatric Pain Rehabilitation, Shaker Campus, Cleveland Clinic; Joint Staff, Center for Neurological Restoration, Cleveland Clinic, Cleveland, Ohio
Chapter 17, Peripheral Nerve Stimulation: Open Technique

Durga Sure, MD
Department of Neurosurgery, LSU Health Sciences Center, New Orleans, Louisiana
Chapter 13, Nerve Root, Sacral, and Pelvic Stimulation

Rebecca J. Taylor, MSC(EXON), MSC(BHAM)
Freelance Health Economist, Exeter, United Kingdom
Chapter 24, Cost-Effectiveness of Neurostimulation

Rod S. Taylor, MSC(LONDON)
Professor in Health Services Research, Scientific Director of
Peninsula Clinical Trials Unit, Peninsula College of Medicine &
Dentistry, University of Exeter, Exeter, United Kingdom
Chapter 24, Cost-Effectiveness of Neurostimulation

I. Elias Veizi, MD, PhD
Clinical Fellow, Department of Anesthesiology, Division of Pain
Medicine, Case Western Reserve University, University Hospitals
Case Medical Center, Cleveland, Ohio
Chapter 9, Neurostimulation in Complex Regional Pain Syndrome

Ashwin Viswanathan, MD
Assistant Professor, Director of Functional Neurosurgery,
Baylor College of Medicine, Houston, Texas; Department of
Neurological Surgery, Oregon Health & Science University,
Portland, Oregon
Chapter 16, Peripheral Nerve Stimulation

Chengyuan Wu, MD, MSBME
Resident Physician, Department of Neurological Surgery, Thomas
Jefferson University Hospitals, Philadelphia, Pennsylvania
Chapter 5, Spinal Cord Stimulation: General Indications

Preface

The use of electricity for painful disorders is not new and has a long and varied history; however, after Melzack and Wall[1] introduced the gate control theory of pain in 1965, it was not too far thereafter that medical innovators introduced modern day neuromodulatory techniques for the control of pain.[2] Today, neuromodulation remains one of the fastest growing fields in modern medicine.[3] Neuromodulation has the ability to help millions of people with varied disorders and diseases that include, but are not limited to, psychiatric disorders such as refractory depression, obsessive compulsive disorder or Tourette syndrome, disorders of movement such as epilepsy, Parkinson's disease or dystonia, diseases of the heart such as angina or disorders of rhythm, autonomic diseases such as congestive heart failure or hypertension, a multitude of chronic painful disorders such as pain from failed back surgery syndrome, atypical face pain, tic douloureux, complex regional pain syndromes, diabetic neuropathy, migraines and many more, dysmotility disorders of the stomach and gut, painful and functional bladder disorders, etc.

In this first volume (Volume 1: *Neurostimulation for the Treatment of Chronic Pain*) of a series of volumes titled, *Interventional and Neuromodulatory Techniques for Pain Management*, Dr. Timothy Deer has put together some of the leading experts of the field to address neurostimulation techniques for the control of chronic painful disorders. This volume is quite extensive and authoritative and includes, to name only a few, chapters on the history of neurostimulation, an overview of spinal cord stimulation, peripheral nerve stimulation techniques, stimulation for spinal disorders, visceral pain syndromes, occipital headaches and angina pectoris and stimulation of the brain. This volume also includes procedural videos of spinal cord, peripheral nerve, and deep brain stimulation that can be viewed on the companion website at www.expcrtconsult.com.

It is my great honor as a student of neuromodulation to recommend this volume to all interested in neurostimulation. This volume should be of interest to medical students, physicians and nurses who treat chronic pain, neurosurgeons, neurologists, bioengineers, device manufacturers and their representatives, insurers and those who invest in devices to improve function in man.

Elliot S. Krames, MD
Medical Director, Pacific Pain Treatment Center,
San Francisco, California
Past Editor in Chief of Neuromodulation: Technology at
the Neural Interface, *Journal of the International*
Neuromodulation Society
Past President, the International Neuromodulation Society

---

1. Melzack R, Wall PD: Pain mechanisms: a new theory. *Science* (150):971-979, 1965.
2. Shealy CN, Mortimer JT, Reswick JB: Electrical inhibition of pain by stimulation of the dorsal columns. Preliminary clinical report. *Anesth Analg* (Cleve) (46):489-491, 1967.
3. Krames ES, Peckham PH, Rezai AR, Aboelsaad F: What is neuromodulation? In Krames ES, Peckham PH, Rezai AR, editors: *Neuromodulation*, London, 2009, Academic Press.

Acknowledgments

I would like to acknowledge Jeff Peterson for his hard work on making this project a reality, and Michelle Miller for her diligence to detail on this and all projects that cross her desk.

I would like to acknowledge Lora Sickora, Pamela Hetherington, and Megan Isenberg for determination, attention to detail, and desire for excellence in bringing this project to fruition. Finally, I'd like to acknowledge Samer Narouze for his diligent work filming and reviewing the procedural videos associated with all of the volumes in the series. Robert Levy would like to acknowledge the editorial assistance of Mary J. Bockman, M.A.

Timothy R. Deer

Contents

I General Considerations

1 History of Neurostimulation

Jeffrey T. B. Peterson

CHAPTER OVERVIEW

Chapter Synopsis: The history of neurostimulation for pain relief reaches back nearly 2000 years to Greece. As with many ancient remedies, healers made use of the natural physiology of an animal—in this case the electrical discharge from a torpedo fish. Since then electrical stimulation devices have come a long way, as has our understanding of the underlying mechanisms. History shows that physicians in Europe and the United States shepherded this development through the 18th and 19th centuries. Even Ben Franklin made a well intended although ill-fated foray into medical research with electrostimulation. The popularity of neurostimulation in the early 20th century seemed to reach its culmination with the advent of a colorfully named and widely used device called the Electreat, an early version of today's more sophisticated transcutaneous electrical nerve stimulation (TENS) devices. With the establishment of Melzack and Wall's gate control theory of pain in the 1960s, clinical neurostimulation underwent a more informed evolution. Norman Shealy's contributions led to both scientific and technological advances. Eventually experiments revealed the efficacy of deep brain stimulation for relief of central pain and other conditions. Although an ancient practice, the benefits of neurostimulation have likely not yet been entirely revealed or appreciated.

Important Points:
- The first documented use of neurostimulation for pain relief occurred around 63 AD.
- The Leyden jar was one of the first methods of harnessing electrical current.
- The Melzack-Wall gate control theory was a defining event in the use of neurostimulation in modern medicine.
- Medtronic received Food and Drug Administration approval in the late 1960s to distribute devices for the treatment of pain.
- Ballard D. Wright[13] described the use of the block-aid monitor in 1969 for nerve stimulation.
- In 1991 Tsubokawa[10] made key advances in motor cortex stimulation for central pain control.

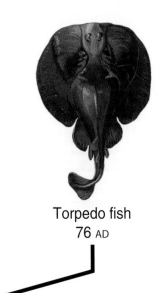

Torpedo fish
76 AD

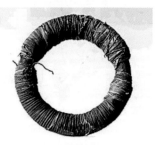

Faraday
transformer
1831

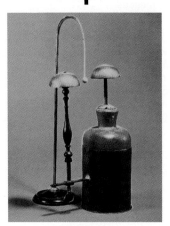

Leyden jar
1745

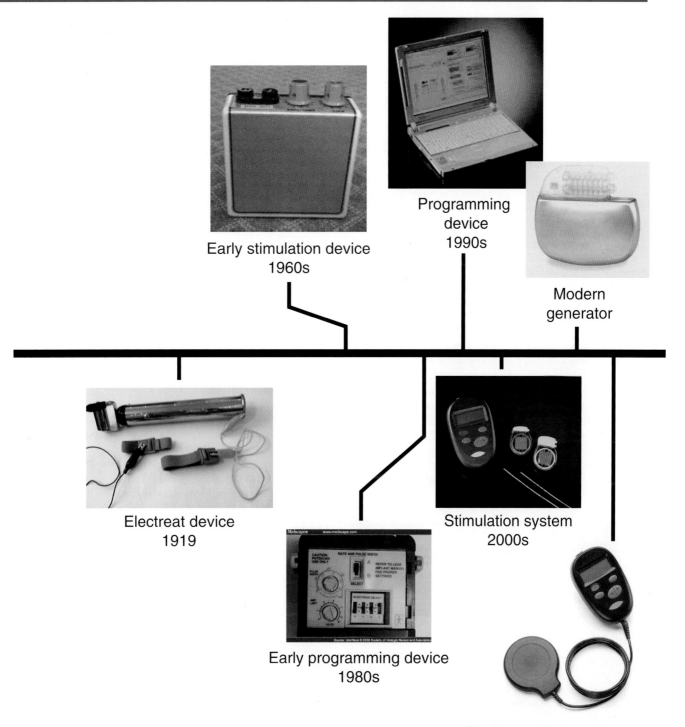

Early stimulation device
1960s

Programming
device
1990s

Modern
generator

Electreat device
1919

Early programming device
1980s

Stimulation system
2000s

Modern patient programmer

Early Discoveries

The first documented use of neurostimulation for pain relief occurred in Greece around 63 AD. It was reported by Scribonius Largus that pain from gout was largely relieved by standing on a torpedo fish (**Fig. 1-1**), and recommended this treatment for pain in general. He said,

> *"For any type of gout, a live black torpedo should, when the pain begins, be placed under the feet. The patient must stand on a moist shore washed by the sea, and he should stay like this until the whole foot and leg up to the knee is numb. This takes away present pain and prevents pain from coming on if it has not already arisen. In this way Ateros, a freedman of Tiberius, was cured."*[1]

In 1771 Luigi Galvani, an Italian physician and physicist, discovered that the leg muscles of a frog twitched when electricity was applied, thereby effectively debuting the study of bioelectricity.[2] Gilbert, a famous 17th century scientist, described the relationship of electromagnetism to pain symptom management on his discovery that a piece of magnetic iron ore could be used in the treatment of headaches, mental disorders, and marital infidelity.[3]

In the years following Gilbert's work, a method of harnessing electrical current was invented that would allow for the development of modern therapies. This device was called the Leyden jar (**Fig. 1-2**). This device was constructed by placing water in a metal container and placing brass wire through a cork top into the water. In 1746, using a Leyden jar, Jean Jallabert discovered the ability to use electricity to stimulate muscle fibers. Jallabert treated a paralyzed limb by causing involuntary contractions leading to regeneration of muscle and increased blood flow.[4] This success led many others in the field to pursue similar methods of treatment.

In 1756 Leopoldo Caldani observed that a Leyden jar could be discharged in the vicinity of a dissected frog's leg and cause it to twitch. This discovery led many scientists to believe that application of electricity was in fact a "miracle cure" and that its use in stimulating the body had far-reaching application.[5] The French physiologist d'Arsonval found that the application of high-frequency current (10,000 oscillations/sec) could reduce pain. In 1890 Hertz demonstrated that when he was able to achieve 1,000,000,000 oscillations/sec, tissue was not stimulated in a painful manner. This initial stimulation was at a low voltage. This was eventually increased by Hertz's spark gap resonator, which allowed the use of a gap in the otherwise complete electrical circuit to discharge current at a prescribed voltage. This increase in voltage control, along with high frequency, led to successful treatment of arthritis, pain, and tumors. The developments of d'Arsonval and Hertz remain critical for modern-day stimulation programming platforms.

Between 1884 and 1886 Sir Victor Horsely introduced the first practical use of intraoperative neurostimulation. Horsley's application of stimulation was used to identify a particular cortical area in a patient with epileptic foci.[6]

Benjamin Franklin

Ben Franklin is credited with being the first American to use neurostimulation. One of Franklin's most important achievements was the discovery that electricity is an ever-present natural force. Franklin is also responsible for developing the theory of positive and negative charges. These discoveries and Franklin's curiosity resulted in experiments that used high voltage stimulation, which unfortunately caused injury and burns to his test subjects. His report to the French Academy of Sciences in the late 1700s concluded that his experiments in neurostimulation were a failure.

Modern Medicine

By the early 1900s many devices, including transcutaneous electrical nerve stimulation (TENS) devices, similar to today's TENS

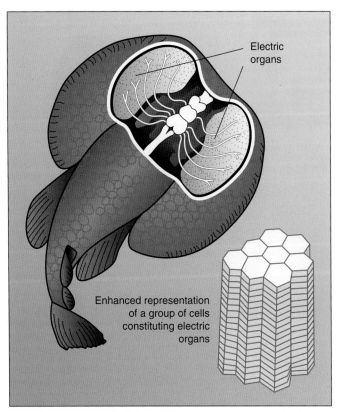

Fig. 1-1 Torpedo fish used for early treatment methods.

Electric organs

Enhanced representation of a group of cells constituting electric organs

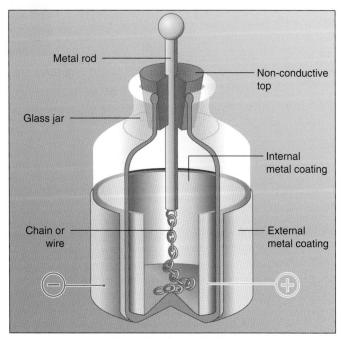

Fig. 1-2 The Leyden jar.

Metal rod

Non-conductive top

Glass jar

Internal metal coating

Chain or wire

External metal coating

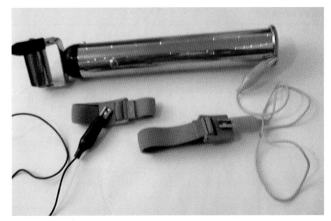

Fig. 1-3   The Electreat device.

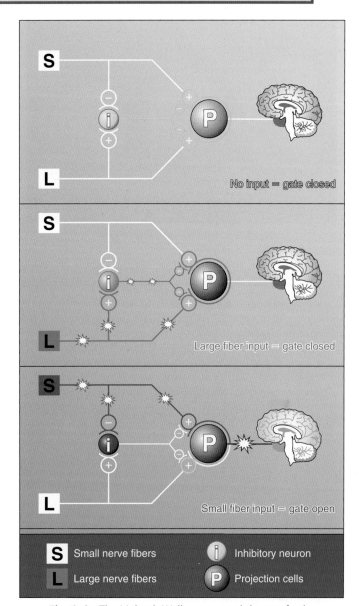

Fig. 1-4   The Melzack-Wall gate control theory of pain.

units, were available to treat all manner of pain conditions. The Electreat (**Fig. 1-3**), patented by Charles Willie Kent in 1919, sold as many as 250,000 units in 25 years. Most physicians' offices had one of these devices, and used it to treat all manner of conditions, including baldness, gout, and rheumatic feet.

The use of neurostimulation in modern medicine had its true beginning in the 1960s. In the 1965 *Science* article, "Pain Mechanisms: A New Theory," Melzak and Wall proposed the gate control theory,[7] which assisted in furthering the understanding of neurostimulation by describing the inhibitory and excitatory relationships in pain pathways (**Fig. 1-4**). Norman Shealy is credited with introducing the neurostimulation in true clinical practice when he and his research assistant developed a stimulating lead to work on the dorsal columns of the spinal cord.[8] The lead consisted of a platinum electrode with positive and negative electrodes. It was used in the treatment of a terminally ill cancer patient, placed in the intrathecal space, and attached to an external cardiac electrical generator. Shealy referred to these devices as *dorsal column stimulators;* they were specifically intended for pain relief. Unfortunately, many serious complications were associated with these early devices, including compression of the spinal cord and spinal fluid leakage. These safety concerns led many to believe that this form of treatment was not a safe alternative to other noninvasive techniques; and, until the development of the extradural placement method, many were wary of its use.

By the late 1960s Medtronic obtained Food and Drug Administration approval to distribute these devices for the treatment of pain. Shealy, Mortimer, and Reswick[8] advanced the technique to stimulate the epidural space with increasing success.

Deep Brain and Motor Cortex Stimulation

In 1973 Hosobuchi, Adams, and Rutkin[9] discovered that these devices could be used in the deep brain to treat facial pain, effectively leading to the discovery of DBS for pain control. In 1991 Tsubokawa and colleagues[10] reported that motor cortex stimulation alleviated pain of central origin. This landmark study introduced the theory and practice of motor cortex stimulation. After some early concerns, DBS was given approval for the treatment of movement disorders in Parkinson disease and dystonia. A number of clinical studies related to depression, obsessive-compulsive disorder, and brain injury are currently underway for deep brain and motor cortex stimulation.

Peripheral Nerve Stimulation

Nerve conduction theory was described in 1826 by Johannes P. Muller, and in 1912 von Perthes was the first to describe the technique of peripheral nerve stimulation to localize a particular nerve.[11] In 1955 Pearson[12] reported success in locating motor nerves by using a transformer, a vacuum tube stimulator, and an electrophrenic stimulator. In 1969 Ballard D. Wright[13] described the usage of the block-aid monitor, a commercially available device, for successful peripheral nerve stimulation; it was one of the first published accounts of success. Wiener, Hassenbusch, Stanton-Hicks and other important research works have shown that devices could be successfully implanted around the peripheral nerve and create paresthesia in the innervation dermatome of the nerve. Older methods of device placement that required surgical dissection have been replaced with percutaneous placement, leading to improved patient satisfaction and patient safety. Many new devices and treatment indications are on the horizon for this type of stimulation.

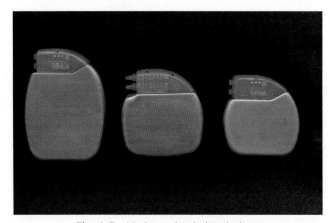

Fig. 1-5   Modern stimulation devices.

Conclusion

Work by Shealy and others in the early development of neuro-stimulation has been followed by steady advances in both the clinical and technological aspects of pain management. The development of smaller implantable devices (**Fig. 1-5**), new lead arrays, battery technology, and programmable devices has advanced treatment options for a wider variety of patients. Studies regarding the clinical effectiveness of neurostimulation have further proven the effectiveness of this technology for treatment of multiple disease states. The future holds promise for additional indications and increased access to technology.

References

1. Stojanovic MP, Andi S: Spinal cord stimulation. *Pain Physician* 5(2):156-166, 2002.
2. Luigi Galvani and animal electricity: two centuries after the foundation of electrophysiology. *Trends Neurosci* 20(10):443-448, 1997,
3. Pumfrey S, Tilley D: William Gilbert: forgotten genius. *Physics World* November 2003.
4. Experiments on electricity with some conjectures on the cause of its effects (Geneva, vol 8, ed 2, Paris, 1749, 12 mo).
5. Cotti Piero: The discovery of the electric current. *Physica B* 204(1-4):367-369, 1995, condensed matter.
6. Sakas D, Simpson A, Krames E: *Operative neuromodulation.* Volume 1: *Functional neuroprosthetic surgery: an introduction*, Verlag, Vienna, 2007, Springer, Volume 1: 482 pages.
7. Melzack R, Wall PD: Pain mechanisms: a new theory. *Science* 150:971-979, 1965.
8. Shealy CN, Mortimer JT, Reswick JB: Electrical inhibition of pain by stimulation of the dorsal columns: preliminary clinical report. *Anesth Analg* 46(4):489-491, 1967.
9. Hosobuchi Y, Adams J, Rutkin B: Chronic thalamic stimulation for the control of facial anesthesia dolorosa. *Arch Neurol* 29(3):158-161, 1973.
10. Tsubokawa T *et al*: Chronic motor cortex stimulation for the treatment of central pain. *Acta Neurochir (Wien)* 52(suppl):137-139, 1991.
11. Pithers C, Raj P, Ford D: The use of peripheral nerve stimulators for regional anesthesia: a review of experimental characteristics, techniques and clinical applications. *Reg Anesth* 10:49-58, 1985.
12. Pearson RB: Nerve block in rehabilitation: a technic of needle localization. *Arch Phys Med Rehabil* 36(10):631-633, 1955.
13. Wright BD: A new use for the block-aid monitor. *Anesthesiology* 30(Issue 2):236-237, 1969.

2 Mechanisms of Spinal Neuromodulation

Robert D. Foreman and Bengt Linderoth

CHAPTER OVERVIEW

Chapter Synopsis: Electrical stimulation of the spinal cord (SCS) improves many forms of neuropathic pain; but, contrary to our early understanding, it can also affect some forms of nonneuropathic nociception. Chapter 2 examines the physiology of these indications. The understanding of SCS is rooted in Melzack and Wall's[5] gate control theory of pain transmission. By spinal stimulation of large-fiber neurons, the gate is activated to reduce transmission of neuropathic pain signals from primary small-fiber afferents. The technique generally does not alleviate acute nociception, but it can reduce certain types of peripheral nociception and can even alleviate underlying conditions. SCS has been shown to affect ischemic limb pain caused by peripheral arterial occlusive disorder (PAOD), angina, and gastrointestinal disorders such as irritable bowel syndrome (IBS).

In addition to modulating pain signals, SCS affects target organs outside the nervous system. In PAOD two theories have been considered; both mechanisms are likely relevant. First, the sympathetic output to peripheral tissues is reduced by SCS, thus alleviating the resulting vasoconstriction. Second, antidromic stimulation of sensory fibers causes release of vasodilators in the periphery, thus alleviating the peripheral ischemia. SCS can also provide relief for intractable angina by inhibiting cardiac nociceptors and again helps to alleviate the underlying ischemia. SCS may result in redistribution of cardiac blood flow or modulation of oxygen demand in the heart. Animal experiments and clinical reports also confirm that SCS can be used to relieve pain originating in the gastrointestinal tract from a variety of conditions, including IBS and its associated somatic hypersensitivity.

Important Points:
- Transmission of nociceptive information from the site of an injury may generate a perception of pain because an imbalance exists between large and small fiber systems (cf. Head and Thompson[1]). This concept eventually evolved into Melzack and Wall's[5] gate control theory.
- The gate control theory was a critical catalyst in the development of various forms of neuromodulation for treating chronic forms of pain.
- Neuromodulation using electrical SCS depends on conductivity of the intraspinal elements relative to the position of the electrode. Electrical conductivity of the dorsal column is anisotropic.
- In several painful syndromes that are suitable candidates for SCS, the effect is mediated via stimulation-induced changes in other organ systems and not necessarily the result of an action onto the neural pain mechanisms per se.
- Ischemic painful conditions of the limbs commonly result from peripheral arterial occlusive diseases (PAODs). Antidromic activation of sensory fibers releasing vasodilators and suppression of sympathetic activity are two mechanisms activated by SCS that may be involved in reduction and prevention of ischemic pain and in cytoprotection. The effect of SCS in vasospastic pain is even more dramatic.
- SCS has been used to treat therapy-resistant angina pectoris since the mid-eighties by applying SCS at the T1-T2 or higher spinal segments in patients. SCS may not only relieve pain but also improve cardiac function.
- Clinical reports and animal studies suggest that SCS might be used to treat various functional bowel disorders.
- Neuropathic pain results primarily from the altered functional characteristics of multimodal wide–dynamic range (WDR) neurons. SCS reduces this pain most likely by reducing hypersensitization of these WDR spinal neurons, to affect other components of the spinal neural network through activation of multiple transmitter/receptor systems.
- Thus spinal neuromodulation acts on various pain syndromes through multiple pathways.
- Improved collaborations between basic scientists and clinicians will greatly hasten the transfer of basic research findings to the clinical setting.

Background

Therapeutic effects of neuromodulation are based on the concept that selective excitation of large afferent fibers activates mechanisms that control pain. This fits well with the idea that pain may occur as a result of an imbalance between large and small fiber systems that transmit nociceptive information from the site of injury. Previous investigators have provided a long history of support for this concept. As early as 1906 Head and Thompson[1] argued that fine discrimination such as touch normally exerts an inhibitory influence on impulses transmitted in fibers mediating nociception, which results in pain. This inhibition or facilitation of sensory impulses has been proposed to occur in the dorsal horn before nociceptive information is relayed onto secondary neurons. Furthermore, clinical trials performed in the early sixties using sensory thalamic stimulation[2,3] were based on the notion that activation of fine discrimination receptors (touch) exerted an inhibitory influence over sensations such as pain, pressure, heat, or cold. It should also be noted that Noordenbos[4] used the descriptive phrase "fast blocks slow" to stress the inhibitory influence of fast on slow fibers.

The concept of excitation of large afferent fibers activating pain control mechanisms advanced very rapidly with the publication of the article proposing the gate control theory; it is one of the most

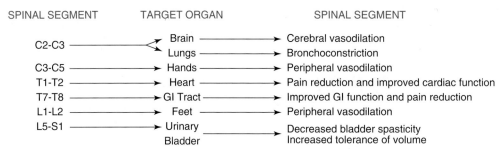

Fig. 2-1   Sites at different segments of the spinal cord where spinal cord stimulation induces functional changes in target organs.

cited papers in modern pain literature.[5] In this article the authors suggested that the therapeutic implication of their model would be to selectively activate large fibers to control pain. Thus even though the basic idea underlying the gate control theory was not completely unknown, it was built on a foundation of creative experiments using modern electrophysiological techniques. The results of these experiments were clearly synthesized and discussed in a form that postulated a new conceptualization of pain and pain control. Subsequently, numerous studies were conducted to criticize the theory, but nevertheless its simplicity has provided a useful frame of reference to explain mechanisms of pain generation and pain control. As Dickenson[6] pointed out in his editorial about the ability of the gate control theory of pain to stand the test of time, the concepts of convergence and modulation changed the focus from destructing pathways for relief of pain to controlling pain by modulation in which excitation is reduced and inhibition is increased. The gate control theory accelerated the pursuit of modern pain research to explore how the pervasive plasticity of the nervous system plays a critical role in the generation, maintenance, and modulation of pain.

The gate control theory served as a critical catalyst in the clinical arena to spawn the development of various forms of neuromodulation that led to new therapies. The insights gained by Shealy and his colleagues[7] and Shealy, Mortimer, and Reswick[8] in animal experiments led them to conduct the first human trials with electrical spinal cord stimulation (SCS) as one form of neuromodulation.[8] Their experimental studies in conscious cats revealed that stimulating the dorsal aspect of the spinal cord blocked responses to nociceptive peripheral stimuli. On the basis of this study and support of the gate control theory, it was assumed that neuromodulation could be used to treat all forms of nociceptive pain. However, several reports pointed out that SCS is ineffective for treating acute nociceptive conditions in contrast to what was predicted from the gate control theory; but eventually it has become the foremost treatment for neuropathic pain originating from the periphery.[9-13] Nevertheless, numerous reports appeared during the eighties to convince clinicians that SCS could also be used to alleviate certain types of nociceptive pain, including selected ischemic pain states such as peripheral arterial occlusive disease (PAOD), vasospastic conditions, and therapy-resistant angina pectoris. The mechanisms of action for SCS are slowly emerging as more solid evidence has revealed some of the underlying physiological mechanisms. Clinical observations coupled with important experimental data clearly demonstrate that SCS applied to different segments of the spinal cord elicits fundamentally different results on various target organs or parts of the body (**Fig. 2-1**).

The purpose of this chapter is to describe the organization of the spinal cord; explain the effects of electrical stimulation on the spinal cord; and discuss the underlying mechanisms activated by neuromodulation, specifically SCS, in ischemic pain, diseases of visceral organs, and neuropathic pain.

Organization and Electrical Properties of the Spinal Cord

The spinal cord is encased within the vertebral canal, which is made up of vertebrae that encircle the spinal cord but limit space for insertion of stimulating electrodes. The spinal cord in an adult human extends from the foramen magnum to the first or second lumbar vertebra and is divided into cervical, thoracic, lumbar, and sacral segments. The naming of the segments is based on the regions of the body innervated by the spinal cord. Examination of a cross section of the spinal cord shows that it is composed of gray matter and surrounded by white matter (**Fig. 2-2**).

The gray matter is comprised of cell bodies with their dendrites and initial segment of the axon, microglia, and astrocytes. It is divided into a posterior horn, intermediate zone, and the ventral horn. The gray matter is further divided into laminae I to X; these divisions are based on the size, shape, and distribution of neurons located in these laminae.[14] The input received by these neurons and the trajectory of the axons from them also help to characterize laminae. Neurons of dorsal and intermediate laminae (I to VII, X) generally receive sensory information originating from peripheral sensory receptors. These neurons integrate this information with input arriving from descending pathways. Some of the cell bodies have short axons and serve as interneurons, whereas others are the cells of origin of ascending sensory pathways. The interneurons may also participate in local reflexes. The ventral laminae (VIII, IX) are generally composed of motoneurons that form the motor nuclei.

The white matter is divided into the posterior, lateral, and anterior funiculi. These funiculi are composed of individual tracts. The posterior funiculi are generally referred to as the dorsal columns. The lateral funiculi contain ascending and descending pathways that transmit information between the spinal cord and the brain. The descending pathways are generally located in the posterolateral region of the lateral funiculi, and the ascending pathways primarily composed of the anterolateral system reside in the anterolateral funiculi. The anterolateral system includes the spinothalamic, spinoreticular, spinomedullary, spinoparabrachial, spinomesencephalic, and spinohypothalamic fibers. The ventral funiculi contain part of the anterolateral system and also pathways that transmit axial muscle control information.

The electrical properties, more specifically the electrical conductivity, of white and gray matter of the spinal cord are not homogeneous. For SCS it is important to know that the electrical conductivity of the dorsal column is anisotropic; that is, current can travel in the direction parallel to the axons more easily than in the direction perpendicular to axons.[15] The electrical properties within the gray matter also vary because neurons and glia have diverse orientations, ubiquitous dimensions, and different dendritic characteristics.

Neuromodulation using electrical stimulation of the spinal cord depends on the conductivity of the intraspinal elements relative to

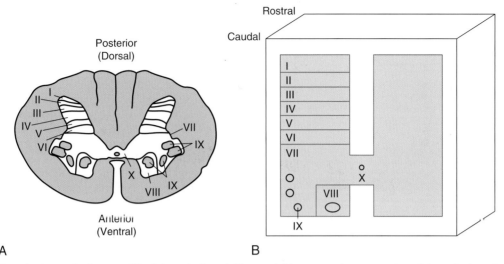

Fig. 2-2   Model **(A)** and schematic diagram **(B)** of the spinal cord. The model is an actual cross section of the spinal cord; the diagram is provided because it will be used in subsequent figures to provide the space to more effectively illustrate neural connections.

the position of the electrode.[16] If an axon is depolarized or made more electrically positive, it produces an action potential that is transmitted orthodromically and antidromically within the axon. The cathode of an external electrode must be negatively charged to generate the action potential in the axon. In contrast, if an axon is hyperpolarized or made more negatively charged, its ability to generate an action potential is reduced because the threshold for depolarization is increased. A positively charged external electrode or anode produces this effect. Thus the active electrode for electrical stimulation serves as the cathode, whereas the anode or positive electrode may serve as a shield to prevent stimulation of neuronal structures such as dorsal roots that might interfere with effective neuromodulation. For SCS the electrode most commonly is placed on the surface of the dura mater. Activation of the electrode releases electric current that is transmitted through the dura mater and the highly conductive cerebrospinal fluid (CSF) before it reaches the dorsal part of the spinal cord. The dura mater has low conductivity, but it is so thin that the current generally is not impeded significantly as it passes through the dura to the CSF. Furthermore, the vertebral bone has the lowest conductivity so it insulates pelvic structures and visceral organs from the electric field generated by SCS. Once the electric current reaches the spinal cord, several factors may determine the neural structure being stimulated. Jan Holsheimer[16] has used computerized models of the spinal cord to study the activation of axons by electrical current. In addition to the fiber diameter, the presence of myelination, and the depth of CSF layer surrounding the cord at the level of an electrode, the axon orientation has important implications for activation thresholds. In general, axons of the dorsal columns have higher activation thresholds than fibers such as the dorsal roots that are oriented laterally or angle as they enter the spinal cord.[16]

The dorsal column is composed primarily of large-diameter afferent nerve fibers with relatively low thresholds for recruitment when cathodal electrical pulses are generated through the epidural electrode that is attached to a spinal cord stimulator. It is important to note that the electrode for SCS needs to be placed near midline to prevent the activation of dorsal root fibers.[17] Stimulation amplitudes are then increased to intensities that recruit large fibers to produce action potentials and produce paresthesias. These action potentials are transmitted orthodromically and antidromically in these axons. The action potentials transmitted antidromically reach the collateral processes that penetrate the gray matter of the spinal cord. Their activation causes the release of transmitters, which activates the "gate." Activation of the gate sets in motion neural mechanisms that reduce pain and improve organ function. The details of these mechanisms are discussed in subsequent paragraphs.

Neuromodulation Mechanisms in Ischemic Pain
Ischemic painful conditions of the limbs commonly results from PAOD, which is caused by obstruction of blood flow into an arterial tree.[18] PAOD is a major cause of disability and loss of work and affects the quality of life.[19,20] Morbidity and mortality are relatively high because effective treatments are very limited. Presently SCS is usually implemented only after vascular surgery and medications fail to slow or prevent the progression of PAOD. Surprisingly the success rate of SCS-treated PAOD is greater than 70%.[21] Since ischemic pain is characterized generally as essentially nociceptive and several studies have indicated that SCS does not alleviate acute nociceptive pain,[9,22,23] SCS-induced pain relief is most likely secondary to attenuation of tissue ischemia that occurs as a result of either increasing/redistributing blood flow to the ischemic area or decreasing tissue oxygen demand.[24,25] Cook and associates[26] were the first to report that SCS increased peripheral circulation of patients suffering from PAOD. Usually SCS is applied to the dorsal columns of lower thoracic (T10-T12) and higher lumbar spinal segments (L1-L2) to increase peripheral circulation in the legs of PAOD patients.

The mechanisms of SCS-induced vasodilation in the lower limbs and feet are not yet completely understood. Since no animal models of PAOD that generate ischemic pain have emerged, normal anesthetized animal models have been used to investigate the physiologic mechanisms of SCS-induced changes in peripheral blood flow (see reference 23 for review). Cutaneous blood flow and calculated vascular resistance in the glabrous skin of ipsilateral and contralateral hindpaws have been determined most commonly by using laser Doppler flowmetry. A thermistor probe placed next to the laser Doppler probe on the plantar aspect of the foot has been used to measure skin temperature. Various interventions such as injections of hexamethonium, administration of adrenergic agonists and antagonists, sympathetic denervation, dorsal rhizotomies, calcitonin gene-related peptide (CGRP) antagonists, nitric oxide synthetase inhibitors, and local paw cooling have been used to explore the underlying mechanisms of peripheral microcirculation. Studies using Doppler flowmetry and interventions for more than

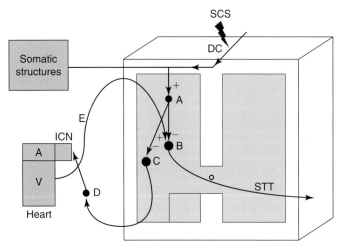

Fig. 2-3 Schematic diagram illustrating how spinal cord stimulation (SCS) (lightning bolt) of primary afferent fibers in the T1-T2 dorsal columns (DC) affects neuronal mechanisms that reduce pain and improves cardiac function resulting from ischemic heart disease. SCS activates interneurons (A) that may reduce activity of spinothalamic tract (STT) cells short term (B); modulate activity of sympathetic preganglionic (C) and postganglionic (D) neurons to stabilize the intrinsic cardiac nervous system (ICN), which reduces ischemia, decreases infarct size, and decreases arrhythmias. In addition, a protective effect associated with local release of catecholamines on ischemic cardiomyocytes has been demonstrated recently (see text). E, A-δ and C fibers transmit innocuous and nociceptive information from the heart to STT cells. A, Atria; V, ventricles; +, excitation; –, inhibition.

30 years of clinical and basic science studies have resulted in the evolution of two theories to explain the mechanisms of SCS-induced vasodilation. One theory is that SCS decreases sympathetic outflow and reduces the constriction of arterial vessels[27,28]; the alternative theory is that SCS antidromically activates sensory fibers, which causes the release of vasodilators[29, 30] (**Fig. 2-3**). The theory for SCS-induced suppression of sympathetic activity was based on results from clinical observations showing that a sympathetic block or sympathectomy produced pain relief and vasodilation imitated effects of treatment with SCS.[31,32] This theory was tested in animal models in which SCS-induced cutaneous vasodilation in the rat hindpaw at 66% of motor threshold was abolished by complete surgical sympathectomy.[33] SCS-induced vasodilation was markedly attenuated after administrating the ganglionic blocker, hexamethonium, or the neuronal nicotinic ganglionic blocker, chlorisondamine. These results led to the suggestion that efferent sympathetic activity, including nicotinic transmission in the ganglia and the postganglionic α_1-adrenergic receptors are suppressed by SCS (see **Fig. 2-3**). The alternative theory of SCS-induced antidromic activation of sensory fibers was confirmed in studies showing that sensory afferent fibers are important for SCS-induced vasodilation and that at higher, but not painful, SCS intensities C-fibers may also contribute to the response[30,34,35] (see **Fig. 2-3**). Thus SCS applied at the spinal L2-L5 segments excites dorsal column fibers that antidromically activate interneurons, which subsequently stimulate spinal terminals of transient receptor potential V1 (TRPV1) containing sensory fibers, which are primarily made up of C-fiber axons.[36,37] These fibers transmit action potentials antidromically to nerve endings in the hindlimb. The action potentials evoke mechanisms that release vasodilators, including the most powerful vasodilator, CGRP, which binds to receptors on endothelial cells. The activation

of these receptors leads to production and subsequent release of nitric oxide (NO), which results in relaxation of vascular smooth muscle cells (see reference 30 for review). The overall result is that relaxation of vascular smooth muscle cells decreases vascular resistance and increases peripheral blood flow. It should be noted that SCS applied at 500 Hz significantly increased cutaneous blood flow and decreased vascular resistance when compared to the responses induced at 50 Hz and 200 Hz; the effects at all of these frequencies depend on the activation of TRPV1-containing fibers and release of CGRP.[38] The clinical use of such findings remains to be determined.

The level of sympathetic nervous system activity may shift the balance between the effects of sympathetic efferent suppression and antidromic activation of sensory afferent fibers. Cooler skin temperatures increase sympathetic activity. A notable observation is that SCS-induced vasodilation of a cooled hindpaw (<25° C) generated an early phase of vasodilation via sensory afferent fibers and a late phase via suppression of the sympathetic efferent activity.[39] However, only sensory afferent activation occurred if SCS-induced vasodilation was performed in a warm paw (>28° C). Thus the balance of these two mechanisms most likely depends on the activity level of the sympathetic nervous system. Furthermore, another study showed that preemptive SCS increased the survival rate of skin flaps that were made ischemic by occluding the blood supply to the tissue for as long as 12 hours.[40] Concomitant administration of the CGRP-1 receptor antagonist CGRP 8-37 markedly attenuated the cytoprotective effect[40]; whereas preoperative administration of antiadrenergic drugs such as guanethidine, reserpine, and 6-hydroxydopamine increased experimental flap survival.[41] Thus the dual mechanisms of the release of vasodilators by antidromic activation of sensory fibers and suppression of sympathetic activity may all be involved in cytoprotection and prevention of vasospasm.

Neuromodulation Mechanisms of Visceral Organs
This section focuses on the heart and gastrointestinal tract because most of the basic research to determine mechanisms underlying the SCS-induced effects has been performed on these organs. Effects of SCS on spasms of bronchi in lungs were examined, but only an abstract was published.[42] To the best of our knowledge the effects of SCS on other visceral organs of animals besides studies of the colon (see section on Gastrointestinal Tract that follows) have not been examined systematically. However, there is abundant evidence of SCS effects on the urinary bladder that were obtained mostly from multiple sclerosis patients.[43]

Heart Ischemic heart disease is often presented as shortness of breath and angina pectoris, which is described clinically as an extremely intense pain and severe discomfort that usually radiates to the chest, shoulder, and left arm and occasionally to the neck and jaw.[44] This pain usually occurs during episodes of vasospasm or occlusion of the coronary vessels that result in decreased blood flow to the heart. The decreased blood flow generally causes an imbalance between the supply and the demand of oxygen in the heart. Ischemic episodes result in the release of prostaglandins, adenosine, bradykinin, and other substances that activate nociceptive spinal sensory afferent fibers innervating the heart.[45] This nociceptive information is transmitted by these sensory afferent fibers, which enter the C7-T5 spinal segments and synapse on spinothalamic tract cells, and cells of other ascending pathways that are also receiving converging cutaneous and muscle input from the overlying somatic structures such as the chest and upper arm.[45] Because of this convergent input, angina pectoris is felt as if it is originating from the chest and left arm. On occasion, angina is referred to the neck and jaw because the ischemic episodes can excite nociceptive vagal afferents that converge on spinothalamic tract cells in the upper cervical segments that also receive somatic convergent input from the neck and jaw.[45]

It is important to note that a large population of patients suffering from chronic angina pectoris does not respond to conventional treatments.[46] This group of patients led clinicians to develop alternative strategies such as neuromodulation to provide pain relief. Thus, following a period of using transcutaneous nerve stimulation for various types of visceral pain, including angina pectoris,[47] SCS has been used to treat such therapy-resistant angina pectoris since the mid-eighties.[48,49] Application of SCS at T1-T2 or higher spinal segments in patients provides pain relief by reducing both the frequency and to some extent the severity of angina attacks; the intake of short-acting nitrates is also reduced.[50-53] Thus SCS improves the quality of life in these patients; however, the mechanisms producing pain relief and improved heart function still remain unclear. An early animal study showed that SCS produced antianginal effects by directly inhibiting spinothalamic tract cell activity resulting from cardiac nociception,[54] but clinical and animal studies have proven that SCS does not solely relieve pain but also improves cardiac function. However, the primary factor appears to be the resolution of myocardial ischemia. Hautvast and colleagues[55] have proposed an SCS-induced flow increase or redistribution of blood supply, whereas Eliasson, Augustinnson, and Mannheimer[56] and Mannheimer and associates[57] interpret the reduction of coronary ischemia (decreased ST changes; reversal of lactate production) as being mainly caused by decreased cardiomyocyte oxygen demand.

Studies have been conducted to determine if blood flow changes relieve angina pectoris with SCS. In a human experimental study, positron emission tomography (PET) was used to show that SCS appeared to redistribute blood.[55] Blood flow and redistribution were also examined in an animal study by determining the distribution of isotope-labeled microspheres in hearts of anesthetized and artificially ventilated adult mongrel dogs.[58] A comparison of occluding the left anterior descending coronary artery with and without SCS showed that local blood flow in the myocardium did not increase and no changes occurred in the pressure-volume relationships during SCS. However, this study was limited because it was performed using acute occlusions in animals with a normal heart. It would have been more appropriate to conduct such studies in canine hearts with previous infarctions and long-term ischemic episodes since patients have long-term coronary ischemic disease.

Clinical and animal studies have been done to determine if SCS produces anti-ischemic effects that contribute to improved cardiac function. In patients whose blood supply in the coronary arteries was reduced, SCS applied during standardized heart workloads, analogous to exercise and rapid cardiac pacing, significantly reduced the magnitude of ST segment changes of the electrocardiogram.[57,59,60] These results support the idea that SCS may affect cardiac function by improving the working capacity of the heart. A canine animal model of myocardial ischemia was used to resemble the development of chronic ischemic heart disease by implanting an ameroid constrictor ring around the proximal left circumflex coronary artery.[61] As the material inside the constrictor ring swells, it gradually reduces arterial blood flow and induces the development of collaterals.[62] After 4 to 6 weeks the chest of anesthetized animals was opened, and the exposed heart was paced at a basal rate of 150 beats/min. A plaque containing 191 unipolar contacts was placed on the left ventricle distal to the left coronary artery occluded by the ameroid constrictor. Recordings were obtained

from unipolar contact sites to determine changes in the ST segments. The heart was stressed by administering angiotensin II via the coronary artery blood supply to the right atrial ganglionated plexus. Hearts stressed with angiotensin II produced elevations of the ST segments; SCS markedly attenuated this ST segment elevation. These data indicate that SCS may counteract the deleterious effects caused by chemical activation of the intrinsic cardiac nervous system that stressors release in a myocardium with reduced coronary reserve. From these results it was concluded that SCS may produce anti-ischemic effects, which in turn contribute to improved cardiac function. In a more recent study Lopshire and associates[63] demonstrated that SCS improved cardiac function in canine heart failure after an experimental myocardial infarction and further stressing the heart by using high-frequency cardiac pacing over 8 weeks.

Further evidence to support the anti-ischemic effects of SCS on the heart is the observation that SCS initiated before the onset of ischemic episodes (preemptive SCS) appears to activate mechanisms that reduce infarct size produced by coronary occlusions.[64] This preemptive SCS treatment reduced infarct size produced by coronary occlusions. This reduction in infarct size depends on adrenergic receptors located in the membrane of cardiac myocytes. Thus preemptive SCS appears to provide protection to the heart during periods of critical ischemia. However, protective effects of SCS therapy are ineffective if SCS is initiated after (reactive SCS) the onset of the ischemic episode.

The intrinsic cardiac nervous system is powerfully activated during ischemic episodes.[65,66] It is located in the cardiac ganglion plexi of epicardial fat pads adjacent to and within the myocardium.[67] This system is composed of interconnecting local circuit neurons and sympathetic efferent, parasympathetic efferent, and sensory afferent fibers. Local circuit neurons have the capacity to produce local interactions and also to connect with neurons arising from other ganglia and higher centers. Thus the intrinsic cardiac nervous system is essential to coordinate regional cardiac function and provide rapid and timely reflex coordination of autonomic neuronal outflow to the heart.[68] An important observation in animal studies is that SCS appears to stabilize activity of these intrinsic cardiac neurons during an ischemic challenge resulting from occlusion of a coronary artery. Thus SCS improves cardiac function to a considerable degree by regulating the intrinsic cardiac nervous system[23] (**Fig. 2-4**).

The stabilizing role of the intrinsic nervous system during SCS may also reduce arrhythmias. These effects have been examined in a canine animal model in which mediastinal nerve stimulation can evoke bradycardias and atrial arrhythmias.[69] SCS significantly reduces these arrhythmias and those evoked by ischemia,[69,70] but bilateral stellectomy eliminated these SCS-induced effects.[69] Thus these results provided evidence that SCS prevents the onset of atrial arrhythmias initiated by excessive activation of intrinsic cardiac neurons (mediastinal nerve stimulation), which depends on intact fibers coursing through the stellate ganglion and subclavian ansae.[69] Thus modulation of the intrinsic cardiac nervous system may be at least one mechanism that provides protection for the heart during more severe ischemic threats caused by generalized arrhythmias.[70] Other mechanisms may also contribute to SCS-induced cardioprotection, including local release of catecholamine in the myocardium[64,65] and an α_1-PKC pathway and a β-PKA pathway that mediates transient myocardial ischemia-induced apoptosis.[64,71] Other neuropeptides such as NO[72] and β-endorphin[73] may also provide cardioprotection. Some of the pathways and proposed mechanisms contributing to the effects of SCS on cardiac function discussed previously are summarized briefly in **Fig. 2-4**.

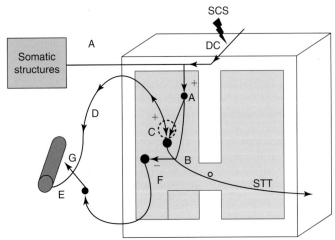

Fig. 2-4 Schematic diagram illustrating how spinal cord stimulation *(SCS)* of primary afferent fibers in the low thoracic-lumbar dorsal columns activates neural mechanisms producing vasodilation of peripheral vasculature. SCS activates interneurons *(A)* that may reduce activity of spinothalamic tract *(STT)* cells *(B)*; activate antidromically by a presynaptic mechanism *(C; dashed circle)* Aδ and C dorsal root afferent fibers *(D)* that releases calcitonin gene-related peptide and nitric oxide *(E)*; and decrease activity of sympathetic preganglionic neurons *(F)* that reduces release of norepinephrine from sympathetic postganglionic neurons *(G)*. +, Excitation; −, inhibition.

Gastrointestinal Tract—Irritable Bowel Syndrome Functional bowel disorders, including irritable bowel syndrome (IBS), are common abnormalities of the gastrointestinal tract that are associated with painful abdominal cramps, abnormal bowel habits, and somatic hypersensitivity.[74,75] Unfortunately no effective therapy is available because mechanisms that contribute to chronic visceral symptoms of IBS are not well understood. This lack of effective therapy led to speculation that SCS might be a means to treat IBS because it effectively reduces hyperexcitable somatosensory and viscerosomatic (bladder) reflexes in patients experiencing spasticity[43] and relieves certain types of visceral pain. This speculation led to the idea of proposing a study that was designed to determine if SCS might be a potential therapy for visceral pain originating from the gastrointestinal tract.[76] To simulate the IBS symptoms observed in patients, an animal model of visceral hypersensitivity was adapted by infusing a small concentration of acetic acid into the colon, which produces hypersensitivity but does not damage the mucosa[77-79] or by producing postinflammatory colonic hypersensitivity with trinitrobenzenesulfonic acid to create the acute inflammatory insult.[80] To quantify the intensity of visceral pain, visceromotor behavioral responses (VMRs) were determined by recording abdominal muscle contractions during noxious colorectal distention.[81] In this model a miniature SCS electrode system was implanted chronically with the techniques used in animal studies on neuropathic pain.[82] After 1 week, animals were anesthetized briefly with isoflurane so a strain gauge force transducer could be sutured on the right external oblique abdominal muscle. A balloon inserted in the colon was then used to distend normal colons and those irrigated with acetic acid, which sensitizes the colon; the number of abdominal contractions recorded from the strain gauge was determined with and without SCS. The results showed that SCS significantly reduced VMR responses generated with colorectal distention in both normal and acutely sensitized colons. The rat model of postinflammatory colonic hypersensitivity also showed that SCS could significantly reduce VMR responses to innocuous

colorectal distention.[80] Thus the ability of SCS to reduce colonic sensitivity raises the possibility that SCS may be used therapeutically to treat abdominal cramping and abdominal spasms that result in visceral pain of gastrointestinal origin. The findings from the animal studies were translated from bench to bedside because subsequently a single case study reported that SCS reduced hypersensitivity and produced relief of diarrhea in a patient suffering from severe IBS.[83] Further support came from Khan, Raza, and Khan,[84] who conducted a retrospective study showing that SCS can be used effectively to treat a variety of visceral pain syndromes such as generalized abdominal pain, chronic nonalcoholic pancreatitis, and pain following posttraumatic splenectomy. Thus the agreement between the clinical reports and animal studies supports the idea that SCS might be used in the future to treat various functional bowel and other visceral disorders. Ongoing randomized cross-over prospective clinical studies indicate that two thirds of patients with IBS can be treated effectively by SCS applied at the T6-T8 segments.[85]

Neuromodulation Mechanisms for Neuropathic Pain

A limitation of the neural mechanisms used to describe the effects of SCS in the previous sections is that they were based on experiments conducted primarily with normal animals. Although these mechanisms provide clues about the mechanisms, the ability to translate that information to the bedside is reduced. The advantage of neuromodulation mechanisms for neuropathic pain is that the studies from the mid-nineties and onward were performed on different models of nerve injury–induced "painlike behavior."[86] After a nerve lesion is generated by manipulating the sciatic nerve, peripheral branches of the sciatic nerve, or spinal roots, the posture of the animals of the nerve-injured limb soon changes; and the sensitivity of the limb to normally innocuous mechanical and thermal stimuli also increases in many cases. These behavioral changes are the visible results of both peripheral and central sensitization.[87] The most common method of evaluating the tactile hypersensitivity is to probe the nerve-injured hindpaw with von Frey filaments and observe the threshold that induces a withdrawal response to innocuous stimuli. This hypersensitivity is the most common behavioral sign in animal models of neuropathy; however, the pathophysiologic mechanisms are still not fully understood.[88,89] This measurable sign of hypersensitivity does resemble a "stimulus-evoked painlike reaction," which can be interpreted as being similar to allodynia observed in patients suffering from painful neuropathic conditions.[90] A notable concern in this context is that tactile hypersensitivity occurs in a much larger proportion of nerve-injured rats but only 20% to 40% of neuropathic pain patients present with mechanical allodynia.[91] Unfortunately, neuropathic pain animal models almost never express behavioral signs indicating the presence of continuous, spontaneous pain. These issues need to be considered when attempting to translate the results of these animal studies to the bedside.

Spinal Neural Networks of the Dorsal Horn Tactile hypersensitivity or allodynia primarily results from the involvement of low threshold Aβ fibers and central sensitization of neural networks in the gray matter of the spinal cord.[92] The central changes in the spinal cord following peripheral nerve injury depend mainly on altered characteristics primarily of multimodal wide–dynamic range (WDR) neurons. The altered characteristics of these neurons are persistent augmented responses to innocuous somatic stimuli and a marked increase in spontaneous activity. These characteristics are amenable to modulation by SCS. Acute experiments conducted in nerve-lesioned rats have shown that SCS elicits a

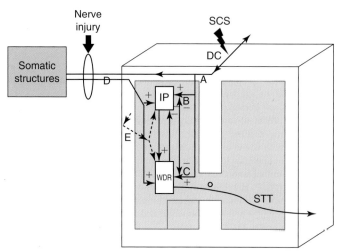

Fig. 2-5 Schematic diagram to explain the possible mechanisms of SCS in neuropathic pain. The mechanisms were discovered primarily from animal (rat) models of mononeuropathy (nerve injury). Spinal cord stimulation (SCS) (lightning bolt) activates dorsal columns orthodromically and antidromically. Antidromic activation activates collaterals (A) of the primary Aβ afferents that excite interneuronal pools (IP) and wide dynamic range cells (WDR). Activation of the IP inhibits the primary afferent afferents (B) and the WDR cells (C). Numerous transmitters and modulators are involved in the modulation exerted by interneurons (IP) as described in the text. (Transmitters in the IP include GABA, adenosine, and acetylcholine). The thin line (D) from somatic structures represents the Aδ and C fibers releasing glutamate, aspartate, and substance P that excite the IP and WDR cells. Orthodromic activation of the primary afferent fibers with SCS evokes supraspinal relays that transmit information in descending pathways (dashed lines, E) that release transmitters (serotonin, norepinephrine) to modulate WDR cells and the IP. Possible supraspinal relays are not included because the organization of a supraspinal loop is still evolving. +, Excitation; −, inhibition.

significant and long-lasting inhibition of the augmented responses to innocuous somatic stimuli and to the after-discharges in WDR cells.[93] Furthermore, studies conducted in freely moving, nerve-lesioned rats have shown that in some of the animals SCS may effectively suppress tactile hypersensitivity, similar to the effect on allodynia observed in neuropathic pain patients.[94-96] In translating this information to the clinical setting, this SCS suppression of dorsal horn neuronal activity may be related to the beneficial effect of SCS not only on the allodynia but also on the spontaneous neuropathic pain.

The ability of SCS to alter the characteristics of WDR spinal neurons, to affect other components of the spinal neural network, and to reduce tactile hypersensitivity most likely requires activation of multiple transmitter/receptor systems. However, very little data are available from human studies to know about systems that are critically involved in the attenuation of chronic, neuropathic pain by SCS. A series of studies performed in nerve-lesioned animals provide important clues about the transmitters that might contribute to central sensitization and the reduction in tactile hypersensitivity (**Fig. 2-5**).

The hyperexcitability of WDR cells in the dorsal horns of nerve-lesioned animals[93] appears to be correlated with increased basal release of excitatory amino acids such as glutamate, and malfunction of the local spinal γ-aminobutyric acid (GABA) system.[97,98] Attenuation of the hyperexcitability of WDR cells by SCS most likely results from an induced release of GABA in

the dorsal and simultaneous decrease of the interstitial glutamate concentration.[93,97]

The GABA-B receptor activation appears to be critical for suppressing release of glutamate.[97,99,100] An early study showed that the release of GABA is only observed in animals when SCS reduces tactile sensitivity, but not in a group of nonresponding animals.[98] However, an intrathecal injection of the GABA-B receptor agonist baclofen administered in these nonresponding animals could transform them into responders to SCS.[100]

In addition to the GABA system, the cholinergic system also plays an important role in producing the antinociceptive effects of SCS. The first indication pointing to the involvement of the cholinergic system came from a study showing that subeffective, intrathecal doses of clonidine transformed animals from nonresponders to responders to SCS.[101] It has also been shown that SCS releases acetylcholine in the dorsal horn; this effect depends on activation of the muscarinic (M4) receptor.[102] Furthermore, a subeffective intrathecal dose of a muscarinic receptor agonist (oxotremorine) could also transform nonresponding animals into responders to SCS.[103]

An exciting development resulting from these studies is that the findings were translated from bench to bedside. Baclofen was developed into a therapeutic benefit to treat neuropathic pain patients who responded inappropriately or did not experience enough relief from SCS. It is also interesting to note that the beneficial effects in patients who responded to this "drug-enhanced spinal stimulation therapy" have been stable for many years.[104,105] In addition to baclofen, intrathecal infusions of clonidine, which depends on the cholinergic system, also proved to be effective as an adjunct to SCS when stimulation alone was ineffective in treating neuropathic pain patients.[106,107]

SCS-induced release of adenosine, serotonin, and norepinephrine into the dorsal horn may also participate in the relief of neuropathic pain.[22,23] In contrast to the cholinergic system that depends on interneurons in the gray matter, serotonin and norepinephrine are released from descending pathways and are involved in inhibition of spinal neuronal activity. El-Khoury and associates[108] and Saadé and Jabbur[109] have conducted a long series of studies showing that neuropathic pain involves spinal and supraspinal mechanisms and that SCS orthodromically excited dorsal column fibers, which in turn activated neural circuits in the brainstem that transmit information in descending pathways that release these transmitters. These results did not agree with previous observations showing that SCS primarily activated local spinal circuits.[110] However, work from the same laboratory showed that serotonin released from the descending tract produces its inhibitory effects via GABA-B receptors in the spinal gray matter.[111] Thus more studies need to be done to understand the local and supraspinal mechanisms that produce the relief of neuropathic pain to resolve these differences.

Concluding Remarks

Two important themes that permeate the literature and the public square are translational research and evidence-based medicine. It is important to find ways that hasten the transfer of basic research to the clinical setting. An important mechanism to facilitate the translation is to improve collaborations between basic scientists and clinicians. These collaborations will help to focus on research that may be clinically relevant, although sometimes new findings that do not seem to be important initially may, through further research, evolve into an important treatment for a specific disease. Therefore it is imperative that scientists and clinicians in this exciting field of neuromodulation make every effort to share their creative ideas that expand the treatments. It is also important that medical therapies are based on a foundation of solid scientific evidence and thereafter tested in well-controlled prospective randomized studies. The cornerstone of solid scientific evidence is research identifying physiologic mechanisms that explain the beneficial effects of SCS. The mechanisms described in this chapter represent the infant stage of studies that need to be performed to provide a tool-box of mechanism-oriented treatments.

References

1. Head H, Thompson T: The grouping of afferent impulses within the spinal cord. *Brain* 29:537-741, 1906.
2. Mazars GJ: Intermittent stimulation of nucleus ventralis posterolateralis for intractable pain. *Surg Neurol* 4:93-95, 1975.
3. Mazars GJ, Merienne S, Cioloca C: Stimulations thalamiques intermittentes antalgiques. *Rev Neurol (Paris)* 128:273-279, 1973.
4. Noordenbos W, editor: *Pain*, Amsterdam, 1959, Elsevier.
5. Melzack R, Wall PD: Pain mechanisms: a new theory. *Science* 150(699):971-979, 1965.
6. Dickenson AH: Gate control theory of pain stands the test of time. *Br J Anaesth* 88(6):755-757, 2002.
7. Shealy CN et al: Electrical inhibition of pain: experimental evaluation. *Anesth Analg* 46:299-305, 1967.
8. Shealy CN, Mortimer JT, Reswick JB: Electrical inhibition of pain by stimulation of the dorsal columns: preliminary clinical report. *Anesth Analg* 46:489-491, 1967.
9. Lindblom U, Meyerson BA: Influence of touch, vibration and cutaneous pain of dorsal column stimulation in man. *Pain* 1:257-270, 1975.
10. Linderoth B, Meyerson BA: Spinal cord stimulation: techniques, indications and outcome. In Lozano AM, Gildenberg PL, Tasker RR, editors: *Textbook of stereotactic and functional neurosurgery*, ed 2, Berlin-Heidelberg, 2009, Springer Verlag, pp 3288 (Chapter 151).
11. Linderoth B, Simpson B, Meyerson BA: Spinal cord and brain stimulation. In McMahon S, Kolzenburg M, editors: *Wall and Melzack's textbook of pain*, ed 5, Philadelphia, 2005, Elsevier; (Chapter 37, pp 563-582).
12. Meyerson BA, Linderoth B: Mechanisms of spinal cord stimulation in neuropathic pain, Invited review. *Neurol Res* 22:285-292, 2000.
13. Meyerson BA, Linderoth B: Therapeutic electrical neurostimulation from a historical perspective. In Merskey H, Loeser JD, Dubner R, editors: *The paths of pain 1975-2005*, Seattle, 2005, IASP Press, (Chapter 21, pp 313-327).
14. Rexed B: A cytoarchitectonic atlas of the spinal cord in the cat. *J Comp Neurol* 100:297-379, 1954.
15. Grill WM: Principles of electric field generation for stimulation of the central nervous system. In Krames ES, Hunter Peckham P, Rezai AR, editors: *Neuromodulation*, Amsterdam, 2009, Elsevier, pp 146-154.
16. Holsheimer J: Computer modelling of spinal cord stimulation and its contribution to therapeutic efficacy. *Spinal Cord* 36:531-540, 1998. Review.
17. Barolat G et al: Mapping of sensory response to epidural stimulation of the intraspinal neural structures in man. *J Neurosurg* 78:233-239, 1993.
18. Garcia LA: Epidemiology and pathophysiology of lower extremity peripheral arterial disease. *J. Endovascular Ther* 13:II3-II9, 2006.
19. Golomb BA, Dang TT, Criqui MH: Peripheral arterial disease: morbidity and mortality implications. *Circulation* 114:688-699, 2006.
20. Hirsch AT et al: Peripheral arterial disease detection, awareness, and treatment in primary care. *JAMA* 1:286:1317-1324, 2001.
21. Cameron T: Safety and efficacy of spinal cord stimulation for the treatment of chronic pain: a 20-year literature review. *J Neurosurg* 100:254-267, 2004.
22. Linderoth B, Foreman RD: Physiology of spinal cord stimulation: review and update: *Neuromodulation* 2(3):150-164, 1999.
23. Linderoth B, Foreman RD: Mechanisms of spinal cord stimulation in painful syndromes: role of animal models. *Pain Med* 7:S14-S26, 2006.
24. Augustinsson LE, Linderoth B, Mannheimer C. Spinal cord stimulation in different ischemic conditions. In Illis LS, editor: *Spinal cord dysfunction III: functional stimulation*, Oxford, 1992, Oxford University Press, Chapter 12, pp 270-293.
25. Linderoth B: Spinal cord stimulation in ischemia and ischemic pain. In Horsch S, Claeys L, editors: *Spinal cord stimulation: an innovative method in the treatment of PVD and angina*, Darmstadt, 1995, Steinkopff Verlag, pp 19-35.
26. Cook AW et al: Vascular disease of extremities: electrical stimulation of spinal cord and posterior roots. *NY State J Med* 76:366-368,1976.
27. Linderoth B, Gunasekera L, Meyerson BA: Effects of sympathectomy on skin and muscle microcirculation during dorsal column stimulation: animal studies. *Neurosurgery* 29:874-879, 1991.
28. Linderoth B, Herregodts P, Meyerson BA: Sympathetic mediation of peripheral vasodilation induced by spinal cord stimulation: animal studies of the role of cholinergic and adrenergic receptor subtypes. *Neurosurgery* 35:711-719, 1994.
29. Croom JE et al: Cutaneous vasodilation during dorsal column stimulation is mediated by dorsal roots and CGRP. *Am J Physiol Heart Circ Physiol* 272:H950-H957, 1997.
30. Wu M, Linderoth B, Foreman RD: Putative mechanisms behind effects of spinal cord stimulation on vascular diseases: a review of experimental studies. *Auton Neurosci* 138:9-23, 2008.
31. Augustinsson L, et al: Epidural electrical stimulation in severe limb ischemia: pain relief, increased blood flow, and a possible limb-saving effect. *Ann Surg* 202:104-110, 1985.
32. Horsch S, Schulte S, Hess S: Spinal cord stimulation in the treatment of peripheral vascular disease: results of a single-center study of 258 patients. *Angiology* 55:111-118, 2004.
33. Linderoth B, Fedorcsak I, Meyerson BA: Peripheral vasodilatation after spinal cord stimulation: animal studies of putative effector mechanisms. *Neurosurgery* 28:187-195, 1991.
34. Tanaka S et al: Role of primary afferents in spinal cord stimulation-induced vasodilatation: characterization of fiber types. *Brain Res* 959:191-198, 2003.
35. Tanaka S et al: Mechanisms of sustained cutaneous vasodilation induced by spinal cord stimulation. *Auton Neurosci* 114(1-2):55-60, 2004.
36. Wu M et al: Sensory fibers containing vanilloid receptor-1 (VR-1) participate in spinal cord stimulation-induced vasodilation. *Brain Res* 1107:177-184, 2006.
37. Wu M: Roles of peripheral terminals of transient receptor potential vanilloid-1 containing sensory fibers in spinal cord stimulation-induced peripheral vasodilation. *Brain Res* 1156:80-92, 2007.
38. Gao J et al: Effects of spinal cord stimulation with "standard clinical" and higher frequencies on peripheral blood flow in rats. *Brain Res* 1313:53-61, 2010.
39. Tanaka S et al: Local cooling alters neural mechanisms producing changes in peripheral blood flow by spinal cord stimulation. *Auton Neurosci* 104:117-127, 2003.
40. Gherardini G et al: Spinal cord stimulation improves survival in ischemic skin flaps: an experimental study of the possible mediation by calcitonin gene-related peptide. *Plast Reconstr Surg* 103:1221-1228, 1999.
41. Jurell G, Jonsson CE: Increased survival of experimental skin flaps in rats following treatment with antiadrenergic drugs. *Scand J Plast Reconstr Surg* 10:169-172, 1976.
42. Gersbach P et al: *Influence of high-cervical spinal cord stimulation on antigen-induced bronchospasm in an ovine model (abstract)*, San Diego, 1999, ALA/ATS International Congress.
43. Illis LS, editor: *Spinal cord dysfunction. III: functional stimulation*, Oxford, 1992, Oxford University Press.
44. Gibbons RJ et al: ACC/AHA/ACP-ASIM guidelines for the management of patients with chronic stable angina: a report of the American College of Cardiology/American Heart Association Task Force on Practice Guidelines (Committee on Management of Patients With Chronic Stable Angina). *J Am Coll Cardiol* 33:2092-2197, 1999.
45. Foreman RD: Mechanisms of cardiac pain. *Annu Rev Physiol* 61:143-167, 1999.

46. DeJongste MJL et al: Effects of spinal cord stimulation on daily life myocardial ischemia in patients with severe coronary artery disease: a prospective ambulatory ECG study. *Br Heart J* 71:413-418, 1994.

47. Mannheimer C et al: Transcutaneous electrical nerve stimulation in severe angina pectoris. *Eur Heart J* Aug;3(4):297-302, 1982.

48. Mannheimer C et al: Epidural spinal electrical stimulation in severe angina pectoris. *Br Heart J* 59:56-61, 1988.

49. Murphy DF, Giles KE: Dorsal column stimulation for pain relief from intractable angina. *Pain* 28:365-368, 1987.

50. Buchser E, Durre, A, Albrecht E: Spinal cord stimulation for the management of refractory angina pectoris. *J Pain Symp Manag* 4(suppl):S36-S42, 2006.

51. Chua R, Keogh A: Spinal cord stimulation significantly improves refractory angina pectoris—a local experience spinal cord stimulation in refractory angina. *Heart Lung Circ* 14:3-7, 2005.

52. Jessurun GA, DeJongste MJ, Blanksma PK: Current views on neurostimulation in the treatment of cardiac ischemic syndromes. *Pain* 66:109-116, 1996.

53. Yu W et al: Spinal cord stimulation for refractory angina pectoris: a retrospective analysis of efficacy and cost–benefit. *Coron Artery Dis* 15:31-37, 2004.

54. Chandler MJ et al: A mechanism of cardiac pain suppression by spinal cord stimulation: implications for patients with angina pectoris. *Eur Heart J* 14:96-105, 1993.

55. Hautvast RW et al: Effect of spinal cord stimulation on myocardial blood flow assessed by positron emission tomography in patients with refractory angina pectoris. *Am J Cardiol* 77:462-467, 1996.

56. Eliasson T, Augustinnson LE, Mannheimer C: Spinal cord stimulation in severe angina pectoris—presentation of current studies, indications, and clinical experience. *Pain* 65:169-179, 1996.

57. Mannheimer C et al: Effects of spinal cord stimulation in angina pectoris induced by pacing and possible mechanism of action. *Br Med J* 307:477-480, 1993.

58. Kingma J et al: Neuromodulation therapy does not influence blood flow distribution or left-ventricular dynamics during acute myocardial ischemia. *Auton Neurosci* 91(1-2):47-54, 2001.

59. Hautvast RW et al: Effect of spinal cord stimulation on heart rate variability and myocardial ischemia in patients with chronic intractable angina pectoris—a prospective ambulatory electrocardiographic study. *Clin Cardiol* 21:33-38, 1998.

60. Sanderson JE et al: Epidural spinal electrical stimulation for severe angina: a study of its effects on symptoms, exercise tolerance and degree of ischaemia. *Eur Heart J* 13:628-633, 1992.

61. Cardinal R et al: Spinal cord activation differentially modulates ischemic electrical responses to different stressors in canine ventricles. *Auton Neurosci* 111(1):34-47, 2004.

62. Tomoike H et al: Functional significance of collaterals during ameroid–induced coronary stenosis in conscious dogs. *Circulation* 67:1001-1008, 1983.

63. Lopshire JC et al: Spinal cord stimulation improves ventricular function and reduces ventricular arrhythmias in a canine postinfarction heart failure model. *Circulation* 120:286-294, 2009.

64. Southerland EM et al: Pre-emptive, but not reactive, spinal cord stimulation mitigates transient ischemia induced myocardial infarction via cardiac adrenergic neurons. *Am J Physiol Heart Circ Physiol* 292:H311-H317, 2006.

65. Armour JA et al: Long-term modulation of the intrinsic cardiac nervous system by spinal cord neurons in normal and ischaemic hearts. *Auton Neurosci* 95:71-79, 2002.

66. Foreman RD et al: Modulation of intrinsic cardiac neurons by spinal cord stimulation: implications for its therapeutic use in angina pectoris. *Cardiovasc Res* 47:367-375, 2000.

67. Ardell JL: Intrathoracic neuronal regulation of cardiac function. In Armour JA, Ardell J, editors: *Basic and clinical neurocardiology*, New York, 2004, Oxford University Press, pp 118-152.

68. Armour JA: Myocardial ischaemia and the cardiac nervous system. *Cardiovasc Res* 41:41-54, 1999.

69. Cardinal R et al: Spinal cord stimulation suppresses bradycardias and atrial tachyarrhythmias induced by mediastinal nerve stimulation in dogs. *Am J Physiol Regul Integr Comp Physiol* 291:R1369-R1375, 2006.

70. Issa ZF et al: Thoracic spinal cord stimulation reduces the risk of ischemic ventricular arrhythmias in a postinfarction heart failure canine model. *Circulation* 111:3217-3220, 2005.

71. Broadley KJ, Penson PE: The roles of alpha- and beta-adrenoceptor stimulation in myocardial ischaemia. *Auton Autacoid Pharmacol* 24:87-93, 2004.

72. Sanada S, Kitakaze M: Ischemic preconditioning: emerging evidence, controversy, and translational trials. *Int J Cardiol* 97:263-276, 2004.

73. Eliasson T et al: Myocardial turnover of endogenous opioids and calcitonin-gene-related peptide in the human heart and the effects of spinal cord stimulation on pacing-induced angina pectoris. *Cardiology* 89:170-177, 1998.

74. Lembo T et al: Symptom duration in patients with irritable bowel syndrome. *Am J Gastroenterol* 91:898-905, 1996.

75. Mayer EA, Gebhart GF: Basic and clinical aspects of visceral hyperalgesia. *Gastroenterology* 107:271-293, 1994.

76. Greenwood-Van Meerveld B et al: Attenuation by spinal cord stimulation of a nociceptive reflex generated by colorectal distention in a rat model. *Auton Neurosci* 104:17-24, 2003.

77. Gunter WD et al: Evidence for visceral hypersensitivity in high-anxiety rats. *Physiol Behav* 69:379-382, 2000.

78. Langlois A et al: Response heterogeneity of 5-HT3 receptor antagonists in a rat visceral hypersensitivity model. *Eur J Pharmacol* 318:141-144, 1995.

79. Plourde V, St-Pierre S, Quirion R: Calcitonin gene-related peptide in viscerosensitive response to colorectal distension in rats. *Am J Physiol* 273:G191-G196, 1997.

80. Greenwood-Van Meerveld B et al: Spinal cord stimulation attenuates visceromotor reflexes in a rat model of post-inflammatory colonic hypersensitivity. *Auton Neurosci* 122(102):69-76, 2005.

81. Ness TJ, Gebhart GF: Colorectal distention as a noxious visceral stimulus: physiologic and pharmacologic characterization of the pseudaffective reflexes in the rat. *Brain Res* 450:153-169, 1988.

82. Linderoth B et al: An animal model for the study of brain transmitter release in response to spinal cord stimulation in the awake, freely moving rat: preliminary results from the periaqueductal grey matter. *Acta Neurochir* 58(suppl [Wien]):156-160, 1993.

83. Krames E, Mousad DG: Spinal cord stimulation reverses pain and diarrheal episodes of irritable bowel syndrome: a case report. *Neuromodulation* 7(2):82-88, 2004.

84. Khan YN, Raza SS, Khan EA: Application of spinal cord stimulation for the treatment of abdominal visceral pain syndromes: case reports. *Neuromodulation* 8:14-27, 2005.

85. Lind G et al: A prospective randomized trial of spinal cord stimulation for treatment of irritable bowel syndrome (abstract), Toronto, May 24-27, 2009, WSSFN Quadrennial Meeting. p 164.

86. Campbell JN, Meyer RA: Mechanisms of neuropathic pain (Review). *Neuron* 5:77-92, 2006.

87. Suzuki R, Dickenson A: Spinal and supraspinal contributions to central sensitization in peripheral neuropathy. *Neurosignals* 14(4):175-181, 2005.

88. Baba H: Removal of GABAergic inhibition facilitates polysynaptic A fiber-mediated excitatory transmission to the superficial spinal dorsal horn. *Mol Cell Neurosci* 24:818-830, 2003.

89. Costigan M, Scholz J, Woolf CJ: Neuropathic pain: a maladaptive response of the nervous system to damage. *Annu Rev Neurosci* 32:1-32, 2009.

90. Harke H et al: Spinal cord stimulation in sympathetically maintained complex regional pain syndrome type I with severe disability: a prospective clinical study. *Eur J Pain* 9:363-373, 2005.

91. Hansson P: Difficulties in stratifying neuropathic pain by mechanisms. *Eur J Pain* 7(4):353-357, 2003.

92. Woolf C, Doubell T: The pathophysiology of chronic pain—increased sensitivity to low threshold A-beta fiber inputs. *Curr Opin Neurobiol* 4:525-534, 1994.

93. Yakhnitsa V, Linderoth B, Meyerson BA: Spinal cord stimulation attenuates dorsal horn neuronal hyperexcitability in a rat model of mononeuropathy. *Pain* 79:223-233, 1999.

94. Meyerson BA, Linderoth B: Spinal cord Stimulation: mechanisms of action in neuropathic and ischemic pain. In Simpson BA, editor: *Electrical stimulation and the relief of pain*, vol 15, New York, 2003, Elsevier, Chapter 11, pp 161-182.

95. Meyerson BA, Linderoth B: Mode of action of spinal cord stimulation in neuropathic pain. *J Pain Symptom Manage* 31:6-12, 2006.

96. Meyerson BA et al: Spinal cord stimulation in animal models of mononeuropathy: effects on the withdrawal response and the flexor reflex. *Pain* 61:229-243, 1995.

97. Cui JG et al: Spinal cord stimulation attenuates augmented dorsal horn release of excitatory amino acids in mononeuropathy via a GABAergic mechanism. *Pain* 73:87-95, 1997.

98. Stiller CO et al: Release of GABA in the dorsal horn and suppression of tactile allodynia by spinal cord stimulation in mononeuropathic rats. *Neurosurgery* 39:367-375, 1996.

99. Cui JG, Linderoth B, Meyerson BA: Effects of spinal cord stimulation on touch-evoked allodynia involve GABAergic mechanisms: an experimental study in the mononeuropathic rat. *Pain* 66:287-295, 1996.

100. Cui JG et al: Effects of spinal cord stimulation on tactile hypersensitivity in mononeuropathic rats is potentiated by GABA-B and adenosine receptor activation. *Neurosci Lett* 247:183-186, 1998.

101. Schechtmann G et al: Intrathecal clonidine potentiates suppression of tactile hypersensitivity by spinal cord stimulation in a model of neuropathy. *Anesth Analg* 99:135-139, 2004.

102. Schechtmann G et al: Cholinergic mechanisms in the pain relieving effect of spinal cord stimulation in a model of neuropathy. *Pain* 139:136-145, 2008.

103. Song Z, Meyerson BA, Linderoth B: Muscarinic receptor activation potentiates the effect of spinal cord stimulation on pain-related behaviour in rats with mononeuropathy. *Neurosci Lett* 436:7-12, 2008.

104. Lind G et al: Intrathecal baclofen as adjuvant therapy to enhance the effect of spinal cord stimulation in neuropathic pain: a pilot study. *Eur J Pain* 8(4):377-383, 2004.

105. Lind G et al: Baclofen-enhanced spinal cord stimulation and intrathecal balofen alone for neuropathic pain: long-term outcome of a pilot study. *Eur J Pain* 12:132-136, 2008.

106. Schechtmann G et al: Intrathecal clonidine and baclofen produce enhancement of pain-relieving effects of spinal cord stimulation: a double blind study. *Acta Neurochir* 150(9):972, 2008 (abstract, ESSFN XVIII Congress, Rimini, Italy October 5-8, 2008).

107. Schechtmann G et al: Drug-enhanced spinal stimulation intrathecal clonidine VS baclofen: a double-blind clinical pilot study. *Pain Pract* 9(Suppl. 1):249-288, 2009 (abstract, Fifth Congress World Institute Of Pain, NY, March 13-19, 2009).

108. El-Khoury C et al: Attenuation of neuropathic pain by segmental and supraspinal activation of the dorsal column system in awake rats. *Neuroscience* 112(3):541-553, 2002.

109. Saadé NE, Jabbur SJ: Nociceptive behavior in animal models for peripheral neuropathy: spinal and supraspinal mechanisms. *Prog Neurobiol* 86:22-47, 2008.

110. Yakhnitsa V, Linderoth B, Meyerson BA: Modulation of dorsal horn neuronal activity by spinal cord stimulation in a rat model of neuropathy: the role of the dorsal funicles. *Neurophysiology* 30(6):424-427, 1998.

111. Song Z et al: Pain relief by spinal cord stimulation involves serotonergic mechanisms: an experimental study in a rat model of mononeuropathy. *Pain* 147:241-248, 2009.

3 Medical Considerations in Spinal Cord Stimulation

Binit J. Shah, Salim M. Hayek, and Al-Amin A. Khalil

CHAPTER OVERVIEW

Chapter Synopsis: Chapter 3 deals with some of the perioperative considerations for surgery for electrical spinal cord stimulation (SCS). The invasive implantation procedure carries inherent risks, but these can be minimized with considerations specific to the patient. We can learn from the technically similar (and far more common) surgeries for implanted cardiac devices (ICDs), including pacemakers and defibrillators.

Surgical site infection (SSI) is perhaps the most common perioperative risk associated with SCS at around 3% to 8%; thus intravenous antibiotics should be used routinely. Implantation at the site of a previous incision increases the risk of infection; therefore previous surgery sites should not be used. Smokers carry a risk of wound infection as high as eight times that of nonsmokers. Smoking cessation within a few weeks before surgery can dramatically reduce the risks. Human immunodeficiency virus (HIV)–positive patients do not intrinsically face higher perioperative risk, but certain members of the population could. Similarly, obesity per se does not increase perioperative morbidity, but it can increase the likelihood of wound infection. Patients with rheumatoid arthritis face specialized risks that should be considered in coordination with their rheumatologist. Patients with diabetes make up a significant component of the implantation population. Surgery can induce a postoperative hyperglycemia that increases SSI risk; therefore postoperative glucose should be maintained below 200 mg/dL. Patients receiving anticoagulation therapy or with ICDs also warrant special consideration. As the population receiving SCS implantation grows, it is important to consider the specific conditions associated with each patient to minimize his or her perioperative risks.

Important Points:

- When considering SCS in a patient on anticoagulation, the implanting physician should have a thorough understanding of the most recent American Society of Regional Anesthesia and Pain Medicine (ASRA) consensus guidelines for patients receiving anticoagulation, while also recognizing that there are no SCS specific guidelines.
- The concern for interaction between SCS and a pacemaker is inability to pace, whereas in defibrillators it is inappropriate shock. To minimize this interaction, the SCS should be set to a bipolar configuration, whereas the cardiac device should be set to bipolar sensing. Coordination should be undertaken with the patient's cardiologist.

Clinical Pearls:

- Preoperative antibiotics should be started 1.5 hours before surgery.
- Obesity alone is not a risk factor for postoperative complications.
- Maintaining *postoperative* blood glucose <200 mg/dL reduces the incidence of SSI.

Clinical Pitfalls:

- Operating through previous incision sites may increase the risk of infection because of decreased vascularity/healing of scar tissue.
- Smokers may have as high as eight times greater risk of perioperative infection.
- HIV+ status alone does not increase surgical complication rates; however, low CD4 count (≤200 cell/mm^3) and high viral load (>10,000 copies/mL) are associated with increased morbidity and mortality.

Background

Electrical stimulation for the treatment of pain has been used for over 4500 years.[1] In 1967 neurosurgeon Dr. C. Norman Shealy and colleagues from Case Western Reserve University were the first to implement spinal cord stimulation (SCS) in the treatment of chronic pain at University Hospitals of Cleveland.[2] Shealy proved the clinical feasibility of SCS, and subsequently there has been tremendous growth in its application. Currently SCS is approved by the Food and Drug Administration (FDA) for chronic pain of the trunk and limbs, pain from failed back surgery syndrome (FBSS), and intractable low back pain. "Off label," SCS has been used for neuropathic painful conditions and vascular and visceral pain, with diverse applications ranging from vulvodynia to cervicalgia. The full range of considerations for SCS is beyond the scope of this chapter.

As the role of SCS has expanded in the treatment of chronic pain conditions, the eligible patient population has grown as well. Patients who previously would not have been candidates are now able to benefit from neurostimulation. It is the responsibility of the implanting physician to consider and maximize the perioperative status of the patient to optimize outcome and minimize risks and complications.

General Considerations

Although an appropriately applied SCS trial and implant can provide significant satisfaction for both the patient and implanting physician, they are invasive interventions and therefore associated with inherent risks. Whether implanting these technologies directly or caring for those with SCS, several factors influencing successful implantation must be considered and are reviewed here: infection risk, tobacco use and smoking cessation, unique issues in those with human immunodeficiency virus/acquired immunodeficiency syndrome (HIV/AIDS), effects of obesity, rheumatoid arthritis (RA) and immunosuppressant therapy, blood glucose control in persons with diabetes, anticoagulation, and other perioperative issues.

Specific Considerations

Surgical Site Infection

Surgical site infection (SSI), in general, has an overall prevalence of 2% to 7%[3]; and, consistent with this, a rate of 3% to 8% has been found with SCS implantation.[4-6] In expert panel recommendations, Kumar and colleagues state that the "use of antibiotics is recommended by the panel and others and should be started intravenously, 1.5 hours prior to surgery."[4]

By comparison, infection rates for implanted cardiac devices (ICDs—pacemakers and defibrillators) were reported as 0.5% to 6% in early studies[7,8] but have more recently been found to be as low as 1%.[9] Although there have been no studies in SCS comparing infection rates in those with and without preoperative antibiotics, a prospective, randomized, double-blind, placebo-controlled trial evaluated infection risk for ICDs in those receiving either prophylactic cefazolin or a placebo.[10] This trial was interrupted early by the safety committee because of the dramatically higher rate of infection in those who did not receive antibiotics vs. those who did (3.28% vs. 0.63%). The authors also found that the presence of postoperative hematoma and procedure duration were positively correlated with infection risk. A recent American Heart Association (AHA) scientific statement also identified ICD infection risk factors to include diabetes mellitus (DM), congestive heart failure (CHF), renal dysfunction, oral anticoagulation, revision surgery, hematoma formation, corticosteroid use, and surgeon inexperience.[11] This statement also notes that "there is currently no scientific basis for the use of prophylactic antibiotics before routine invasive dental, gastrointestinal, or genitourinary procedures." Although these findings are in the setting of ICDs, the similarity between minimally invasive surgeries such as these and SCS may provide guidance. There are no similar studies in the SCS population and until such a time this literature may be used as a prudent reference.

Gaynes and colleagues[12] have also found that American Society of Anesthesiologists' (ASA) classification, the National Nosocomial Infection Surveillance (NNIS) wound classification, and prolonged operative time—defined as ≥75th percentile compared to average duration of the operation—are associated with SSI. In a retrospective review of >10,000 patients over 6 years, Haridas and Malangoni[13] identified several other significant risk factors for SSI: hypoalbuminemia (≤3.4 mg/dL), anemia (Hgb ≤10 g/dL), excessive alcohol use (not defined), history of chronic obstructive pulmonary disease, history of CHF, infection at remote site, and current operation through a previous incision (**Box 3-1**). Most of these risk factors can be identified through an appropriate history and physical examination and preoperative laboratory work and can be addressed in conjunction with the patient's primary care physician or appropriate specialist. However, operation through a previous incision site may be of greater concern. One of the most common indications for SCS use is FBSS. Many times old scars are used as an entry points for the new procedure, either because they provide adequate anatomic access or to prevent further cosmetic disfiguration. Haridas and Malangoni[13] suggest that using a previous incision may predispose to SSI because of the decreased vascularity of scar tissue.

The pathogen most commonly involved in SSI is *Staphylococcus aureus*, which is responsible for more than 50% of infections,[14-16]

Box 3-1: Postoperative Risk Factors in General Surgery

Alcohol use (excessive)
Anemia (Hgb ≤10 g/dL)
ASA Classification: I-VI
Chronic obstructive pulmonary disease
Congestive heart failure
Hypoalbuminemia (≤3.4 mg/dL)
Infection at remote site
NNIS Wound classification
- Clean
- Clean-contaminated
- Contaminated
- Dirty/infected
Operation through previous incision
Prolonged operation (≥75th percentile)
Smoking status

ASA, American Society of Anesthesiologists; *Hgb*, hemoglobin; *NNIS*, National Nosocomial Infection Surveillance.

---

with most cases occurring in patients who are themselves carriers of the organism. The carriage site is most often the anterior nares,[17] and multiple studies have shown that nasal carriage is one of the most important risk factors for the development of surgical site infection.[14,18,19] Given this, there is a new body of research specifically focused on identifying and treating nasal carriers of *Staphylococcus aureus*, with resultant dramatic decreases in SSI. Studies in cardiothoracic,[14] orthopedic,[20-22] and dialysis[23,24] populations have shown that treatment is feasible and cost-effective, decreases infection rates by 57% to 93%, and reduces morbidity and mortality. A recent, randomized, double-blind, placebo-controlled, multicenter trial showed that treatment with mupirocin nasal ointment and chlorhexidine soap reduced the infection rate to 3.4%, compared to 7.7% in the placebo control group.[25]

Although different treatment protocols have been used, there is accumulating evidence for a combination of intranasal mupirocin and chlorhexidine showers preoperatively, and vancomycin intraoperatively. When patients are seen in presurgical screening (or during a routine office visit for potential SCS patients), a polyester (Dacron) nasal swab of the nasal passage may be taken. Polymerase chain reaction (PCR)-based rapid testing is used to identify methicillin-resistant *Staphylococcus aureus*, and standard cultures are used to identify methicillin-sensitive *Staphylococcus aureus*. If patients test positive for either strain, they are treated with 2% intranasal mupirocin (Bactroban) twice daily for a five-day treatment course prior to implant date and continued for two days post-implant. Additionally, a shower wash of 2% chlorhexidine (Hibiclens) is taken the evening prior to surgery.[20] A combination of vancomycin and cefazolin dosed for weight can be used intraoperatively, as β-lactam antibiotics may provide better coverage for methicillin-sensitive *Staphylococcus aureus* strains.[26,27] SSI can be particularly devastating and difficult to treat in patients with implanted hardware, and, although the ideal regimen has yet to be determined, these developments allow another opportunity to minimize patient morbidity.

Finally a great deal of research has been done about the increased risk of SSI with smoking, as discussed in the following paragraphs.

Tobacco Use/Smoking Cessation

It is now clear that smoking is an important and significant factor in perioperative complications.[28-31] Although there are no SCS studies that have looked at the increased risk of SSI in smokers, there is an abundance of evidence in the general surgery literature from which to draw conclusions. Smokers have up to eight times the risk of wound infection (≈8% vs. 1%) after surgery.[32] Although the exact etiologic mechanism is unclear, carbon monoxide and the hypoxemic state it creates are likely important factors. The role of nicotine itself is unclear. It is a known vasoconstrictor that impairs tissue revascularization.[33] However, nicotine replacement therapy (NRT) does not increase infection rates in experimental or clinical studies and there is no evidence that it adversely affects wound healing.[34-36]

The risks of smoking have been unequivocally shown, and evidence continues to accumulate that smoking cessation can drastically reduce perioperative morbidity. In one study preoperative smoking cessation before joint replacement surgery reduced wound infection rates from 27% in smokers to 0% in those who quit,[37] At this time there is no consensus on the duration of smoking cessation for maximum benefit before surgery. Increased length of abstinence is certainly beneficial for a patient's overall health, and the ideal situation would be for this to continue permanently after surgery. However, given the difficulty most patients experience with quitting smoking, the search continues for the shortest amount of time that will still yield clinical benefit operatively. Initial studies showed clear benefit from smoking cessation for 6 to 8 weeks before surgery, consistent with physiological improvements in pulmonary and cardiac function.[32,38,39] Moller and associates[37] found a 65% decrease in postoperative complications with 6 to 8 weeks of preoperative smoking cessation before orthopedic surgeries. Even 4 weeks of smoking cessation reduced wound infection rates to that of nonsmokers in those having skin biopsies.[34] The 3-week mark may be the cutoff point to see benefit from smoking cessation. One study found that the complication rate for colorectal surgery was unchanged with smoking cessation ≤3 weeks,[40] whereas two separate studies found a reduction in complications in head and neck and breast reduction surgery with cessation ≥3 weeks.[41,42]

With the clear and proven increased risks from continued smoking, discussing smoking cessation with patients considering SCS may be an important part of preoperative education and teaching. Perioperative intervention can directly and dramatically decrease complication rates and can lead to sustained smoking cessation for up to 1 year after surgery.[43,44] Peters and colleagues[45] gave important perspective to the need for smoking cessation: "the adverse effect of failing to quit smoking is similar to that of omitting antibiotic prophylaxis." Unfortunately, despite this overwhelming increase in risks, many patients still continue to smoke.

Human Immunodeficiency Virus+

Advances in the treatment of human HIV/AIDS in the last 20 years have changed the disease course from a rapid and progressive affliction to a manageable chronic illness. With HIV/AIDS patients living longer and a general paradigm shift away from the focus on acute management, a greater percentage of HIV/AIDS patients are being seen for chronic pain states, whether specific to the condition or similar to those of the general population.

Currently there is the misperception that HIV-positive status alone increases the risk of postoperative complications. With the exception of certain transoral procedures,[46,47] review of the literature does not support this belief.[48-51] The most important risk factor for postoperative complications in the HIV+ patient is the one routinely assessed in *all* patients: ASA classification.[49] However, there are markers used to monitor disease status that are predictive of increased risk (**Box 3-2**). Increased morbidity and mortality rates are associated with CD4 count ≤200 cell/mm^3 and viral load

---

Box 3-2: Operative Risk Factors in Human Immunodeficiency Virus+ Patients

ASA Classification
CD4 <200 cells/mm^3
Viral load >10,000 copies/mL
Postoperative CD4% ≤18 ± 3
↓ in CD4% of ≥3

ASA, American Society of Anesthesiologists.

>10,000 copies/mL.[50,52-55] In addition, a postoperative CD4 percent of ≤18 ± 3 and a decrease in percent CD4 of ≥3 are associated with increased morbidity.[54] All these values can easily be tested for, and any physician operating on an HIV+ patient should strongly consider ordering these laboratory values routinely. If there are abnormalities, both SCS trial and implant should be delayed, and the patient referred to an infectious disease specialist. To date there are no SCS studies that have specifically looked at the increased risk of infection in HIV+ patients.

Thrombocytopenia (platelets <50,000/µL) is a frequent finding in HIV+ patients, with prevalence rates from 9% to 37% in various study populations.[56] Therefore thorough preoperative evaluation of platelet count and correction of a possible coagulation disorder is mandatory before proceeding with surgical intervention. Most implanters believe that an implant should be delayed until platelets are above 50,000 by either disease correction or platelet infusion.

Obesity

There is considerable stigma associated with obesity (body mass index [BMI] >30 kg/m^2), and outcomes are impacted in many areas of medicine. Most physicians are aware of the deterioration of cardiac, pulmonary, and immunological function associated with obesity.[57-59] Obesity is also associated with decreased quality of life and life expectancy.[60,61] The co-morbidities of obesity are well known, and the list of associated disease states continues to grow annually. Given this, there is the commonly held deduction that obesity is a significant risk factor for perioperative complications. Although there is an increased risk of wound infections,[62,63] Dindo and colleagues[64] have shown that obesity alone is not a risk factor for postoperative complications. Further, their prospective study of >6000 patients over 10 years showed no significant difference in median operation time or need for blood transfusions. The latter results are especially encouraging given the high prevalence of obesity among chronic pain patients. However, the increased risk of wound infection is particularly worrisome. With implantable technologies, simple wound infections can lead to significant morbidity, often requiring explanation of an otherwise well-functioning device. To date there have been no SCS studies specifically assessing the increased risk of wound infection in obese patients and whether obesity leads to increased rates of explantation or further morbidity in SCS. At this time it is appropriate to counsel the obese patient of his or her increased risk of infection. At worst this allows the patient to make a better-informed decision; at best it may provide further motivation toward weight loss. Anecdotal data suggest that, with improved pain control, patients may be able to engage in the behavioral modifications necessary for weight loss.

Rheumatoid Arthritis

Compared to the general population, patients with RA have an increased incidence of SSI, as high as 15%. Concomitant steroid use has been associated with increased risk, whereas continued methotrexate use has been linked to decreased risk.[65-67] den Broeder

---

Box 3-3: Recommendations for Management of Persons with Type I Diabetes Undergoing Spinal Cord Stimulation

- Patients should not administer any insulin the morning of surgery.
- Blood glucose, serum electrolytes, and ketones (urine or blood) measured morning of surgery.
- Begin an infusion of 10% dextrose in ½ NS. Flow rate should be consistent with fluid maintenance for the patient (≈100 mL/hr in an average adult). Add 20 mEq of KCl to each liter if no renal failure.
- If blood glucose is 100 to 200 mg/dL, proceed with surgery.
- If blood glucose is >200 mg/dL, rapid-acting insulin is administered subcutaneously using the Rule of 1500 to determine dose (see Box 3-4).
- Check blood glucose every hour. Rapid-acting insulin is administered if >200 mg/dL as stated previously.

Adapted from Bergman S: Perioperative management of the diabetic patient, *Oral Surg Oral Med Oral Pathol Oral Radiol Endod* 103:731-737, 2007.
NS, Normal saline.

Box 3-4: Rule of 1500

1. 1500 is divided by the patient's daily dose of insulin to determine the correction factor (e.g., if the patient is taking 30 units of insulin/day, 1500/30 = 50). This indicates that each unit of insulin is expected to lower the blood glucose by 50 mg/dL.
2. 150 is subtracted from measured blood glucose. The remainder is the amount the blood glucose must be lowered using the correction factor. (In the previous example, if the patient's blood glucose is 300 mg/dL, 300 − 150 = 150. The blood glucose must be lowered by 150. Using the correction factor in the previous example, each unit of insulin would decrease blood glucose by 50; therefore 3 U of rapid-acting insulin is given.)

Adapted from Bergman SA: Perioperative management of the diabetic patient, *Oral Surg Oral Med Oral Pathol Oral Radiol Endod* 103:731-737, 2007.

Box 3-5: Recommendations for Management of Patients With Type II Diabetes Undergoing Spinal Cord Stimulation

1. Patients well controlled with diet and exercise require no special intervention.
2. Patients taking oral diabetic medication should not take usual AM dose.
   a. Patients taking a long-acting second-generation sulfonylurea medication should not take their daily dose *the day before* surgery: glimepiride (Amaryl), glipizide (Glucotrol), glyburide (DiaBeta, Micronase).
   b. Patients taking chlorpropamide (Diabinese) should stop taking the medication *2 days before* surgery.
3. Blood glucose should be measured before surgery:
   a. 100 to 250 mg/dL: Proceed with surgery.
   b. >250 mg/dL: Begin an infusion of 5% or 10% dextrose in ½ normal saline. Flow rate should be consistent with fluid maintenance for the patient (≈100 mL/hr in an average adult). Add 20 mEq of KCl to each liter if no renal failure. Rapid-acting insulin lispro (Humalog) or aspart (NovoLog) 0.1 U/kg is given subcutaneously.

Adapted from Bergman SA: Perioperative management of the diabetic patient, *Oral Surg Oral Med Oral Pathol Oral Radiol Endod* 103:731-731, 2007.

---

and associates[68] examined the risk of SSI in those using anti–tumor necrosis factor (TNF) therapy and found no effect on SSI. However, the patients on anti-TNF therapy did have higher rates of wound dehiscence and bleeding. Interestingly, they found sulfasalazine to have a strong protective effect against SSI and hypothesized that this may be because of the bactericidal effect of the sulfapyridine component. Currently it would seem prudent to withhold anti-TNF medications before surgery. This would require stopping anti-TNF treatment for at least four drug half-lives before surgery (12 days for etanercept [Enbrel], 39 days for infliximab [Remicade], 56 days for adalimumab [Humira]).[69] Changes in the patient's disease-modifying agents are best coordinated with their rheumatologist.

Diabetes Mellitus

As the rate of DM increases,[70] the proportion of patients who are candidates for SCS with diabetes will likewise grow. Currently pain from peripheral diabetic neuropathy shows excellent response to SCS.[71,72] The stress from surgery induces the release of counter-regulatory hormones, which leads to insulin resistance, increased glucose production, decreased insulin secretion, and ultimately hyperglycemia.[73] Subsequently this hyperglycemic state inhibits leukocyte function[74] and collagen formation, decreasing wound tensile strength.[75,76] Perioperative hyperglycemia is known to be an independent risk factor for the development of SSI.[77] Interestingly, in a retrospective review of over 38,000 surgeries by Acott, Theus, and Kim,[78] there was no correlation between hemoglobin A1c levels and risk of complication, type of complication, or death.

Although the terms "strict" and "optimal" glycemic control are used in the management of DM, there is no consensus definition of these terms in the surgical patient. There is evidence that maintaining *postoperative* blood glucose <200 mg/dL reduces the incidence of SSI,[79] but there is no clear guide as to what an ideal *preoperative* blood glucose range is. Bergman[80] has developed guidelines for the management of persons with type I diabetes (**Boxes 3-3 and 3-4**) and those with type II diabetes undergoing minor surgery (**Box 3-5**). He further recommends that persons with type II diabetes should take their oral medication as soon as they resume eating/drinking. There are no recommendations for the discontinuation of rosiglitazone (Avandia) or pioglitazone (Actos) before surgery. With their long duration of action, it is

unclear if there is a reason to stop them at all.[81] After surgery persons with type I diabetes should monitor their blood glucose every 2 hours; persons with type II diabetes should monitor every 4 hours. To date no SCS studies have specifically addressed the increased risk of infection in patients with diabetes.

Anticoagulation

One of the most devastating complications involving SCS procedures in the patient with a compromised coagulation status is epidural hematoma. There are no figures to cite regarding epidural hematoma following SCS trial/implant; however, the anesthesia literature shows the rate to be <1 in 150,000 following epidural anesthesia.[82] As dimensions of a percutaneous lead are similar to an epidural catheter, familiarity with guidelines in regional anesthesia are necessary until such time that there are studies specifically applicable to SCS. A synthesis of recommendations from the 2010 American Society of Regional Anesthesia and Pain Medicine (ASRA) consensus guidelines for patients receiving anticoagulation is presented in **Table 3-1**.[83] A patient on warfarin (Coumadin) should stop it for at least 5 days before the procedure and have their

Table 3-1: 2010 ASRA Precautions and Recommendations in Anticoagulated Patients

Medication	Recommendation
Aspirin	May continue. There are no specific timing concerns of administering neuraxial anesthesia or catheter removal.
Clopidogrel (Plavix)	Discontinue 7 days before surgery.
Fondaparinux (Arixtra)	Neuraxial techniques can be considered if single-needle pass, atraumatic technique is used. However, authors favor to wait >3 half-lives (3-5 days) after discontinuation. Avoid indwelling catheters.
Glycoprotein IIb/IIIa inhibitors Abciximab (ReoPro), eptifibatide (Integrilin), tirofiban (Aggrastat)	Discontinue eptifibatide, tirofiban 8 hours before surgery. Discontinue abciximab 24-48 hours before surgery.
Heparin, unfractionated (UFH)	Perform procedure immediately before next dose of SQ heparin or 2 hours after last dose. No contraindication with twice-daily dosing or total daily dose <10,000 U. Safety is unknown in those receiving >10,000 U daily or with more than BID dosing. Remove catheter (trial lead) 1 hour before next scheduled dose. In patients receiving heparin >4 days, check platelet count given risk of heparin-induced thrombocytopenia (HIT).
Heparin (systemic heparinization)	Heparinize 1 hour after technique. Discontinue heparin 2-4 hours before catheter (trial lead) removal. Check coagulation status before removal. Continue neurological assessment for 12 hours after catheter removal.
Herbals (garlic, ginkgo, ginseng)	May continue. No specific timing concerns of administering neuraxial anesthesia or catheter removal
Low-molecular-weight heparin (LMWH) Enoxaparin (Lovenox), dalteparin (Fragmin)	Monitoring anti-Xa levels is not recommended. Wait 10-12 hours after last dose if patient is taking prophylactic doses. Wait ≥24 hours after last dose if patient is taking therapeutic doses. Resume 24 hours after surgery if on BID dosing. Indwelling catheter must be removed before first dose of LMWH. Administer LMWH 2 hours after catheter removal. Resume 6-8 hours after surgery if on daily dosing. Indwelling catheter can be maintained. When catheter is removed, it should be done 10-12 hours after last dose of LMWH. Next dose of LMWH is at least 2 hours after removal.
NSAIDs	May continue. There are no specific timing concerns of administering neuraxial anesthesia or catheter removal.
Thrombin inhibitors Argatroban (Acova), bivalirudin (Angiomax), desirudin (Iprivask/Revasc), lepirudin (Refludan)	There are no recommendations at this time because of lack of information.
Ticlopidine (Ticlid)	Discontinue 14 days before surgery.
Warfarin (Coumadin)	Discontinue warfarin 5 days before surgery. Recommend against concurrent use of aspirin, NSAIDs, clopidogrel, ticlopidine, UFH or LMWH. Check preoperative PT/INR. If INR <1.5, proceed. Resume warfarin on first postoperative day.

Adapted from Horlocker TT et al: Regional anesthesia in the patient receiving antithrombotic or thrombolytic therapy, *Reg Anes Pain Med* 35(1):64-101, 2010.
ASRA, American Society of Regional Anesthesia and Pain Medicine; *INR*, international normalized ratio; *LMWH*, low-molecular-weight heparin; *NSAID*, nonsteroidal antiinflammatory drug; *PT*, prothrombin time; *UFH*, unfractionated heparin.

prothrombin time (PT)/international normalized ratio (INR) checked before surgery. The INR should be <1.5 before proceeding with regional anesthesia per ASRA guidelines. For those patients in whom stopping warfarin poses too high a risk without continued anticoagulation, low-molecular-weight heparin (LMWH) should be used as a bridge (**Box 3-6**).[84] Clopidogrel (Plavix), an antiplatelet agent that binds to the cysteine residue of platelet receptor P2Y12, is commonly used in conjunction with aspirin to attenuate platelet aggregation. However, unlike warfarin, there is no drug with a shorter half-life that can be adequately substituted before surgery.[85,86] Although heparin "bridge" therapy has been advocated for those on clopidogrel and considered high risk for thrombotic

events, there is no literature to support this.[87] In this case, when the risk of thrombosis is so high that any interruption of antiplatelet therapy could result in significant morbidity, elective surgery should be reconsidered. Arguably, with both SCS trial and implant, the greater concern is bleeding rather than thrombotic risk: the procedure is short and performed on an outpatient basis, and many patients have improved mobility after it is completed. In this situation stopping clopidogrel 7 days before the procedure and resuming 12 to 24 hours after surgery are logical.[88,89] When weighing the decision to stop clopidogrel, it is recommended that there be no interruption in therapy for the first year after it is initiated.[88,90] Physicians should strongly consider coordinating changes in the patient's anticoagulant medications with the prescribing physician and/or a hematologist.

Other Considerations

At this time the only SCS that are approved for use with magnetic resonance imaging (MRI) are those produced by Medtronic. Only an MRI of the head with a magnet strength ≤1.5 Tesla is considered safe. MRI can only be conducted in completely implanted systems and can*not* be conducted during a trial. Even following these precautions, there is still a risk of permanent damage to the SCS requiring revision or explant.[91] Given the considerable risk to the patient and necessary precautionary steps, including reprogramming the SCS to manufacturer recommended specifications, these changes are best made in conjunction with a representative from the company.

Previously the combination of SCS and ICDs (pacemaker, defibrillator) was contraindicated. However, review of the manufacturers' prescriptive information shows that their stance is softening, no doubt based on the successful use of these devices together in case reports.[92-94] Nonetheless, the official statements for the three manufacturers are as follows:

1. Boston Scientific: "Spinal cord stimulators may interfere with the operation of implanted sensing stimulators such as pacemakers or cardioverter defibrillators. The effects of implanted stimulation devices on neurostimulators are unknown."[95]
2. Medtronic: "An ICD (e.g., pacemaker, defibrillator) may damage a neurostimulator, and the electrical pulses from the neurostimulator may result in an inappropriate response of the cardiac device."[96]
3. St Jude Medical: Identifies "demand-type cardiac pacemakers" as a contraindication and cardioverter defibrillators under "warnings/precautions."[97]

The concern for interaction between SCS and pacemaker is inability to pace, whereas in defibrillators it is inappropriate shock. To minimize this interaction the SCS should be set to a bipolar configuration, and the cardiac device should be set to bipolar

sensing. Coordination should be undertaken with the patient's cardiologist involved in all aspects of perioperative evaluation. Regardless of device, the physician should request the presence of the company representative from the pacemaker manufacturer to be present in the perioperative period to evaluate any interaction between the SCS and the pacemaker. In many cases these devices are used in combination without problems. The successful use of SCS in this patient group is very important since the use of these devices for patients with ischemic pain, peripheral vascular disease, and diabetic peripheral neuropathy will most likely increase over time. Each of these groups has a propensity toward cardiovascular disease and may require ICD placement.

Is Spinal Cord Stimulation Disease-Modifying?

Despite our current neuroanatomical knowledge, conditions such as complex regional pain syndrome prove that there is still much more to be learned and deciphered. Most chronic pain states almost certainly have a neuropathic component and some degree of central sensitization, and it is these features that can be exploited via SCS. As SCS use expands and it is used for a greater variety of patients with multiple medical conditions, there is evidence that it modulates more than just pain. Krames and Mousad[98] describe a case in which reductions in diarrheal episodes were found in a patient initially implanted for the pain of irritable bowel syndrome. In those with critical limb ischemia, a long-term outcome study in Italy showed that those implanted with SCS had statistically significant improved limb survival at 1 year.[99] Kapural and associates[100] describe a patient with complex regional pain syndrome (CRPS), type 1 of the left lower extremity and type 2 DM who had ≈50% decrease in insulin requirement after successful SCS implantation. It has also been found that, even in FBSS cases in which SCS provides only minimal pain relief, there can still be improvements in leg muscle strength and gait.[101]

Conclusion

As the safety and efficacy of SCS expand, a greater number of patients may benefit from its use. Although many patient factors are now considerations rather than contraindications,[102,103] there are still many questions left unanswered. As the use of SCS grows, there may be evidence to direct clinicians as to how specific disease processes affect and in turn are affected by SCS. Until that time, knowledgeable physicians will continue to rely on and synthesize information from a variety of fields to best treat their patients—a familiar situation for any of us who treat those in pain.

References

1. Kane K, Taub A: A history of local electrical analgesia. *Pain* 1:25-138, 1975.
2. Shealy CN, Mortimer JT, Reswick JB: Electrical inhibition of pain by stimulation of the dorsal columns: preliminary clinical report. *Anesth Analg* 46(4):489-491, 1967.
3. Culver DH et al: Surgical wound infection rates by wound class, operative procedure, and patient risk index. *Am J Med* 91(S):152-157, 1991.
4. Kumar K et al: Spinal cord stimulation versus conventional medical management for neuropathic pain: a multicentre randomized controlled trial in patients with failed back surgery syndrome. *Pain* 132:179-188, 2007.
5. Stojanovic MP, Abdi S: Spinal cord stimulation. *Pain Phys* 5:156-166, 2002.
6. Rosenow JM et al: Failure modes of SCS hardware. *J Neurosurg* 100(3):254-267, 2004.

7. Hill PE: Complications of permanent transvenous cardiac pacing: a 14-year review of all transvenous pacemakers inserted at one community hospital. *Pacing Clin Electrophysiol* 10:564-570, 1987.

8. Kearney R, Eisen HJ, Wolf JE: Nonvalvular infections of the cardiovascular system. *Ann Intern Med* 121:219-230, 1994.

9. Nery PB, Fernandes R, Nair G: Device-related infection among patients with pacemakers and implantable defibrillators: incidence, risk factors, and consequences. *J Cardiovasc Electrophysiol* 21(7):786-790, 2010.

10. Cesar de Oliveira J et al: Efficacy of antibiotic prophylaxis before the implantation of pacemakers and cardioverter-defibrillators: results of a large, prospective, randomized, double-blinded, placebo-controlled trial. *Circ Arrhythmia Electrophysiol* 2:29-34, 2009.

11. Baddour LM et al: Update on cardiovascular implantable electronic device infections and their management. *Circulation* 121:458-477, 2010.

12. Gaynes RP et al: Surgical site infection (SSI) rates in the United States, 1992 1998: the National Nosocomial Infections Surveillance System basic SSI risk index. *Clin Infect Dis* 33(S2):S69-S77, 2001.

13. Haridas M, Malangoni MA: Predictive factors for surgical site infection in general surgery. *Surgery* 144:496-503, 2008.

14. Walsh EE, Greene L, Kirshner L: Sustained reduction in methicillin-resistant *Staphylococcus aureus* wound infections after cardiothoracic surgery. *Arch Intern Med* 171(1):68-73, 2011.

15. Sharma M, Berriel-Cass D, Baran J, Jr: Sternal surgical-site infections following coronary artery bypass graft: prevalence, microbiology, and complications during a 42-month period. *Infect Control Hosp Epidemiol* 25(6):468-471, 2004.

16. Filsoufi F, Castillo JG, Rahmanian PB et al: Epidemiology of deep sternal wound infection in cardiac surgery. *J Cardiothorac Vasc Anesth* 23(4):488-494, 2009.

17. Boucher HW, Corey GR: Epidemiology of methicillin-resistant *Staphylococcus aureus*. *Clin Infect Dis* 46(Suppl 5):S344-S349, 2008.

18. Perl TM, Golub JE: New approaches to reduce *Staphylococcus aureus* nosocomial infection rates: treating *S. aureus* nasal carriage. *Ann Pharmacother* 32:S7-16, 1998.

19. Wenzel RP, Perl TM: The significance of nasal carriage of *Staphylococcus aureus* and the incidence of postoperative wound infection. *J Hosp Infect* 31:13-24, 1995.

20. Kim DH, Spencer M, Davidson SM et al: Institutional prescreening for detection and eradication of methicillin-resistant *Staphylococcus aureus* in patients undergoing elective orthopedic surgery. *J Bone Joint Surg Am* 92:1820-1826, 2010.

21. Rao N, Cannella B, Crossett LS et al: A preoperative decolonization protocol for *Staphylococcus aurues* prevents orthopaedic infections. *Clin Orthop Relat Res* 466:1343-1348, 2008.

22. Kalmeijer MD, Coertjens H, van Nieuwland-Rollen PM et al: Surgical site infections in orthopedic surgery: the effect of mupirocin nasal ointment in a double-blind, randomized, placebo-controlled study. *Clin Infect Dis* 35:353-358, 2002.

23. Herwaldt LA: Reduction of *Staphylococcus aureus* nasal carriage and infection in dialysis patients. *J Hosp Infect* 40(Suppl B): S13-S23, 1998.

24. Kluytmans JA, Manders MJ, van Bommel E et al: Elimination of nasal carriage of *Staphylococcus aureus* in hemodialysis patients. *Infect Control Hosp Epidemiol* 17:780-785, 1996.

25. Bode LGM, Kluytmans JAJW, Wertheim HFL et al: Preventing surgical-site infections in nasal carriers of *Staphylococcus aureus*. *N Engl J Med* 362:9-17, 2010.

26. Engelman R, Shahian D, Shemin R et al: Workforce on Evidence-Based Medicine, Society of Thoracic Surgeons. The Society of Thoracic Surgeons practice guideline series: antibiotic prophylaxis in cardiac surgery, II: antibiotic choice. *Ann Thorac Surg* 83(4):1569-1576, 2007.

27. Stevens DL: The role of vancomycin in the treatment paradigm. *Clin Infect Dis* 42(suppl 1):S51-S57, 2006.

28. Schwilk B et al: Perioperative respiratory events in smokers and non-smokers undergoing general anaesthesia. *Acta Anaesthesiol Scand* 41:348-355, 1997.

29. Morton HJV: Tobacco smoking and pulmonary complications after operation. *Lancet* 1:368-370, 1944.

30. Bluman LG et al: Preoperative smoking habits and postoperative pulmonary complications. *Chest* 113:883-889, 1998.

31. Wetterslev J et al: PaO$_2$ during anaesthesia and years of smoking predict late postoperative hypoxaemia and complications after upper abdominal surgery in patients without preoperative cardiopulmonary dysfunction. *Acta Anaesthesiol Scand* 44:9-16, 2000.

32. Padubidri AN et al: Complications of postmastectomy breast reconstructions in smokers, ex-smokers, and nonsmokers. *Plast Reconstr Surg* 107:342-349, 2001.

33. Krueger JK, Rohrick RJ: Clearing the smoke: the scientific rationale for tobacco abstention with plastic surgery. *Plast Reconstr Surg* 108:1063-1073, 2001.

34. Sorensen LT, Karlsmakr T, Gottrup F: Abstinence from smoking reduces incisional wound infection: a randomized controlled trial. *Ann Surg* 238:1-5, 2003.

35. Glassman SD et al: The effect of cigarette smoking and smoking cessation on spinal fusion. *Spine* 25:2608-2615, 2000.

36. Bennett-Guerrero E et al: The use of a postoperative morbidity survey to evaluate patients with prolonged hospitalization after routine, moderate-risk, elective surgery. *Anesth Analg* 89:514-519, 1999.

37. Moller AM et al: Effect of preoperative smoking intervention on postoperative complications: a randomized clinical trial. *Lancet* 359:114-117, 2002.

38. Buist AS et al: The effect of smoking cessation and modification of lung function. *Am Rev Respir Dis* 114:115-122, 1976.

39. Kinsella JB et al: Smoking increases facial skin flap complications. *Ann Otol Rhinol Laryngol* 108:139-142, 1999.

40. Sorensen JT, Jorsengen T: Short-term pre-operative smoking cessation intervention does not affect postoperative complications in colorectal surgery: a randomized clinical trial. *Colorectal Dis* 5:347-352, 2003.

41. Kuri M et al: Determination of the duration of preoperative smoking cessation to improve wound healing after head and neck surgery. *Anesthesiology* 102:892-896, 2005.

42. Chan L, Withey S, Butler P: Smoking and wound healing problems in reduction mammoplasty: is the introduction of urine nicotine testing justified? *Ann Plast Surg* 56:111-115, 2006.

43. Azodi OS et al: The efficacy of a smoking cessation programme in patients undergoing planned surgery—a randomized clinical trial. *Anaesthesia* 64:259-265, 2009.

44. Villebro NM et al: Long-term effects of a preoperative smoking cessation programme. *Clin Resp J* 2:175-182, 2008.

45. Peters MJ, Morgan LC, Gluch L: Smoking cessation and elective surgery: the cleanest cut. *Med J Aust* 180:317-318, 2004.

46. Reilly MJ, Burke KM, Davison SP: Wound infection rates in elective plastic surgery for HIV-positive patients. *Plast Reconstr Surg* 123:106-112, 2009.

47. Rose DN, Collins M, Kleban R: Complications of surgery in HIV-infected patients. *AIDS* 12:2243-2251, 1998.

48. Ayers J, Howton M, Layon J: Postoperative complications in patients with human immunodeficiency virus disease. *Chest* 103:1800-1807, 1993.

49. Jones S et al: Is HIV infection a risk factor for complications of surgery? *Mt Sinai J Med* 29:329-333, 2002.

50. Horberg M et al: Surgical outcomes of HIV+ patients in the era of HARRT (Abstract 82). Presented at the 11th Conference of Retroviruses and Opportunistic Infections, San Francisco, California. February 8-11, 2004.

51. Dodson TB: HIV status and the risk of post-extraction complications. *J Dent Res* 76:1644-1652, 1997.

52. Emparan C et al: Infective complications after abdominal surgery in patients infected with human immunodeficiency virus: role of CD4 lymphocytes in prognosis. *World J Surg* 22(8):778-782, 1998.

53. Saltzman DJ et al: The surgeon and AIDS: twenty years later. *Arch Surg* 140:961-967, 2005.

54. Tran HS et al: Predictors of operative outcome in patients with human immunodeficiency virus infection and acquired immunodeficiency syndrome. *Am J Surg* 180(3):228-233, 2000.

55. Consten EC et al: Severe complications of perianal sepsis in patients with human immunodeficiency virus. *Br J Surg* 83(6):778-780, 1996.

56. Sullivan P et al: Surveillance for thrombocytopenia in persons infected with HIV. *J Acquir Immune Defic Syndr Hum Retrovirol* 14:(4):374-379, 1997.

57. Berkalp B et al: Obesity and left ventricular diastolic dysfunction. *Int J Cardiol* 52:23-26, 1995.

58. Pi-Sunyer FX: Medical hazards of obesity. *Ann Intern Med* 119:655-660, 1993.

59. Tanaka S et al: Impaired immunity in obesity: suppressed but reversible lymphocyte responsiveness. *Int J Obes Relat Metab Disord* 17:631-636, 1993.

60. Manson JE et al: Body weight and mortality among women. *N Engl J Med* 333:677-685, 1995.

61. Allison DB et al: Meta-analysis of the effect of excluding early deaths on the estimated relationship between body mass index and mortality. *Obes Res* 7:342-354, 1999.

62. Moulton MJ et al: Obesity is not a risk factor for significant adverse outcomes after cardiac surgery. *Circulation* 94(S):II87-92, 1996.

63. Shapiro M et al: Risk factors for infection at the operative site after abdominal or vaginal hysterectomy. *N Engl J Med* 307:1661-1666, 1982.

64. Dindo D et al: Obesity in general elective surgery. *Lancet* 361:2032-2035, 2003.

65. Grennan DM et al: Methotrexate and early postoperative complications in patients with rheumatoid arthritis undergoing elective orthopedic surgery. *Ann Rheum Dis* 60:214-217, 2001.

66. Hamalainen M, Raunio P, Von Essen R: Postoperative wound infection in rheumatoid arthritis surgery. *Clin Rheumatol* 3:329-335, 1984.

67. Bongartz T et al: Incidence and risk factors for prosthetic joint infections in patients with rheumatoid arthritis following total knee and total hip replacement. *Arthritis Rheum* 52(S):1449, 2005.

68. den Broeder AA et al: Risk factors for surgical site infections and other complications in elective surgery in patients with rheumatoid arthritis with special attention for anti-tumor necrosis factor: a large retrospective study. *J Rheumatol* 34:689-695, 2007.

69. Nederlandse Vereniging voor Reumatologie: *Medicijnen: het toepassen van TNF blokkade in de behandeling van reumatoïde artritis.* Utrecht, November 2003, Dutch Society for Rheumatology.

70. Shaw JE, Sicree RA, Zimmet PZ: Global estimates of the prevalence of diabetes for 2010 and 2030. *Diabetes Res Clinic Pract* 87(1):4-14, 2010.

71. Daousi C, Benbow SJ, MacFarlane IA: Electrical spinal cord stimulation in the long-term treatment of chronic painful diabetic neuropathy. *Diabet Med* 2005;22(4):393-398.

72. Tesfaye S et al: Electrical spinal-cord stimulation for painful diabetic peripheral neuropathy. *Lancet* 348(9043):1698-1701, 1996.

73. Shamoon H, Hendler R, Sherwin RS: Synergistic actions among anti-insulin hormones in pathogenesis of stress hyperglycemia in humans. *J Clin Endocrinol Metab* 52:1235-1241, 1981.

74. Marhoffer W et al: Impairment of polymorphonuclear leukocyte function and metabolic control of diabetes. *Diabetes Care* 15:256-260, 1992.

75. Gottrup F, Andreassen TT: Healing of incisional wounds in stomach and duodenum: the influence of experimental diabetes. *J Surg Res* 31:61-68, 1981.

76. McMurray JFJ: Wound healing with diabetes mellitus: better glucose control for better wound healing in diabetes. *Surg Clin North Am* 64:769-778, 1984.

77. Golden SH et al: Perioperative glycemic control and risk of infectious complications in a cohort of adults with diabetes. *Diabetes Care* 22:1408-1414, 1999.

78. Acott AA, Theus SA, Kim LT: Long-term glucose control and risk of perioperative complications. *Am J Surg* 198(5):596-599, 2009.

79. Zerr KJ et al: Glucose control lowers the risk of wound infection in diabetics after open heart operations. *Ann Thorac Surg* 63:356-361, 1997.

80. Bergman SA: Perioperative management of the diabetic patient. *Oral Surg Oral Med Oral Pathol Oral Radiol Endod* 103:731-737, 2007.

81. Marks JB: Perioperative management of diabetes. *Am Fam Phys* 67:93-100, 2003.

82. Tryba M: Ru ckmarksnahe regionalana sthesie und niedermolekulare heparine. *Pro Ana sth Intensivmed Notfallmed Schmerzther* 28:179-181, 1993.

83. Horlocker TT et al: Regional anesthesia in the patient receiving anti-thrombotic or thrombolytic therapy. *Reg Anes Pain Med* 35(1):64-101, 2010.

84. Jaffer AK, Brotman DJ, Chukwumerije N: When patients on warfarin need surgery. *Cleve Clin J Med* 70(11):973-984, 2003.

85. Gonzalez-Correa JA et al: Effects of dexibuprofen on platelet function in humans: comparison with low-dose aspirin. *Anesthesia* 106(2):218-225, 2007.

86. Samama CM: Preoperative nonsteroidal anti-inflammatory agents as substitutes for aspirin: already too late? *Anesthesia* 106(2):205-206, 2007.

87. Collet JP, Montalescot G: Premature withdrawal and alternative therapies to dual oral antiplatelet therapy. *Eur Heart J Suppl* 8(suppl G):G46-G52, 2006.

88. Thacil J, Gatt A, Martlew V: Management of surgical patients receiving anticoagulation and antiplatelet agents. *Br J Surg* 95:1437-1448, 2008.

89. Di Minno MND et al: Perioperative handling of patients on antiplatelet therapy with need for surgery. *Intern Emerg Med* 4:279-288, 2009.

90. O'Riordan JM et al: Antiplatelet agents in the perioperative period. *Arch Surg* 144(1):69-76, 2009.

91. Medtronic: *MRI guidelines,* accessed February 13, 2010, from http://professional.medtronic.com/interventions/spinal-cord-stimulation/mri-guidelines/index.htm#anchor1.

92. Kosharskyy B, Rozen D: Feasibility of spinal cord stimulation in a patient with a cardiac pacemaker. *Pain Phys* 9:249-252, 2006.

93. Hoelzer BC, Burgher AH, Huntoon MA: Thoracic spinal cord stimulation for post-ablation cardiac pain in a patient with permanent pacemaker. *Pain Prac* 8(2):110-113, 2008.

94. Andersen C, Pedersen HS, Scherer C: Management of spinal cord stimulators in patients with implantable cardioverter-defibrillators. *Neuromodulation* 5(3):133-136, 2002.

95. Boston Scientific: *Precision plus SCS system,* accessed February 26, 2010, from http://www.bostonscientific.com/Device.bsci?page=ResourceDetail&navRelId=1000.1003&method=DevDetailHCP&id=10068931&resource_type_category_id=1&resource_type_id=91&pageDisclaimer=Disclaimer.ProductPage.

96. Medtronic: *Spinal cord stimulation—indications, safety and warnings,* accessed February 26/2010 from http://professional.medtronic.com/interventions/spinal-cord-stimulation/indications-safety-and-warnings/index.htm.

97. St. Jude Medical: *Eon mini rechargeable IPG system,* accessed February 26, 2010, from http://www.sjmneuropro.com/Products/US/Eon-Mini-Rechargeable-IPG-System.aspx.

98. Krames E, Mousad D: Spinal cord stimulation reverses pain and diarrheal episodes of irritable bowel syndrome: a case report. *Neuromodulation* 7(2):82-88, 2004.

99. Tedesco A, D'Addato M: Spinal cord stimulation for patients with critical limb ischemia: immediate and long-term clinical outcome from the prospective Italian register. *Neuromodulation* 7(2):97-102, 2004.

100. Kapural L et al: Decreased insulin requirements with spinal cord stimulation in a patient with diabetes. *Anesth Analg* 98:745-746, 2004.

101. Buonocore M, Demartini L, Bonezzi C: Lumbar spinal cord stimulation can improve muscle strength and gait independently of analgesic effect: a case report. *Neuromodulation* 9(4):309-313, 2006.

102. Segal R: Spinal cord stimulation, conception, pregnancy, and labor: case study in a complex regional pain syndrome patient. *Neuromodulation* 2(1):41-45, 1999.

103. Saxena A, Eljamel S: Spinal cord stimulation in the first two trimesters of pregnancy: case report and review of the literature. *Neuromodulation* 12(4):281-283, 2009.

4 Patient Selection: Psychological Considerations

Daniel M. Doleys

CHAPTER OVERVIEW

Chapter Synopsis: Chapter 4 addresses the *mind* of the recipient of electrical spinal cord stimulation (SCS), beyond considerations strictly of the nervous system. A brief history of the prevailing views of the mind-body connection—or lack thereof—illustrates the historical dismissal of the psyche in pain management. Today the forthcoming fifth edition of the *Diagnostic and Statistical Manual of Mental Disorders* (DSM-V) leaves behind mind-body dualism by excluding hypochondriasis and other such disorders. We now realize that psychological factors are the predominant reason behind failure of SCS treatment and that technical success by no means ensures clinical success. Both the patient's and the clinician's expectations—and their beliefs about the very nature of pain—can influence the success of SCS. It is clear by now that a preimplantation psychological assessment is a nontrivial component of SCS treatment. Moreover, SCS should not be used as a treatment in isolation; clinicians need to recognize their role as long-term facilitators of the patient's experience. A patient's understanding of the SCS device and technique seems to positively impact outcome, as does his or her appreciation of pain as a multifactorial experience with sensory, affective, and cognitive components. Some mood and personality disorders can be contraindications for SCS. Psychological assessments should be conducted by a pain-oriented psychologist and should not be left to computerized questionnaires. This vague and diverse array of psychological factors should not be underestimated. Further study may provide ways to standardize our assessment before SCS treatment to optimize outcomes.

Important Points:
- Do not underestimate the effect of psychosocial factors on the outcome of SCS.
- Obtain the psychological consultation early in the treatment process.
- Seek out a description of the relevant patient characteristics and not just a prediction.
- Whenever appropriate, emphasize a 'functionally-oriented' trial and outcome.
- Develop a working relationship with your psychological consultant.

Clinical Pearls:
- Chronic pain is a multidimensional, multifactorial, and dynamic experience.
- A pre-implant psychological evaluation, including a clinical interview and appropriate testing, can yield information relevant to patient selection and long-term management.
- Significant numbers of patients passing a screening trial report the loss of benefit within 24 months, despite a functional SCS system.

Clinical Pitfalls:
- Ignoring the impact of psychosocial factors on chronic pain
- Assuming the screening trial is the sole and best predictor of long-term treatment outcome
- Focusing only on pain relief without attending to quality of life (QoL) and functional outcomes

Introduction

Electrical stimulation for the treatment of pain dates back to 46 AD when Scribonius Largus described the use of torpedoes, a fishlike animal capable of emitting an electric discharge, placed over the area of pain for relief from intractable headache and arthritis. In 1745 the Leyden jar allowed physicians to control electrical current, and its use spread rapidly. Electrical stimulation of the brain was noted in 1950. Shealy, Mortimer, and Reswick[1] reported on the use of cardiac pacemaker technology to deliver electric current to the spinal cord via surgically implanted electrodes in 1967. Remarkable surgical and technological advances over the ensuing half century have resulted in various types of percutaneous and surgically implanted paddle leads capable of delivering thousands of different stimulating patterns using totally internalized, radiofrequency coupled, or rechargeable pulse generators. This technological flexibility has dramatically broadened the horizon of clinical application. The emphasis in this chapter is on the use of electrical stimulation in the treatment of chronic pain.

Descartes' explanation of pain mechanisms and processing[2] put forth in his 1664 book *Treatise of Man* held sway from the 1600s until Melzack and Wall presented their gate control theory in 1965.[3] The latter theory, which has now undergone many revisions, allowed for the role of psychological factors in the modulation of pain. The ingenious model of chronic pain put forth by Apkarian, Baliki, and Geha[4] provides for even greater clarification of the role of psychological factors. Spawned by the revealing work on pain mechanisms and system reorganization,[5] pain processing,[6,7] and neuroimaging,[8,9] the model is neurophysiological in nature. It highlights the brain as a "…dynamical network wherein detailed connectivity is consistently modified by the instantaneous experience of the organism."[4(p95)] Although the involvement of the nociceptive transmission system (i.e., spinal thalamic pathways) is acknowledged, activity at the cortical level is central to the theory.

Along with changes in our understanding of the neurophysiological aspects of "pain" (I use pain inside quotation marks because its definition and our understanding of its nature [i.e., disease vs. symptom vs. syndrome vs. emergent phenomenon] continue to evolve), the psychological/psychiatric conceptualization has changed as well. Psychoanalytical theories of pain based on the work of Sigmund Freud were popular in the psychiatric and psychological communities in the 1960s.[10] The psychodynamic approach of Freud held pain to be a means of controlling the expression of unwanted and unconscious desires or motivations. Engel[11] followed by detailing the "pain-prone personality." The essential features of the psychodynamic approach included (a) pain as a common conversion system, often with symbolic meaning; (b) unpleasant affect, usually guilt, hostility, resentment, or conflict is converted to bodily pain; (c) the choice of the symptom is determined by precipitating events; and (d) frequently there is a hereditary influence, most always a physical substrate, if only muscular.[10,12]

Although largely replaced by psychological approaches based on learning theory, the legacy of psychodynamic theory lives on in the classifications of Somatization Disorder and Pain Disorder found in the revised fourth edition of the *Diagnostic and Statistical Manual of Mental Disorders* (DSM-IV-TR) of the American Psychiatric Association.[13] Because of the tendency of such terms to continue to invigorate the notion of pain as a psychogenic phenomenon, Merskey[14] has called for their removal from the DSM. In fact, the term *Complex Somatic Symptom Disorder* has been proposed to replace Somatization Disorder, Pain Disorder, Hypochondriasis, and Undifferentiated Somatoform Disorder in the upcoming DSM-V[13a] and eliminate "medically unexplained symptoms" as a diagnostic criterion (www.dsm5.org/ProposedRevisions). The DSM Working Group is hopeful that this change will eliminate any unintended reference to mind-body dualism and believe that it is more in keeping with the identification of somatic symptoms and cognitive distortions as shared features among the four existing disorders listed.

Early on, C. Norman Shealy[15] recognized the importance of psychological factors in the treatment of pain as illustrated by his recommendation of (a) the absence of elevations on the Minnesota Multiphasic Personality Inventory (MMPI), except on the depression scale; (b) emotional stability; and (c) involvement in a rehabilitation program such as patient selection criteria in the application of spinal cord stimulation (SCS). Indeed, the psychological status of the patient was noted by Long[16] to be the most common reason for failure of stimulation therapy. One would be hard pressed to find any reputable publication on the subject that does not put forth psychological factors as important to the outcome of SCS therapy for the treatment of pain. In fact, the National Institute for Health and Clinical Excellence (NICE)[17] strongly recommends that SCS therapy for chronic pain be carried out within a multidisciplinary setting.

On surveying the outcome studies from the 1970s to the1980s, Bedder[18] concluded an estimated 40% success rate for SCS therapy. In a 2005 article Taylor, van Buyten, and Bucher[19] noted a significant pain reduction in 62% of patients with 40% returning to work, 53% discontinuing their use of opioids, and 70% expressing satisfaction with SCS therapy. Any concern over significant activity restrictions in patients with a properly secured SCS device appears

resolved by reports, including one in 2009, documenting the return to active duty in combat zones of military personnel following internalization of SCS.[20]

Less encouraging are the results of a prospective controlled study that compared SCS therapy, pain clinic, and usual care for failed back surgery syndrome (FBSS) in patients under worker compensation. By way of summarizing their data, the authors concluded that "…the SCS group did not differ from the other groups at 12 or 24 months on any outcome, including leg pain intensity, physical function, back pain intensity, and mental health. Outcomes were poor in all groups … fewer than 6% of patients achieved success on the primary outcome (a composite index of improvement in pain, function, and medication use); fewer than 10% were working; and more than twice as many patients reported a decline as report improvement in ability to perform everyday tasks."[21(p23)]

May, Banks, and Thomson[22] reported that, of the 100% of patients reporting success 16 months after implantation, only 59% did so at 58 months. Disease progression, adaptation, or tolerance to the stimulation; "a regression to the mean"; misinterpretation of the screening trial; and psychological variables may be contributing factors. These very disparate results combined with the loss of effect over time suggests that factors other than those related to surgical technique and device function are contributing to therapeutic outcomes. Indeed, North and Shipley emphasized that, "Technical success, however, is not sufficient to ensure clinical success."[23(pS202)]

Psychological Evaluation

In performing a psychological evaluation, it is important to consider several basic assumptions of pain management. First, persistent pain, regardless of its associated physical pathology (e.g., malignant tumor, degenerative disc disease, or osteoarthritis), is multidimensional and therefore influenced by psychosocial factors. Second, these psychosocial factors can influence the outcomes of pain relief–oriented therapies; in addition, co-use of behavior/psychological therapies along with somatic therapies can enhance pain relief and functioning. Finally, the prominence and priority of psychosocial factors can vary according to the type and degree of pain and pain-related pathology.[24]

Several years ago my colleagues and I examined the literature and, along with our own experience, listed a number of hypothesized positive patient characteristics thought to indicate an appropriate patient to proceed to a screening trial.[25] These positive indicators included (a) generally stable psychologically; (b) cautious, sufficiently defensive, self-confident; (c) self-efficacy, ability to cope with setbacks without responding in emergent fashion; (d) realistic concerns regarding illness often associated with a congruent mild depression; (e) generally optimistic regarding outcome, with the patient and significant other having appropriate expectations; (f) comprehends instructions and has a demonstrated history of compliance with previous treatments; (g) appropriately educated regarding procedure and device, supportive and treatment-educated family/support member(s); (h) behavior and complaints consistent with pathology and a behavioral/psychological evaluation consistent with the patient's complaints and reported psychosocial status; and (i) able to tolerate electrical stimulation, perhaps evidenced by a trial of transcutaneous electrical nerve stimulation (TENS).

Patient beliefs which were thought to be associated with a less positive outcome include (a) pain is a purely physical phenomenon, (b) psychosocial factors play little role in pain and treatment outcome, (c) chronic pain means loss of productive life, (d) pain can only be relieved if the medical cause (e.g., arthritis, scar tissue) is eliminated, and (e) medical technology holds the solution. Those appearing to correlate with a positive outcome are: (a) pain is multidimensional and multi-factorial, (b) attitudes and behaviors can affect treatment outcomes, (c) coping skill (e.g., relaxation, distraction, goal setting) can be helpful, (d) an active participant in therapeutic decision, (e) support systems that reinforce positive behavioral change are useful, and (f) proper expectations influence outcomes.

In addition, we proposed a set of clinician beliefs and attitudes thought to be more closely linked to a negative or positive outcome:

Negative: (a) Pain generators are sensory/physical phenomena; (b) failure of intervention is usually the patient's fault (i.e., poorly motivated); (c) long-term management is someone else's responsibility; (d) trial outcome is the primary predictor of success; (e) the more reversible or nondestructive a procedure is, the greater is the flexibility in patient selection; (f) and relief of subjective pain underlies all other areas of concern (e.g., psychological well-being, increased function, general quality of life).

Positive: (a) Pain is multidimensional and multifactorial; (b) treatment of psychosocial factors can be as effective as medical treatment, (c) the patient's concept of pain can profoundly affect treatment outcome, (d) patients are capable of change, (e) treatment is a long-term process, and (f) the clinician's role is facilitative as much as prescriptive.

Assessing and ensuring that the perspective SCS patient has proper, realistic, and appropriate expectations is seen as part of the evaluation process. The term *expectation* is often used in somewhat of a parochial manner, perhaps because its clinical impact may tend to be underestimated. Imaging studies have examined the effect of both positive and negative expectations. Expectancies have been demonstrated to affect the activity of the pain modulatory system, including the anterior cingulated cortex (ACC), thalamus, prefrontal cortex, and insula cortex.[26,27] Expectations related to anticipated good or bad motor performance influenced the outcome of subthalamic nucleus stimulation in patients undergoing deep brain stimulation.[28]

Furthermore, expectations contribute to the placebo effect. Price, Finiss, and Benedetti[29] noted the average placebo effect to be 2 U on a 0 to 10 pain scale in their total study population. However, it was as high as 5 U in the placebo responders (which varied from 20% to 55%, depending on the study). Expectations accounted for 49% of the variance. A series of studies by Dolce and associates[30-32] reported the impact of self-efficacy and expectancy on pain and exercise tolerance. It might be of interest to study the relationship between patient expectations and the reported loss of analgesia over time, despite a functioning SCS device. The author is unaware of any validated psychological instrument designed to evaluate expectations, particularly as they related to neuromodulation. However, the meeting of patient expectations has been shown to be central to good clinical outcomes.[33] This highlights the importance of appropriate expectations. Here again one encounters the necessity of the clinical interview.

How might the awareness of the patient's expectations and the possibility of the placebo effect influence the screening trial? For one, the clinical interview could obtain information regarding the level of pain acceptable to the patient, allowing him or her to be more active (i.e., the functional pain level). The patient could then be encouraged to outline their functional goals (e.g., sitting longer, walking further, traveling more), which can be individualized for each patient, depending on his or her particular anatomical limitations. Second, the screening trial might then examine both cognitive or perceptual effects of SCS (i.e., pain ratings) and functional changes. The pleasure gained from being able to perform reinforcing activities again and the accolades from others may be important to long-term improvement. It is likely to be more difficult for a patient to perceive himself or herself as more functional, especially if one involves and solicits observations from a significant other in the screening process, than it is to experience a reduction in pain. In a sense the preimplant screening trial can function as an extension of the interview. Agreed on therapeutic goals can be addressed during the trial and used as a means to determine the desirability or appropriateness of proceeding to implantation. Logic would suggest that the more closely the trial circumstances mimic the final outcome, the less chance there is of a false positive trial. This type of a screening trial mimics the N-of-1 approach illustrated by Cepeda and colleagues.[34]

North and Shipley[23] published what might arguably be one of the most comprehensive reviews of the SCS literature. Over 20 participating experts reviewed some 300 articles spanning 40 years from 1967 to 2007. The document summarized some psychologically relevant information. Regarding psychological predictors, it was noted that, "We lack sufficient information to predict SCS outcome from the result of a pretreatment psychological evaluation, but SCS, as is the case for every interventional pain treatment, is reserved for patients with no evident unresolved major psychiatric co-morbidity."[23(pS233)] Concerning the benefits of a psychological evaluation, they stated that it "…provides patient selection information by identifying the small percentage of patients who might benefit from psychological treatment before undergoing SCS therapy or in whom SCS therapy might be complicated by psychological factors."[23(pS234)] The literature was interpreted to suggest that the psychological evaluation be conducted before the screening trial when a surgical lead was being used, before anchoring if percutaneous leads are used, and before internalization. The various tests that had been used in the studies reviewed included the MMPI with Wiggins content scales[35-37]; Symptom Checklist-90-R[38]; Derogatis Affects Balance Scale[39]; Chronic Illness Problem Inventory[40]; Spielberger State-Trait Anxiety Inventory (STAI) Scale and State-Trait Anger Scale[41-44]; Beck Depression Inventory (BDI)[45-47]; Locus of Control Scale[48-49]; Absorption Scale[50]; McGill Pain Questionnaire (MPQ)[51-52]; Social Support Questionnaire[53]; Sickness Impact Profile (SIP)[54]; Oswestry Disability Index (ODI)[55]; Roland Morris Questionnaire[56]; and Fear-Avoidance Beliefs Questionnaire[57](Table 4-1). Interestingly, the authors noted Conversion Disorder to be a condition that could escape detection.

An unresolved major psychiatric co-morbidity; unresolved possibility of secondary gain; an active and untreated substance abuse disorder; inconsistency among the patient's history, pain description, physical examination, and diagnostic studies; abnormal or inconsistent pain ratings; and/or a predominance of nonorganic signs (e.g., Waddell signs) were listed as psychological factors that should cause the clinician to defer, delay, or modify the screening trial.[23(pS238)] The inability to control the device was considered an absolute contraindication. A successful screening trial, which tended to range from 3 to 8 days, was defined by (a) 50% or greater reduction in pain, (b) decreased pain despite provocative physical activity, (c) stable or reduced analgesic consumption, and (d) patient satisfaction. A 7- to 14-day postimplantation follow-up visit with monthly visits fading to annual visits was recommended.

The specifics and parameters of the evaluation process and what it means to psychologically clear a patient for SCS trial or

Table 4-1: Advantages and Disadvantages of Various Psychological Tests

Test	Description	Comment
McGill Pain Questionnaire	Measures subjective pain experience. Consists of 78 adjectives organized into 20 sets covering sensory, affective, and cognitive domains. Patients select best descriptor in each set. Each descriptor is assigned a score. Sum of ranked scores yields a pain-rating index.	*Advantages* Reliable, valid, and easy to administer; helps evaluate treatment outcomes; available in many languages. *Concerns* Limited to patient's experience of pain; does not ask about behavior or reinforcement factors; pain descriptors are culturally bound.
Minnesota Multiphasic Personality Inventory-2	Measures psychological traits and overall psychological status. Considered the gold standard. Consists of 180, 370, or 566 true-false questions, depending on the form. Describes patients in terms of 10 clinical scales, three validity scales, content scales, and numerous other subscales. Scored by computer.	*Advantages* Well normed and extensively researched; provides data about patient's test-taking approach. *Concerns* Not normed on pain patients; scales 1-3 often elevated in pain patients (this may unfairly label patients as neurotic); lengthy (long test form may take 2 hr to complete, short form takes about 45 min); highly skilled evaluator necessary to interpret test results.
Symptom Checklist-90-R	Screens for psychological symptoms and overall distress level. Consists of 90 items that measure intensity in nine symptom areas (e.g., somatization depression, anxiety, anger, paranoia). Yields three global distress scores measuring current depth of pain disorder (Global Severity Index), intensity of symptoms, and number of patient-reported symptoms.	*Advantages* Takes 12-15 min; yields an overall measure of psychological distress; well normed; can be used for screening and evaluation of treatment outcomes. *Concerns* Limited in scope; not a diagnostic tool; no correction scales.
Beck Depression Inventory	Assesses level of depression. Consists of 21 items ranked by severity. Patient chooses best statement. Includes two subscales (somatic-performance, cognitive-affective). Yields depression severity score.	*Advantages* Has a 30-year history; easy to take (10 min) and score. *Concerns* No validity scales (diagnosis may require confirmation); limited in scope.
Spielberger State-Trait Anxiety Inventory	Assesses state and trait anxiety. Consists of 40 multiple-choice items.	*Advantages* Good reliability and validity; easy to administer and score; can be used as treatment outcome measure. *Concern* No validity scales.
Chronic Illness Problem Inventory	Assesses coping ability, functioning, and patient's perception of problems. Consists of 65 self-report items related to pain behaviors, physical dysfunctions, health care behaviors, finances, sleep, and relationships. Yields a problem severity rating.	*Advantages* Provides useful information for treatment planning and evaluation; contains an illness focus scale; easy to score; excellent face-validity. *Concerns* May oversimplify problem; no correction scales.
Oswestry Disability Questionnaire	Assesses patient's daily functioning and activity level. Contains 10 multiple-choice items covering nine aspects of daily living and use of pain medication.	*Advantages* Correlates with functional tests of impairment; can be used as outcome measure; easy to take (10 min). *Concerns* No validity scales; generally applies to low back conditions; has not been validated in other patient conditions.
Multidimensional Pain Index	Evaluates patient's ability to cope. Includes nine clinical scales covering pain ratings, distress level, social support, and response by significant others. Yields probability of patient fitting one of three profiles (dysfunctional, interpersonally distressed, or adaptive coper).	*Advantages* Test is pain-specific; includes information about perceived responses of significant others; has greater focus on behavioral factors. *Concern* No validity scales.

From Raj PP, editor: *Practical management of pain*, ed 3, Mosby, 2000, p 414.

internalization remains ill defined. One main reason may be the tendency for authors to merely state that their patients had been cleared psychologically without revealing, or being required to reveal, the screening process and outcomes. This observation becomes particularly poignant when considered in light of the fact that some 25% to 50% of implanted SCS patients report the loss of analgesia 12 to 24 months after implant, despite a functional SCS unit and continued concordant paresthesias.[58-60] Nevertheless, Long and associates[61] reported a 70% "success" rate in patients who were screened and only 33% in those who were not.

In 2004 an Expert Panel Report incorporating input from clinicians in Europe and the United States[62] addressed the issue of psychological assessment for SCS therapy in managing chronic pain. The pretrial assessment was to have two objectives: (1) to determine the presence of psychological and social characteristics that could increase the probability of benefit; and (2) to help the physician identify the small number of patients in whom this treatment would result in uncertainty, failure, or medicolegal consequences.[62(p214)] The panel recommended evaluating (a) the present status and knowledge of the pain and it sensation, (b) painful behaviors and moods of the patients, (c) the patient's premorbid personality structure, (d) environmental factors affecting the pain, and (e) the patient's personal strengths and internal resources. The evaluation should include a clinical interview, structured inventory for pain, and psychometric testing. Specific measures of depression, anxiety, personality, and coping skills were reviewed. The panel did not provide a list of inclusion or exclusion criteria but rather a review of the literature. In their recent review of the intrathecal therapy literature from 1990 to 2005, Raffaeli and colleagues[63] concluded that the psychological evaluation should explore: (a) patient expectations, (b) quality and meaning of the patient's pain, (c) psychological disease, and (d) barriers to patients and family compliance with treatment. The European Federation of the International Association for the Study of Pain Chapters (EFIC) goes a step further. In its 1998 *Consensus Document on Neuromodulation Treatment of Pain,* the panel states that, given the intricate relationship between psychological and physiological factors in chronic pain, neuromodulatory procedures "are not to be considered as standalone treatments."[64(p208)]

In the United States a psychological evaluation is mandated by the Centers for Medicare and Medicare Services (CMS: Medicare Insurance). The policy states, "Patients must undergo a careful screening, evaluation and diagnosis, by a multidisciplinary team prior to implantation. (Such screening must include psychological as well as physical evaluation)" (Medicare Guidelines: SCS. Psychological evaluation. Medicare Coverage Issues Manual: Section 65-08: Electrical Nerve Stimulators). The American Psychological Association (APA)[64a] has outlined ethical guidelines regarding psychological assessment. Section 9.01b states, "Psychologists provide opinions of the psychological characteristics of individuals only after they have conducted an examination of the individual adequate to support their statement or conclusions"; and Section 9.06 states, "When interpreting assessment results, including automated interpretations, psychologists take into account the purpose of the assessment and various factors, test-taking abilities, and other characteristics of the person being assessed such as situational, personal, linguistic, and cultural differences that might affect the psychologists' judgment or reduce the accuracy of their interpretation."[64a]

Deyo and associates[65] have recommended assessing pain, mood, personality, and function when treating chronic pain conditions. Consistent with their suggestion, the authors have relied on the MPQ, BDI, MMPI, ODI, and clinical interviews in the evaluation

of SCS candidates. The total patient/family time required for the evaluation is approximately 3 to 4 hours at a cost of about $500.00 U.S. dollars or less, depending on insurance coverage. One or more preparation/educational sessions[66] may be involved, depending on the particular patient's needs. In recent years increased attention has been given to psychological factors vs. diagnosis/states (e.g., depression, anxiety) and statistically derived cutoff scores. The latter represent a sterile, deterministic, and statistical approach to the chronic pain patient for which there is little clinical and theoretical support. Do those espousing this approach really believe that patients are incapable of change? Their readiness-for-change is obviously an issue to be considered. In addition, we are also focusing more on patient expectations (functional pain level), functionally oriented trials (patient specific goals), conscientiousness (committing to and accepting obligations), and activity engagement (active despite pain).

As recommended by North and Shipley,[23] the evaluation should be conducted before the final determination is made about a temporary SCS trial. Whenever possible, the clinical interview should include a significant other, given the reported discrepancy between the patient and significant-other interpretation of treatment effectiveness.[67,68] The patient's goal(s), expectations, current coping strategies, level of readiness for change, degree of acceptance of the realities of his or her situation and projected outcome, and potential complications and side effects can be measured informally via the interview or by the use of questionnaires designed for that particular purpose.[69] Information should be sought regarding (a) any untreated or undertreated major affective disorder; (b) presence of any personality disorder (PD) and how it may affect the patient's perception of pain, compliance, or cooperation; (c) any undertreated or untreated drug or alcohol abuse problems, present or past; (d) the contribution of nonphysical factors to the patient's pain perception and behavior, (e.g., spousal reinforcement, secondary gain); and (e) the type and degree of social support.

Block and associates[70] have created an algorithm containing a number of risk factors obtained from the clinical interview, psychological testing, and the patient's medical background. These factors include personality types, mood states, and insurance status. Each factor is assigned a value of 0, 1, or 2 on the basis of how strongly it has been associated with outcomes, predominantly in the spine surgery literature. The total score is combined with the number of adverse clinical features, (e.g., deception, PD, medication seeking). Patients are then classified as having a good, fair, or poor prognosis.

This presurgical behavioral medicine evaluation (PBME) has only recently been applied in the field of neuromodulation.[71] The usefulness of this scheme might be enhanced by adding variables derived from the preimplantation trial, an advantage not available with spinal surgery, creating a pretrial and a posttrial score.

Areas of patient responsibility such as exercise and increased functional activity accompanying a reduction in pain should be emphasized to minimize an overdependence on the SCS technology as the sole source of clinical efficacy. Patients should be encouraged to understand that there may be a hierarchy of symptom improvement. For example, improved functioning and quality of life do not always accompany a reduction in pain but may need to be treated as a separate targeted problem. Similarly, I have recently encountered several patients with sacral stimulators wherein improvement in bladder functioning preceded significant reduction in pelvic pain. As noted previously, appreciating pain as an experiential, multifactorial symptom, the components (sensory, affective, cognitive) of which interact in a dynamic fashion, at times rendering pain intensity and unpleasantness (affect) somewhat independent but related aspects, should influence the assessment. Instruments emphasizing this multidimensional approach should be favored.

Allowing the patient to examine and manipulate the hardware to be used may be beneficial, as can be the viewing of audiovisual materials. Assessing as best one can the patient's acceptance and willingness to cope with persistent concordant paresthesias and the potential for electrode migration and positional sensitivity is a priority. Although these matters are often reviewed by the implanter, the repetition can be useful.

The information presented to the patient, level of understanding and comprehension of the patient and significant other, degree of discussion/agreement, and acknowledgment of awareness of complications and side effects should be documented in the chart note. The ill-prepared or uncertain patient and significant other may benefit from additional educational/orientation sessions. Projected outcomes should be based on evidence-based literature.

Levels of patient anxiety and depression can be assessed via the BDI and STAI. These tests can provide a measure of baseline depression and anxiety. Those patients exhibiting a significant amount of apprehension may benefit from cognitive behavioral therapy, relaxation, or other stress management pretrial. A certain amount of anxiety and depression is to be expected and should be appreciated as such. The MMPI and Symptom Checklist 90 (SCL 90) can yield a measure of the patient's general psychological status and personality tendencies. Patients manifesting manipulative or strongly maladaptive PDs should be identified and approached with caution.

The role of PDs is sometimes overshadowed by the emphasis on the mood disorders. PDs make up a large part of the Axis II diagnoses in DSM-IV scheme and are marked by "...behavior that deviates markedly from the expectations of the individual's culture" and leads to distress and impairment.[72(p287)] A personality trait represents a pattern of perceiving or relating to one's environment and presents as less pathological compared to PDs. The incidence of PDs in chronic pain has been estimated to be as high as 50%.[73,74] The PDs have been conveniently ordered into three clusters. Cluster A (i.e., paranoid, schizotypal) are characterized by individuals with odd or eccentric behavior. Cluster B includes the more dramatic, emotional, and manipulative individuals such as borderline, histrionic, narcissistic, and antisocial PDs. The anxious, fearful, and depressive PDs (i.e., dependent, avoidant, and obsessive-compulsive) make up cluster C.

As discussed by Doleys,[24] cluster A patients are more prone to unusual somatic experiences. They may perceive the hardware or stimulation as producing some psychological or somatic distortions. In extreme cases there may be associated hallucinations or somatic delusions. Cluster B–type patients often pose the greatest management problem. They tend to be noncompliant, challenging of authority, and demanding. They may have hidden agendas and pose significant management problems. Cluster C patients may benefit from behavioral therapies to address their fears, anxieties, and depression, any of which can influence their perception of pain and degree of disability. In our experience these patients are more likely to have a better short-term vs. long-term result and pose a risk of a false-positive trial (i.e., they have good response to the preimplant trial but report decreased effect over time).

The use of psychophysiological scaling might prove useful during the screening trial. This would involve several, perhaps four or five, trials wherein the SCS intensity is gradually increased (ascending trials) to establish detection threshold, analgesia, and tolerance. Descending trails (i.e., starting at tolerance and decreasing the SCS intensity to the level of stimulus detect) can be interspersed among the ascending trials. An overall average for stimulus threshold, analgesia, and tolerance can then be calculated. This information would yield a usable range, which is the difference between the average threshold intensity and the tolerance intensity of the SCS stimulation. The characteristics of this usable range and the location of the analgesic intensity within the usable range could be evaluated every 6 months after implant. Comparing changes in these characteristics with pain relief (i.e., magnitude of the useable range) may give additional information to use during the screening trial. In addition, certain psychological states or personality characteristics such as hysteria and hypochondriasis may be associated with certain patterns. For example, highly anxious and emotionally reactive patients may have a much more narrow usable range and thus be more prone to loss of analgesia after implant despite a positive trial.

A significant percentage of patients report the negative impact of pain and related psychological distresses on their quality of life. Although this technically defines a somatoform disorder, it does not necessarily exclude the patient as an appropriate candidate. The greater concern is for those patients meeting the DSM-IV-TR[13] criteria for somatization disorder, indicating a lifelong pattern likely to be unaltered by an intervention. The evaluation process should also focus on identifying the presence of any substance abuse or addiction problem. Most feel that an active, especially untreated, drug abuse or addiction disorder to be an absolute contraindication SCS therapy.

One frequently asked question is how to find a pain-oriented psychologist to perform these evaluations. There are several ways: (1) contact universities granting a doctoral degree in psychology; (2) obtain the membership rosters of the American Pain Society (APS) and International Society for the Study of Pain (IASP) as they list members by degree and geographical location; (3) contact the state board of examiners in psychology; and (4) discuss with your local technology representative. Not all psychologists, even those already practicing in the area of pain psychology, are familiar with the nuances of SCS therapy. However, a growing amount of reading material, conferences/workshop, and proctorships is available. A discussion with the prospective evaluator should take place to emphasize that the evaluation for SCS therapy be objective and not biased by concerns over potential referrals.

Some pain physicians have chosen to bypass this process by ordering and administering computer-scored tests to their patients and relying on the interpretation of the computer. No matter how much effort has gone into the development of such questionnaires (and I have no doubt as to their validity), to use them in the absence of a clinical interview/examination is tantamount to performing surgery on the basis of radiologist interpretation of magnetic resonance imaging without examination of the patient. Although more expedient, this approach may be doing a disservice to the patient, and I question its potential benefit and ethics.

Brief Review of the Literature

Although obviously finite, there are an ever growing, and perhaps inestimable, number of psychosocial factors capable of influencing a patient's experience of pain and pain-related disability on quality of life. These psychological factors may be mediators, moderators, or maintainers of the outcomes. Indeed, their influence may vary over time in accordance with the patient's circumstances (e.g., resolution of insurance claim, effectively treated depression or anxiety, degree or pain acceptance, progression through the stages of change). Gender, sex, ethnicity, culture, and type of pain interact with psychological factors in ways that are only beginning to be understood. Our speculations (and that is about all that we can call them at this time) about these relationships, interactions, and/or associations are based on the assumption that we are measuring the right things in the right way.[75]

The following is a brief summary of some of the studies examining psychological variables in SCS. The information presented should be interpreted with the preceding in mind. Most studies have used preimplantation or preimplantation and postimplantation psychological evaluations in an effort to determine which psychological variables tend to be associated with or predict the outcomes. More detailed reviews can be found elsewhere.[76-79]

Several studies have used the MMPI. Patients with elevations on hypochondriasis (scale 1), depression (scale 2), and hysteria (scale 3), up to two standard deviations (SDs), were thought to be appropriate for SCS trial; but those with elevations on four scales or more not.[78] Long and Erickson[80] recommended including patients with evidence of depression (scale 2) and anxiety (scale 7). However, elevation of hypochondriasis (scale 1) and depression (scale 2) have been associated with negative outcomes.[81,82] North and colleagues[83] found that patients with higher scores on hypochondriasis (scale 1) and hysteria (scale 3) tended to have successful trials resulting in internalization, but those with high scores on hysteria (scale 3) reported diminished effect at 3-month follow-up. The appearance of a conversion V pattern, as represented by elevations in hypochondriasis (scale 1) and hysteria (scale 3) relative to depression (scale 2), is thought to suggest the presence of a conversion disorder. Somewhat surprisingly, and perhaps contrary to conventional wisdom, patients with similar profiles have demonstrated successful preimplantation trials and/or long-term outcomes.[82-86] Lower scores on depression (scale 2) and mania (scale 9) correlated with a positive outcome in the Olson and associates' study.[87] Meilman, Leibrock, and Leong[88] failed to find any correlation between MMPI scores and SCS outcomes. However, they noted the accuracy of prediction to be greater for simple mononeuropathies (71%) compared to the more complex arachnoiditis (32%). This observation suggests a possible interaction between the complexity or the underlying pathology and psychological factors.

Depression and anxiety are among the more common psychological co-morbidities found in chronic pain patients. Using the BDI (scoring range 0 to 63), Olson and colleagues[87] found that patients having a successful outcome had an average score of 12.4 (SD 6.9), whereas those who were determined to have a poor outcome averaged 16.4 (SD 6.5). Although the average BDI score decreased after implant, the change was not statistically significant. Daniel and associates[89] claimed an 80% accuracy rate when combining the results of the MMPI with the BDI. Burchiel and colleagues[85,86] noted that the BDI emerged as predictor, but their average score was only 13, considered to be in the mild range of depression. The average prereduction/postreduction was 2 points. This relatively small effect raises the question as to whether the finding is of any clinical significance or merely a statistical anomaly.

The STAI (scoring range 0 to 80) was used by Olson and colleagues[87] as a measure of anxiety. Patients proceeding to SCS trial scored an average of 23.5 and 19.3 on State and Trait anxiety respectively, whereas those who did not go on to a trial scored 25.1 and 21.1. The average STAI scores in Long, BenDebba, and Tirgerson[90] were 39 SAI and 37 TAI. A sample of patients in the author's day treatment program had average SAI of 51 and TAI of 47. These different STAI scores could represent three different chronic pain populations. Therefore the relationship of STAI scores in the lower range, as in the Olson and associates' study,[87] with SCS outcomes might not hold for groups scoring in the higher range. Thus the correlation between the degree of anxiety and long-term outcome

with SCS remains unclear. The relationship between an anxiety disorder and SCS also remains uncertain. However, Verdolin, Stedje-Larasen, and Hickey[91] reported on the treatment of neuropathic pain by SCS in war veterans also diagnosed with posttraumatic stress disorder (PTSD). The presence of PTSD did not affect, nor was it affected by, successful SCS therapy.

One area often overlooked is that of the consequence of SCS therapy on psychological conditions. Panic attacks beginning after SCS implantation were noted by Sheu and colleagues,[92] which resolved only when the unit was explanted. Han and associates[93] sighted the brief occurrence of "locked-in syndrome" (i.e., defined as quadriplegia and anarthria), thought to indicate a conversion disorder following implantation SCS. Parisod, Murray, and Cousins[94] also reported the appearance of a conversion disorder in a complex regional pain syndrome patient following internalization, which required additional treatment. This latter case highlighted the potential advantages of combining a more comprehensive cognitive behavioral functional restoration program with SCS therapy. Indeed, Molloy and colleagues[95] demonstrated improved outcomes when both approaches were used. In addition, they did not find an order effect. Of interest was the association of improvement in functional and psychological variables with multidisciplinary therapy and pain ratings with SCS treatment.

A recent review by Celetin, Edwards, and Jamison[96] of 753 articles relating to pretreatment psychological screening for lumbar surgery and SCS found that only four SCS-related studies (1981, 1995, 1995, 1996) met the criteria for analysis. Psychological factors (e.g., depression, coping, anxiety, somatization, hypochondriasis) were more predictive than other variables but mostly for short-term vs. long-term outcomes. Kumar and Wilson[97] suggested that patients manifesting psychological factors such as fear avoidance, depression, secondary gain, refusal to be weaned off narcotics, or currently under workers' compensation should be avoided. Although a number of psychological factors have been identified as potentially associated with outcome of SCS therapy, there is yet to be any consensus as to which have the most reliable and predicable impact (i.e., may be considered predictors).[24]

One of the more recent tools for examining the patient's response during the screening trial is neuroimaging. One report by Nagamachi and associates[98] used SPECT technology before and after SCS. They compared patients reporting a four point or greater reduction in pain on a 0 to 10 scale (good response, GR) to those reporting a decrease of three points or less (poor response, PR). The authors noted a distinctive pattern of activity before and after SCS for the GR and PR groups involving thalamic structures and the anterior cingulate gyrus. Others have documented activation of pain and emotional processing cortical structures in response to occipital nerve stimulation in normal volunteers. As yet there have been no attempts to correlate data collected from the psychological evaluation with that of neuroimaging. Whether or not neuroimaging becomes a reliable and practical tool for evaluating patient response to SCS trail screening remains to be seen. The possibilities at least are intriguing.

Summary

The search for one or more optimal psychological variable(s) or test scores that will predict the outcome of SCS therapy continues. This more-or-less statistical approach assumes the existence of one or more psychological states or variables compatible or not with SCS therapy and which can be detected by the psychological evaluation process. The emergence of an interest in narrative analysis[99] and other qualitative approaches calls this assumption into question. Models that profess to predict the outcomes of SCS therapy on the basis of pretrial or preimplantation evaluation are, at least in part, predicated on the assumption that the circumstances present at the time of evaluation (a) will persist; or (b) if changed, will not alter the predicted relation; or (c) if altered, the effect will not be clinically or statistically meaningful (i.e., not strong enough to invalidate the prediction). A possible alternative to attempts to predict outcomes is to emphasize developing a detailed description of the particular patient, pain, and therapeutic variables thought to influence the outcome and create a somewhat dynamic therapeutic algorithm that is adjusted according to the patient circumstances and response to treatment.

Each clinician is likely to have his or her favorite tests. For the efforts to distill meaningful information from the evaluation and treatment process to advance, there needs to be some standardization of the process, if not the particulars. Doleys[24] proposed the following process suggestions. (1) Well-known and validated tests should be used. (2) Ideally the test(s) should have validity scale(s) or some mechanism for detecting dissimilation. (3) Tests should be used in the context of an overall evaluation, including clinical interview. (4) The assessment should be done by a knowledgeable and experienced, preferably doctoral level, provider. (5) The evaluator should have contact with the patient, or at least the outcome data, from the preimplant trial and follow up to determine the correlation between the evaluation and outcome. (6) Screening tests should be readministered on follow-up. (7) Both disease-specific and generic measures should be obtained.

Dr. Timothy Deer kindly invited me to give a talk entitled, "The psychology of implantable devices: avoiding mental land-mines and achieving great outcomes," at the 2010 American Academy of Pain Medicine annual meeting. The following were presented as recommendations, albeit not necessarily experimentally verified but a result of 25 years' experience with implantable devices. First, follow the 3 Ps: pain *pattern*, pain *pathology*, and *psychological* status (i.e., stick to the basics, especially new implanters or less experienced clinicians). There is significant evidence to support the use of SCS in patients with extremity pain, with or without back pain (pain pattern), having a neuropathic component (pain pathology), and presenting as psychologically intact and stable (psychological status). That is not to say that exploring new applications should be avoided, but it should be undertaken by those few with extraordinary skills and technical and clinical support. Second, at least moderately stringent criteria should be applied when evaluating the screening trial. Those outlined by North and Shipley[23] as a result of their review of the literature seem very appropriate, especially continued pain relief despite provocative physical activity. Finally, consistent with the growing emphasis of chronic pain as a disease, regular follow-up visits to reinforce/stimulate psychological/behavioral changes should be required. More often then not, patients are essentially ignored until there is a complication or mechanical failure.

It would be difficult to find a publication from the United States, Canada, Europe, or Australia relating to the use of SCS with chronic pain that does not call for its use in the context of a multidisciplinary framework.[17,23,97] Unfortunately, with the possible exception of very few works such as that of Molloy and colleagues,[95] which examined the effects of combining an intensive cognitive-behavioral program with SCS therapy, it has largely been more rhetoric then reality. Enormous amounts of time and money have been devoted, and justifiably so, to developing new and more advanced technology (i.e., building a better mouse trap). Ironically, especially when considered in the context of the relative lack of emphasis on regular postimplantation follow-up visits, these efforts encourage the patient to interpret success or failure as beyond their influence and solely dependent on the procedure and technology. This is precisely the message we do not want to convey. I wonder what would happen if the technology companies devoted even 1% of their research and development funds to examining how to make what works work better by supporting multidisciplinary research. A simple beginning point would be the random assignment of SCS patients to X number of postimplantation cognitive-behavioral therapy sessions or usual care. Hopefully the profession has not already arrived at a point where the fascination for gadgetry is betraying sound sense.

References

1. Shealy CN, Mortimer J, Reswick J: Electrical inhibition of pain by stimulation of the dorsal columns: preliminary clinical report. *Anesth Anal* 46:489-499, 1967.
2. Descartes R: *Description of the human body*, 1647. (Translation ©George MacDonald Ross).
3. Melzack R, Wall PD: Pain mechanisms a new theory. *Science* 150:971-979, 1965.
4. Apkarian AV, Baliki MN, Geha PY: Toward a theory of chronic pain. *Progr Neurobiol* 87:81-97, 2009.
5. Woolf CJ, Salter MW: Neural plasticity: increasing the gain in pain. *Science* 288:1765-1769, 2000.
6. Price DD: *Psychological mechanisms of pain and analgesia*, Seattle, Wash, 1999, IASP Press.
7. Price DD: Psychological and neural mechanisms of the affective dimension of pain. *Science* 288:1769-1772, 2000.
8. Casey KL, Bushnell MC, editors: *Pain imaging*, Seattle, Wash, 2000, IASP Press.
9. Tracey I, Bushnell MC: How neuroimaging studies have challenged us to rethink: is chronic pain a disease? *J Pain* 10:1113-1120, 2009.
10. Merskey H: History of psychoanalytic ideas concerning pain. In Gatchel RJ, Weisberg JN, editors: *Personality characteristics of patients with pain*, Washington DC, 2000, American Psychological Press, pp 25-35.
11. Engel GL: "Psychogenesis" pain and the pain-prone patient. *Am J Med* 26:899-918, 1959.
12. Spear FG: An examination of some psychological theories of pain. *Br J Med Psychol* 39:349-351, 1966.
13. American Psychiatric Association: *Diagnostic and statistical manual of mental disorders* (revised 4th edition), Washington DC, 2000, APA.
13a. American Psychiatric Association: Proposed draft revisions to DSM disorders and criteria. *American Psychiatric Association DSM-5 development*, accessed from www.dsm5.org/ProposedRevisions, October 2008.
14. Merskey H: Somatization: or another God that failed. *Pain* 145:4-5, 2009.
15. Shealy CN: Dorsal column stimulation: optimizing of application. *Surg Neurol* 4:142-145, 1975.
16. Long D: Psychological factors and outcomes of electrode implantation for chronic pain. *Neurosurgery* 7:225-229, 1980.
17. National Institute for Health and Clinical Excellence: *Spinal cord stimulation for chronic pain of neuropathic of ischemic origin*, NICE technology appraisal guidance 159, London, 2008, National Institute for Health and Clinical Excellence, accessed from www.nice.org.uk, November 2008.
18. Bedder M: Spinal cord stimulation and intractable pain: patient selection. In Waldman S, Winnie A, editors: *Interventional pain management*, Philadelphia, 1996, Saunders, pp 412-418.
19. Taylor RS, Van Buyten JP, Bucher E: Spinal cord stimulation for chronic low back and leg pain and failed back surgery syndrome: a systematic review and analysis of prognostic factors. *Spine* 30:152-160, 2005.
20. Dragovich A et al: Neuromodulation in patients deployed to war zones. *Anesth Analg* 109:245-248, 2009.
21. Turner JA et al: Spinal cord stimulation for failed back surgery syndrome: outcomes in workers compensation setting. *Pain* 148:14-25, 2010.

22. May MS, Banks C, Thomson SJ: A retrospective, long-term, third-party follow-up of patients considered for spinal cord stimulation. *Neuromodulation* 5(3):137-144, 2002.

23. North R, Shipley J: Practice parameters for the use of spinal cord stimulation in the treatment of chronic neuropathic pain. *Pain Med* 8(suppl 4):S200-S275, 2007.

24. Doleys DM: Psychological issues and evaluation for patients undergoing implantable technology. In Krames E, Peckman PA, Rezai A, editors: *Textbook of Neuromodulation*, Oxford, England, 2009, Blackwell Publishing, pp 69-80.

25. Doleys DM: Psychologic evaluation for patients undergoing neuro augmentive procedures. *Neurosurg Clin North Am* 14:409-417, 2003.

26. Keltner JR et al: Isolating the modulatory effect of expectation on pain transmission: a functional magnetic resonance imaging study. *J Neuroscience* 16:4437-4443, 2006.

27. Koyama T et al: The subjective experience of pain: where expectations become reality. PNAS, Sept 6, 2055, 102, 36, 12950-12955, accessed from www.pnas.org/cgi/doi/10.1073/pnas.o4o8576102, October 2008.

28. Pollo A et al: Expectation modulates the response to subthalamic nucleus stimulation in Parkinson patients, *Cognitive Neurosc Neuropsychol* (Neuro Report) 13(1):1383-1386, 2002.

29. Price D, Finniss DG, Benedetti F: A comprehensive review of the placebo effect: recent advances and current thought. *Annu Rev Psychol* 59:565-590, 2008.

30. Dolce JJ et al: The role of self-efficacy expectancies in the prediction of pain tolerance. *Pain* 27:261-272, 1987.

31. Dolce JJ et al: Exercise quotas, anticipatory concern, and self-efficacy expectancy in chronic pain: a preliminary report. *Pain* 24:365-372, 1986.

32. Dolce JJ et al: Exercise quotas, anticipatory concern and self-efficacy expectations in chronic pain: a preliminary report. *Behav Res Ther* 28:289-299, 1986.

33. Mannion AF et al: Great expectations: really the novel predictor of outcome after spinal surgery? *Spine* 34(15):1590-1599, 2009.

34. Cepeda MS et al: An N-of-1 trial as an aid to decision-making prior to implanting a permanent spinal cord stimulator. *Pain Med* 9:235-239, 2008.

35. Minnesota Multiphasic Personality Inventory, Brandwin MA, Kewman DG: MMPI indicators of treatment response to spinal epidural stimulation in patients with chronic pain and patients with movement disorders. *Psychol Rep* 51:1059-1064, 1982.

36. Fordyce WE et al: MMPI scale 3 as a predictor of back injury report: what does it tell us? *Clin J Pain* 8:222-226, 1992.

37. Moore J et al: Empirically derived pain-patient's MMPI subgroups: prediction of treatment outcome. *J Behav Med* 9:51-63, 1986.

38. Derogatis LR: *Symptom-Checklist-90-R: Scoring and Procedures Manual I for the Revised Version*, Eagan, NM, 1977, Pearson Assessments.

39. Derogatis LR: *Derogatis affects balance scale*, Baltimore, Md, 1975, Clinical Psychometric Research.

40. Kames LD et al: The Chronic Illness Problem Inventory: problem-oriented psychosocial assessment of patients with chronic illness. *Int J Psychiatry Med* 14(1):65-75, 1984.

41. Romano JM, Turner JA, Jensen MP: The Chronic Illness Problem Inventory as a measure of dysfunction in chronic pain patients. *Pain* 49(1):71-75, 1992.

42. Spielberger C: *State-Trait Anxiety Scale and State-Trait Anger Scale: the State-Trait Anxiety Inventory*, New York, 1970, Academic Press.

43. Spielberger C: *Manual for the State-Trait Anxiety Inventory (STAI)*, Palo Alto, Calif, 1983, Consulting Psychologists Press.

44. Spielberger CD et al. The experience and expression of anger: construction and validation of an anger expression scale. In Chesney MA, Rosenman RH, editors: *Anger and hostility in cardiovascular and behavioral disorders*, Washington, DC, 1985, Hemisphere Publishing Corp, pp 5-30.

45. Beck A, Steer RA, Garbin M: Beck Depression Inventory psychometric properties of the BDI: twenty-five years of evaluation. *Clin Psychol Rev* 8(1):77-100, 1988.

46. Beck AT et al: An inventory for measuring depression. *Arch Gen Psychiatry* 4:561-571, 1961.

47. Novy DM: What does the Beck Depression Inventory measure in chronic pain?: a reappraisal. *Pain* 61:261-271, 1995.

48. Lau RR, Ware JF, Jr: Refinements in the measurement of health-specific locus-of-control beliefs. *Med Care* 19(11):1147-1158, 1981.

49. Wallston BS et al: Development and validation of the Health Locus of Control (HLC) Scales. *J Consult Clin Psychol* 44:580-585, 1976.

50. Tellegren A, Atkinson G: Openness to absorbing and self-altering experiences ("absorption"), a trait related to hypnotic susceptibility. *J Abnorm Psychol* 83:268-277, 1974.

51. McGill Pain Questionnaire, Melzack R: The McGill Pain Questionnaire: major properties and scoring methods. *Pain* 1:277-299, 1975.

52. Turk DC, Rudy TE, Salovey P: The McGill questionnaire reconsidered: confirming the factor structure and examining appropriate uses. *Pain* 21:385-397, 1985.

53. Sarason IG et al: Assessing social support: the Social Support Questionnaire. *J Pers Soc Psychol* 44:127-139, 1983.

54. Bergner M et al: The Sickness Impact Profile: Development and final revision of a health status measure. *Med Care* 19:787-805, 1981.

55. Fairbank JC et al: The Oswestry low back pain disability questionnaire. *Physiotherapy* 66:271-273, 1980.

56. Gronbald M et al: Relationship of the Pain Disability Index (PDI) and the Oswestry Disability Questionnaire (ODQ) with three dynamic physical tests in a group of patients with chronic low back and leg pain. *Clin J Pain* 10:197-203, 1994.

57. Waddell G et al: A Fear-Avoidance Beliefs Questionnaire (FABQ) and the role of fear-avoidance in chronic low back pain and disability. *Pain* 52:157-168, 1993.

58. Cameron T: Safety and efficacy of spinal cord stimulation for the treatment of chronic pain: a.20-year literature review. *J Neurosurg Spine* 100(suppl 3):254-267, 2004.

59. May MS, Banks C, Thomson SJ: A retrospective, long-term, third-party follow-up of patients considered for spinal cord stimulation. *Neuromodulation* 5(3):137-144, 2002.

60. Mailis-Gagnon A et al: Spinal cord stimulation for chronic pain, *Cochrane Database Syst Rev* CD003783, 2004.

61. Long DM et al: Electrical stimulation of the spinal cord and peripheral nerves for pain control: a 10-year experience. *Appl Neurophysiol* 44(4):207-217, 1981.

62. Beltrutti D et al: The psychological assessment of candidates for spinal cord stimulation for chronic pain management. *Pain Pract* 4(3):204-221, 2004.

63. Raffaeli W et al: Intraspinal therapy for the treatment of chronic pain: a review of the literature between 1990-2005 and suggested protocol for its rational safe use. *Neuromoduation* 9:290-308, 2006.

64. Gybels J, Erdine S, Maeyaert J, et al: Neuromodulation of pain: a consensus statement prepared in Brussels 16-18, January 1998, by the following task force of the European Federation of IASP Chapters (EFIC). *Eur J Pain* 2:203-209, 1998.

64a. American Psychological Association (APA): Ethics principles of psychologists and code of conduct, 2000, accessed from www.apa.org/ethics/code2002html, March 2007.

65. Deyo RA et al: Outcome measures for low back pain research: a proposal for standardized use. *Spine* 23:2003-2013, 1998.

66. Doleys DM: Preparing patients for implantable technology. In Turk D, Gatchel RJ, editors: *Psychological aspects of pain management*, New York, 2002, Guilford Press, pp 334-347.

67. Tutak U, Doleys DM: Intrathecal infusion systems for treatment of chronic low back and leg pain of noncancer origin. *Southern Med J* 89(3):295-300, 1996.

68. Willis KD, Doleys DM: The effect of long-term intrathecal infusion therapy with noncancer pain patients: evaluation of patient, significant-other, and clinic staff appraisals. *Neuromodulation* 2:241-253, 1999.

69. Doleys DM, Doherty DC: Psychological and behavioral assessment. In Raj PP, editor: *Practical management of pain*, ed 3, St Louis, 2000, Mosby, pp 408-426.

70. Block AR et al: *The psychology of spine surgery*, Washington, DC, 2003, American Psychological Association Press.

71. Schocket KG et al: A demonstration of a presurgical behavioral medicine evaluation for categorizing patients for implantable therapies: a preliminary study. *Neuromodulation* 11:237-249, 2008.

72. American Psychiatric Association: *Diagnostic and statistical manual of mental disorders, Fourth Edition, Text Revision*, Washington DC, 1994, American Psychiatric Association Press.

73. Polatin PB et al: Psychiatric illness and low back pain. *Spine* 18:66-71, 1993.

74. Fishbain DA et al: Male and female chronic pain patients categorized by DSM III psychiatric diagnostic criteria. *Pain* 26:181-197, 1986.

75. Wittink H et al: Are we measuring what we need to measure. *Clin J Pain* 24(4):316-324, 2008.

76. Doleys DM: Psychological factors in spinal cord stimulation therapy: brief review and discussion. *Neurosurg Focus* 21:1-6, 2006.

77. Doleys DM, Klapow J, Hammer M: Psychological evaluation in spinal cord stimulation therapy. *Pain Rev* 4:189-207, 1997.

78. Doleys DM: Psychological assessment for implantable therapies. *Pain Digest* 10:16-23, 2000.

79. Shealy CN: Dorsal column stimulation: optimization of application. *Surg Neurol* 4(1):142-145, 1975.

80. Long DM, Erickson DE: Stimulation of the posterior columns of the spinal cord for relief of intractable pain. *Surg Neurol* 4:134-141, 1975.

81. Blumetti AE, Modesti LM: Psychological predictors of success and failure of surgical intervention for intractable back pain. In Bonic JJ, Albe-Fessard B, editors: Adv Pain Ther Res, vol 1, New York, 1976, Raven Press, pp 233-247.

82. Brandwin MA, Kewman DG: MMPI indicators of treatment response to spinal epidural stimulation in patients with chronic pain and patients with movement disorders. *Psychol Rep* 51:1059-1064, 1982.

83. North RB et al: Failed back surgery syndrome: 5-year follow-up after spinal cord stimulator implantation. *Neurosurgery* 28(5):692-699, 1991.

84. North et al: Prognostic value of psychological testing in patients undergoing spinal cord stimulation: a prospective study. *Neurosurgery* 39(2):301-310, 1996.

85. Burchiel KJ et al: Prospective, multicenter study of spinal cord stimulation for relief of chronic back and extremity pain. *Spine* 21(23):2786-2794, 1996.

86. Burchiel KJ et al: Prognostic factors of spinal cord stimulation for chronic back and leg pain. *Neurosurgery* 36(6):1101-1110, 1995.

87. Olson KA et al: Psychological variables associated with outcome of spinal cord stimulation trials. *Neuromodulation* 1(1):6-13, 1998.

88. Meilmen PW, Leibrock LG, Leong FT: Outcome of implantable spinal cord stimulation in the treatment of chronic pain: arachnoiditis versus single nerve root injury and mononeuropathy. *Clin J Pain* 5:189-193, 1989.

89. Daniel MS et al: Psychological factors and outcomes of electrode implantation for chronic pain. *Neurosurgery* 17:773-777, 1985.

90. Long D, BenDebba M, Tirgerson WS: Persistent back pain and sciatica in the United States: patient characteristics. *J Spinal Disorders* 40-58, 1996.

91. Verdolin MH, Stedje-Larasen ET, Hickey AH: Ten consecutive cases of complex regional pain syndrome of less than 12 months' duration in active duty United States military personal tested with spinal cord stimulation. *Anesth Analg* 104:1557-1562, 2007.

92. Sheu R et al: Panic Attacks after spinal cord stimulator implantation. *Anesth Analg* 103:1334-1335, 2006.

93. Han D et al: Conversion locked-in syndrome after implantation of a spinal cord stimulator. *Anesth Analg* 104:163-165, 2007.

94. Parisod E, Murray RF, Cousins MJ: Conversion disorder after implant of a spinal cord stimulator in a patient with a complex regional pain syndrome. *Anesth Analg* 96(1):201-206, 2003.

95. Molloy AR et al: Does the combination of intensive cognitive-behavioral pain management and spinal implantable devices confer any advantages? a preliminary examination. *Pain Pract* 6(2):96-103, 2006.

96. Celestin J, Edwards RR, Jamison RN: Pretreatment psychosocial variables as predictors of outcomes following lumbar surgery and spinal cord stimulation: a systematic review and literature synthesis. *Pain Med* 10:639-653, 2009.

97. Kumar K, Wilson JR: Factors affecting spinal cord stimulation outcome in chronic benign pain with suggestions to improve success rate. *Acta Neurochir* 97(suppl 1):91-99, 2007a.

98. Nagamachi S et al: Alteration of regional cerebral blood flow in patients with chronic pain-evaluation before and after epidural spinal cord stimulation. *Ann Nuclear Med* 20:303-310, 2006.

99. Carr DB, Loeser JD, Morris DB, editors: *Narrative, pain and suffering*, Seattle, Wash, 2005, IASP Press, pp 362.

II Spinal Cord Stimulation

5 Spinal Cord Stimulation: General Indications

Chengyuan Wu, Steven M. Falowksi, and Ashwini Sharan

CHAPTER OVERVIEW

Chapter Synopsis: Spinal cord stimulation (SCS) is an adjustable, nondestructive, mode of neuromodulation that delivers therapeutic doses of electrical current to the spinal cord for the management of neuropathic pain. Stimulation can be provided by both implanted paddle electrodes and percutaneous electrodes. Although a large body of work has been published, the exact mechanisms of action of SCS remain unclear. Overall SCS has been shown to have an approximately 50% improvement in pain relief that persists over years of follow-up, which is superior to many other invasive modalities.

Important Points: It is important to remember that the goal of neurostimulation is to reduce pain rather than to completely eliminate it. It can be applied reliably to patients with postlaminectomy syndrome/failed back surgery syndrome (FBSS), complex regional pain syndrome (CRPS), chronic critical limb ischemia (CCLI), and pain.

Clinical Pearls: Growing experience with SCS and improvement of available hardware have not only improved the reliability of this modality but have also allowed for its use in other disease processes. Other applications of SCS include its use in patients with angina, abdominal/visceral pain syndromes, brachial plexitis/neurogenic thoracic outlet syndrome, phantom limb pain, intractable pain secondary to spinal cord injury, mediastinal pain, cervical neuritis, and postherpetic neuralgia.

Clinical Pitfalls: Although results are largely beneficial, appropriate patient selection is imperative; psychological screening is needed to detect mood disorders, which can alter pain reporting and perception by a patient. In addition, coverage of low back pain alone is often difficult and has a lower rate of success. Complications of SCS include electrode migration or breakage, other hardware failure, infection, epidural hematoma, cerebrospinal fluid leak, and rarely neurologic deficit.

Establishing Diagnosis

Spinal cord stimulation (SCS) is an adjustable, nondestructive, mode of neuromodulation that delivers therapeutic doses of electrical current to the spinal cord for the management of neuropathic pain. The most common indications include postlaminectomy syndrome, complex regional pain syndrome (CRPS), ischemic limb pain, and angina (**Table 5-1**); but it has been applied to other causes of intractable pain.

Anatomy

The spinal canal contains several neural and nonneural structures that can be stimulated electrically. The properties of the intraspinal contents are similar to an inhomogeneous conductor. Knowledge of the different type of responses and their correlation with the underlying anatomical substrate is extremely important in implementing strategies for SCS.

Stimulation of large myelinated afferent fibers may occur in four different areas: the dorsal root, the dorsal root entry zone (DREZ), the dorsal horn, or the dorsal columns (**Fig. 5-1**). Electrical stimulation of these structures results in an ipsilateral tingling paresthesia, but changes to discomfort and pain with increasing stimulation voltage. Particularly, activation of the dorsal roots causes a radicular paresthesia at a particular dermatomal level, whereas stimulation of the dorsal columns causes paresthesia in areas of the body caudal to the level of the electrode. In the cervical and thoracic cord the dorsal columns are usually about 3 to 5 mm wide, largest at the level of the cervical enlargement, and smallest in the midthoracic spine.

The single most important factor in determining stimulation parameters is the width of the cerebrospinal fluid (CSF) space dorsal to the spinal cord (**Fig. 5-2**). Increasing thickness of the dorsal CSF (dCSF) layer leads to early stimulation of the dorsal root fibers instead of the dorsal column fibers. This is largely because rootlet fibers, which are immersed in well-conducting CSF, have high conductivity at the DREZ. Therefore the stimulation threshold for the segmentary system ranges from 0.1 V to 0.5 V, whereas activation of the dorsal columns occurs at a threshold that is at least 0.5 V to 1 V higher.

Differentiating between stimulation of the dorsal root, DREZ, or dorsal horn can be exceedingly difficult. One can expect dorsal root stimulation with laterally placed electrodes; stimulation of the DREZ or dorsal horn is more likely if the electrode is placed near midline. In the latter group stimulation leads to segmentary paresthesias that are rapidly followed by activation of the dorsal columns with a small voltage increment. Interestingly, minute changes in mediolateral position of the electrode have been shown to lead to movement of the paresthesias in a W two-dimensional pattern[1] as shown in **Fig. 5-3**.

If electrical stimulation reaches the ventral cord, motor structures are affected, and consequently muscle contractions are seen. Much like dorsal cord stimulation, activation of the ventral root or motor neurons causes muscular contractions in a myotomal distribution, whereas activation of the descending corticospinal pathways results in diffuse muscle contractions caudal to the level of the electrode. In the vast majority of patients stimulation over the dorsal columns is not complicated by simultaneous activation of the motor system unless a significantly higher voltage is

Table 5-1: Spinal Cord Stimulation Indications and Probability of Success

Indications	Probability of Success
Postlaminectomy syndrome/failed back surgery syndrome (FBSS)	50%-60% with >50% pain relief
Complex regional pain syndrome (CRPS)	67%-84%
Chronic critical limb ischemia (CCLI) and pain	70%-80% with >75% pain relief
Angina Abdominal/visceral pain syndromes Brachial plexitis/neurogenic thoracic outlet syndrome Phantom limb pain Intractable pain secondary to spinal cord injury Mediastinal pain Cervical neuritis Postherpetic neuralgia	No data available

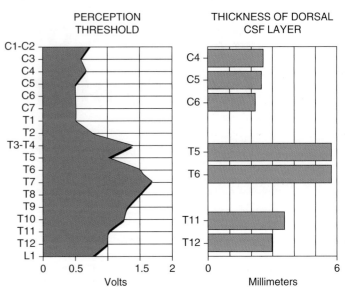

Fig. 5-2 Relationship between spinal level and perception threshold/dorsal cerebrospinal fluid thickness.

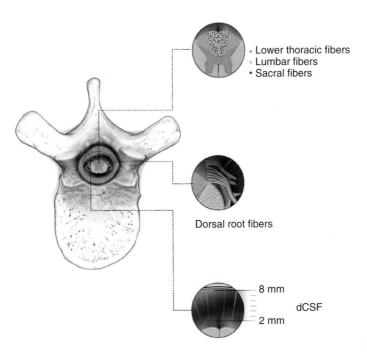

Fig. 5-1 Anatomy of the spinal canal. At T9 the lower thoracic fibers are located laterally within the dorsal columns. Some of these fibers are in close proximity to the dorsal root entry zones. Dorsal root fibers are larger, curved, and more easily activated than dorsal column fibers. Within the lower thoracic spine, the highly conductive dorsal cerebrospinal fluid (dCSF) layer is thickest where spinal cord stimulation leads are typically placed for back pain therapy. The dCSF can diffuse the stimulation field, increasing the likelihood that the dorsal roots will be inadvertently stimulated.

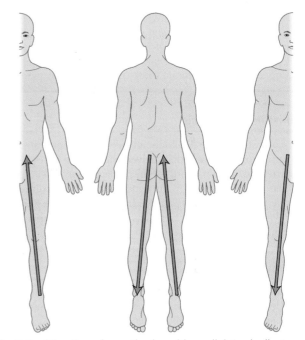

Fig. 5-3 Migration of paresthesias with mediolateral adjustment of stimulation. Modified from Oakley JC et al: Transverse tripolar spinal cord stimulation: results of an international multicenter study, *Neuromodulation* 9(3):192-203, 2006.

implemented. Nevertheless, there have been cases in which activation of the motor structures has been seen to occur at the same threshold as the sensory system; therefore selective stimulation of the dorsal column could not be successfully maintained.[2]

Understanding the somatotopy of the spinal cord is paramount to knowing the technical aspects of implantation. A basic tenet of SCS is to create an area of paresthesia that overlaps the patient's region of pain.[3] Therefore correlation of the somatotopy and the level of the spinal cord is necessary. Barolat and colleagues[4] have published extensively on the mapping of the spinal structures, which led to a database correlating areas of sensory response to levels dorsal SCS.[4]

High cervical regions such as C2 can cover regions of the posterior occiput and occasionally the lower jaw. C2-C4 stimulation provides coverage of the neck, shoulder, and upper extremities, as well as the face as a result of involvement of the descending nucleus of the trigeminal nerve. As one moves to the lower cervical region such as C5-C6, stimulation affects the entire hand. To cover the anterior chest wall or the axilla, an electrode placed toward C7-T1 is necessary.

More commonly an implanter seeks coverage of the lower extremities. Lateral placement at T11-T12 covers the anterior thigh, whereas placement at T11-L1 can cover the posterior thigh. Although coverage of the foot as a whole can be achieved by stimulating these same areas, it is difficult to cover the sole of the foot, which may require insertion on the lumbar L5 or S1 nerve roots. Low back pain is very difficult to cover because midthoracic stimulation can also affect the chest and abdominal wall. In general, midline placement of the electrode at T8-T10 seems to provide the best outcomes.

Recently this paradigm has been challenged by case series demonstrating successful four-limb paresthesia in patients receiving only cervical stimulation.[5] In general, this effect was achieved with stimulation with longer pulse widths and lower frequencies. Although the mechanism is not yet well understood, some have hypothesized that thinner dorsal CSF thickness in the cervical spine may allow for the stimulation of deeper medial and midline fibers that correspond to the lower extremities.

Basic Science

The enthusiasm with SCS began with the introduction of the gate control theory for pain control by Melzack and Wall[6] in 1965. They noted that stimulation of large myelinated fibers of peripheral nerves resulted in paresthesia and blocked the activity in small nociceptive projections. In other words, appropriate stimulation of a competing afferent signal can effectively block an existing pain signal.

Although a large body of work has been published, the exact mechanisms of action of SCS remain unclear. The computer modeling work of Coburn,[7,8] Coburn and Sin,[9] Holsheimer and associates,[10] Holsheimer and Struijk,[11] and Holsheimer and Wesselink[12] have shed some light, at least theoretically, on the distribution of the electrical fields within the spinal structures. It is clear that stimulation on the dorsal aspect of the epidural space creates complex electrical fields that affect a large number of structures, including afferents within the peripheral nerve, dorsal columns, or supralemniscal pathways. Mechanisms at distinct levels of the central nervous system apart from the spinal cord are believed to contribute to the effects of SCS. Such mechanisms include antidromic action potentials that pass caudally in the dorsal columns to activate spinal segmental mechanisms in the dorsal horns and action potentials ascending in the dorsal columns activating cells

in the brainstem, which in turn might drive descending inhibition. Recent work by Schlaier and associates[13] demonstrated changes in cortical excitability with SCS, which is believed to be N-methyl-D-aspartate (NMDA)-related neuroplasticity at the supraspinal level. At the chemical level, animal studies suggest that SCS triggers the release of serotonin, substance P, and γ-aminobutyric acid (GABA) within the dorsal horn.[14-16]

Indications/Contraindications

As mentioned previously, SCS has been used for a variety of pain conditions and is particularly indicated for pain of neuropathic origin rather than for nociceptive pain. It is important to realize that neurostimulation is a treatment option along the continuum of pain control.

Another important consideration is the need for careful psychological screening in the selection of candidates for SCS procedure.[17-24] This becomes particularly important because mood disorders can alter pain reporting and perception by a patient. Patients who have frank psychiatric disorders, excessive depression, anger, or unrealistic expectations may be inappropriate for SCS; however, some of these patients may become favorable candidates for SCS after appropriate psychiatric therapy. The most common indications for SCS follow.

Postlaminectomy Syndrome/Failed Back Surgery Syndrome

Postlaminectomy syndrome is vaguely defined. The term has included pain localized to the center of the lower lumbar area, pain in the buttocks, persistent radicular pain, or diffuse lower extremity(s) pain. Arachnoiditis, epidural fibrosis, radiculitis, microinstability, recurrent disc herniations, and infections have been perpetrated in the etiology of this syndrome. Although SCS is accepted in the treatment of leg pain, its widespread use for relief of pain in the lower lumbar area still remains to be defined.

Complex Regional Pain Syndrome

CRPS is characterized by gradually worsening severe pain, swelling, and skin changes of the hands, feet, elbows, or knees. It may be secondary to injury (CRPS type II) or may not have a clear etiology (CRPS type I). Implementation of SCS in these patients may be more difficult than with any other patient group, partly because of the ill-defined nature of the pain. In addition, there is an increased possibility of aggravating the original pain or causing new pain or allodynia at the site of implanted hardware. Furthermore, the pain may also spread to other body parts, thus making lasting coverage extremely challenging.

Chronic Critical Limb Ischemia and Pain

In 1973 Cook and Weinstein[25] were the first to suggest that the indications for SCS might extend beyond intractable pain control. They observed a group of patients with multiple sclerosis who underwent SCS to treat their chronic pain. Unexpectedly the patients experienced not only pain relief but also an improvement in mobility and sensory and bladder function. They incidentally found an apparent improvement in lower limb blood flow and subsequently used SCS in patients whose primary problem was peripheral vascular disease (PVD).[26] These patients were found to have relief of rest pain, increased skin temperature, improved plethysmographic blood flow, and healing of small cutaneous ulcers.

Similarly, it is believed that SCS benefits patients with pain secondary to Raynaud phenomenon[27] and diabetic neuropathy[28] as well.

Angina

The role of SCS in the management of refractory angina pectoris seems to be very promising. There are well-documented reports in the literature revealing uniformly good results in the relief of angina pain.[29-33] Further, the results have been maintained in long-term follow-up and have been substantiated by a reduction in the intake of nitrates as well. Interestingly, other findings have supported the evidence that SCS has effects that go beyond pain relief. The observations that there is less ST segment depression and that the exercise capacity, the time to angina, and the recovery time all improve with stimulation may suggest that there is a reduction in ischemia. In a positron emission tomography study, a redistribution of myocardial flow in favor of ischemic parts of the myocardium has been demonstrated as a long-term effect of SCS, both at rest and after pharmacological stress induction.[34]

Moreover, since the relation between pain and myocardial ischemia has not been fully clarified, we do not know whether the pain relief is caused by direct depression of nociceptive signals in the spinal cord or whether there is secondary gain from a reduction in the ischemia.[35,36] On the one hand, a significant amount of work by Foreman[14] has shown that dorsal column stimulation inhibits the activity of spinothalamic tract cells, which are typically activated by cardiac sympathetic afferents or intracardiac bradykinin. On the other hand, the effects of stimulation might be equivalent to those of a sympathectomy in that it inhibits a hyperactive sympathetic system. This latter mechanism has been shown experimentally in the rat by Linderoth and associates.[37]

Brachial Plexitis/Neurogenic Thoracic Outlet Syndrome

SCS has also been described for pain secondary to either brachial plexitis or neurogenic thoracic outlet syndrome. Most of these patients complain of pain that affects the upper extremity, the shoulder, the trapezius, the axilla, and/or the anterior upper chest wall. Unfortunately literature is relatively lacking for this indication.

Other Indications

Early studies in the 1980s demonstrated benefits of SCS for urinary incontinence, with consequent increases in continence and substantial reduction in residual urine volumes.[38-42] These effects were found with stimulation of ventral sacral roots, a method that has also been shown to improve bowel function in patients with spinal cord injury.[43] Trials in the 1970s reported initial benefits of this modality for phantom limb pain, but few of these patients experienced lasting results with long-term follow-up.[44] Scattered reports also exist demonstrating the benefit of SCS in the treatment of intractable pain secondary to spinal cord injury pain, mediastinal pain, cervical neuritis, and postherpetic neuralgia.

Equipment

Electrical stimulation consists of rectangular pulses delivered to the epidural space through an implanted electrode via a power source. Electrodes were initially all unipolar in nature, but subsequently bipolar and tripolar arrays were developed. The initial radio-frequency (RF)-driven passive receivers have given way to implantable pulse generators (IPGs), which were first introduced in the mid-1970s. In 1980 the first percutaneous quadripolar electrode was produced; it could be reprogrammed noninvasively through an external transmitter.[45] Subsequently IPGs that can be both transcutaneously charged and programmed have been developed. This most recent advance is now leading a renewed interest in the possibility of using special electrode arrays in the delivery of electrical stimulation to the spinal cord.

Percutaneous Electrodes

Percutaneous electrodes, otherwise known as wire electrodes, are particularly appealing because they can be inserted without much dissection and are more appropriate for performing a trial to assess candidacy for a permanent implant. During implantation these electrodes can be advanced over several segments in the epidural space, allowing testing of several spinal cord levels to assess for optimal electrode position. After the trial period these electrodes can easily be removed in the physician's office. Contemporary percutaneous electrodes are slim (i.e., only a few millimeters in diameter) and contain four (quadripolar) or eight (octipolar) contacts with various spacings. These percutaneous electrodes also come in varying lengths, which differ by manufacturer. Last, extension cables are occasionally necessary to bridge the distance from the spinal entry point to the pocket in which the battery will reside.

Electrode choice generally depends on how many segments of the spinal cord are to be covered. Although electrodes with larger spacing allow for broader coverage, closer spacing permits better steering and electric field shaping. The general trend is to use one or two quadripolar electrodes for limb pain and one or two octipolar electrodes for axial pain. Even insertion of three electrodes is being explored for better steering of current.[46]

A major disadvantage of percutaneous electrodes is their tendency to migrate—secondary to their inherent flexibility, which is necessary for their insertion through a Tuohy needle and their cylindrical shape. These factors can lead to migration even months after implantation. As a result, patients with percutaneous leads have reported a greater positional variance in their paresthesia. To address this issue, some percutaneous electrodes have been introduced that require a stiffening stylet for introduction. Another disadvantage is that percutaneous electrodes are less energy efficient than plate electrodes. The electrical current is distributed circumferentially around the electrode and consequently results in greater shunting of current.

Recently ANS (A St. Jude company, Plano, Tex) has introduced a slim-line plate type electrode that can be inserted percutaneously. The broader electrode base provides a surface in which fibrosis should lessen the risk of caudal electrode migration. The slimmer profile of the electrode might also have advantages in the cervical spine where spinal cord compression might be an issue. Finally, the design emulates that of a miniplate lead since the contacts are on one side with the other side being insulated, leading to a more energy efficient system (**Fig. 5-4**).

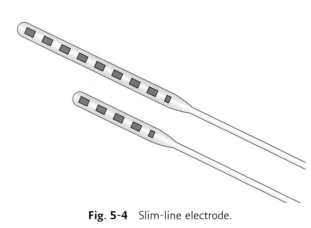

Fig. 5-4 Slim-line electrode.

Paddle Electrodes

Paddle or laminotomy electrodes are offered in many sizes, shapes, lengths, spacing, and configurations of electrodes. They are primarily offered as single- and dual-column configurations; with three (tripole)- and five-column models being introduced more recently (**Figs. 5-5** and **5-6**). With regard to their shape, these electrodes may come with curved or hinged leads to help facilitate insertion.

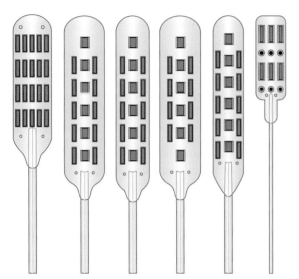

Fig. 5-5 Tripole and Pentad electrode paddles.

The main advantage of these electrodes resides in their more inherent stability in the dorsal epidural space and lesser propensity to migrate. Some preliminary data by North and associates[47] also suggest a broader stimulation pattern and lower stimulation requirements. As alluded to previously, paddle electrodes are also energy efficient in delivering electrical stimulation.

There is some theoretical evidence that shaping of the electrical field is possible with more complex electrode arrays. Current available tripole electrodes and their dimensions are shown in **Table 5-2**. Holsheimer and colleagues[48] concluded that the transverse tripolar system enabled finer control of paresthesia because of its ability to more accurately shape the stimulating electromagnetic field. Specifically the transverse tripolar configurations allow for stimulation of the dorsal columns at higher amplitudes before the dorsal roots begin experiencing clinically significant stimulation. These electrodes are composed of a central cathode flanked by lateral anodes, which modulate the field medially or laterally, depending on their programmed voltage. In other words, the current delivered to the spinal cord can be steered not by moving the electrode but instead by simply modifying the voltage ratio between the central cathode and two flanking anodes.[1] The lateral anodes create a shielding effect such that the dorsal roots are protected from stimulation; deeper activation of the dorsal columns is achieved with higher voltages (**Fig. 5-7**). This feature ultimately results in a wider therapeutic range, wider paresthesia coverage, and a greater probability to fully cover the painful area with paresthesia. Possible programming configurations of these tripole electrodes are shown in **Fig. 5-8**.

Although increasing the number of contacts allows for finer control of the electromagnetic field, there is also a significant

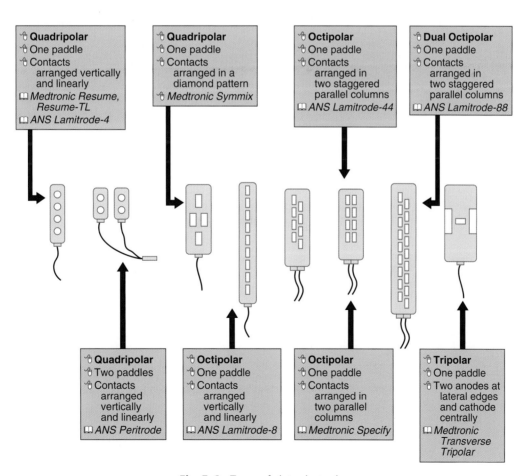

Fig. 5-6 Types of plate electrodes.

increase in power consumption and an even greater increase in the complexity of programming. The number of possible configurations is $n2n$, where n is the number of electrodes. Therefore with two contacts the total number of configurations possible is eight; with four contacts, sixty-four; and with sixteen contacts, it increases exponentially to reach a number in the millions.

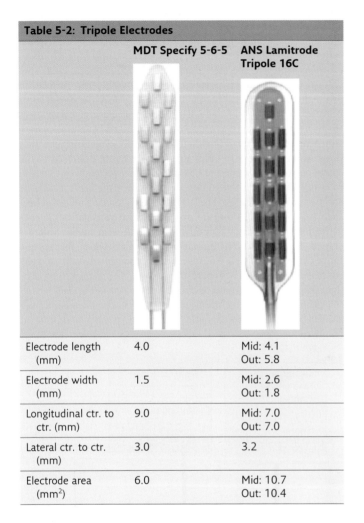

Table 5-2: Tripole Electrodes		
	MDT Specify 5-6-5	**ANS Lamitrode Tripole 16C**
Electrode length (mm)	4.0	Mid: 4.1 Out: 5.8
Electrode width (mm)	1.5	Mid: 2.6 Out: 1.8
Longitudinal ctr. to ctr. (mm)	9.0	Mid: 7.0 Out: 7.0
Lateral ctr. to ctr. (mm)	3.0	3.2
Electrode area (mm^2)	6.0	Mid: 10.7 Out: 10.4

Implantable Pulse Generators

The totally implantable pulse generator contains its own lithium battery. Activation and modification of stimulation parameters can occur through an external transcutaneous telemetry device, which the patient can carry. More extensive programming of the system can be achieved through a small portable unit that can be managed by the physician. These generators allow stimulation with fine resolution increments of 0.05 V and with varying rates and pulse widths.

Some systems also use multiple channels, which allow for treatment of multiple, distinct areas of the body using a single IPG. Once programmed, the patient can also select a particular channel at any particular time to best cover his or her symptoms.

Battery life varies with usage and with the used parameters such as voltage, rate, and pulse width. These factors, particularly voltage, are affected by patient factors such as epidural scarring and accommodation to stimulation. With typical use these batteries last between 2.5 to 4.5 years. Replacement of the battery requires a surgical procedure, which is usually performed on an outpatient basis.

IPG selection is based on many variables. From a practical standpoint, the first and foremost reason might be the size of the patient. Although larger batteries have a longer life, they obviously have more bulk and can often become the source of significant patient complaints. Although the IPG can be implanted into the buttock, abdomen, or subclavicular area, implantation in the buttock has multiple advantages. This location makes it easier to tunnel the electrode leads to the battery; with a patient placed prone, repositioning is not required to reach the buttock region.

Rechargeable Implantable Pulse Generators

Rechargeable systems have now become available. Medtronic's device, known as the *Restore Rechargeable Neurostimulation System*, uses a battery with an estimated 9-year total life span and takes about 6 hours to fully recharge. Advanced Neuromodulation Systems' Eon device has a battery life that is currently estimated to be 7 years. Boston Scientific's Precision device has a battery life estimated to be 5 years. A detailed comparison of the features of these rechargeable batteries is shown in **Table 5-3**.

In an analysis of cost between rechargeable and nonrechargeable systems, Hornberger and associates[49] found that the former would require 2.6 to 4.2 fewer replacement procedures, resulting

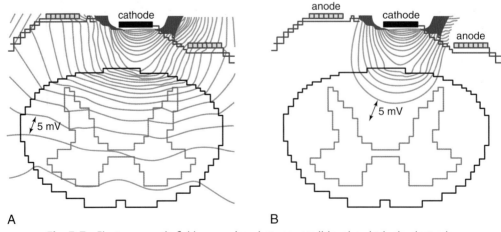

Fig. 5-7 Electromagnetic field comparison between traditional and tripole electrodes.

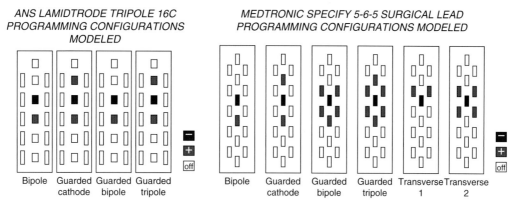

Fig. 5-8 Tripole programming configurations.

Table 5-3: Rechargeable Batteries	Eon	Restore	Precision
Dimensions (mm)	59 × 58 × 16	65 × 49 × 15	55 × 45 × 11
Volume	42 mL	39 mL	22 mL
Weight	75 g	72 g	36 g
IPG engine	Constant current	Constant voltage	Constant current
Battery chemistry	Rechargeable Li+	Rechargeable Li+	Rechargeable Li+
Battery capacity	340 mA-hrs	300 mA-hrs	2000 mA-hr
Electrodes	Up to 16	Up to 16	Up to 16
Amplitude	0-25.5 mA	0-10.5 V	0-20 mA
Frequency	2-1200 Hz	2-130 Hz (260 Hz)	0-1200 Hz
Pulse width	50-500 μs	60-450 μs	20-1000 μs
No. of programs	1 to 24	1 to 26	1 to 4
Multiplexed channels per program	Up to 8 1 set @ ≤ 1200 Hz 2 set @ ≤ 600 Hz 4 set @ ≤ 300 Hz 8 set @ ≤ 150 Hz	Up to 4 1 set @ ≤ 130 Hz 2 set @ ≤ 130 Hz 4 set @ ≤ 65 Hz	Up to 4 1 set @ ≤ 1200 Hz 2 set @ ≤ 130 Hz 4 set @ ≤ 80 Hz
Programmer communication	Near-field	Near-field	Far-field
Device life	7 yrs @ high settings	Up to 9 yrs @ medium settings	5 yrs @ medium settings
Compatible perc leads	5	3	1
Compatible surgical leads	11	1	1
Maximum implantation depth	1 in (2.5 cm)	4/10 in (1 cm)	¾ in (2 cm)

in a total lifetime savings ranging from $104,000 to $168,833. With regard to overall efficacy, a 12-month study looking specifically at the Restore rechargeable IPG demonstrated that the system was easy to use and that all patients were able to recharge it successfully. Moreover, both patient and physician satisfaction was high, with significant improvements in pain, quality of life, and functional status.[50]

Technique

In 1967 Shealy and Cady[51] and Shealy, Mortimer, and Reswick[52] inserted the first dorsal column stimulator in a human suffering from terminal metastatic cancer. Subsequently electrodes have been implanted using a variety of techniques: via a laminectomy in the subarachnoid space[52]; between the two layers of the dura, or in the epidural space, either dorsal or ventral to the spinal cord.[53-55] Subsequently less invasive percutaneous techniques were introduced.[56] Current practice indicates the placement of electrodes in the dorsal epidural space and connecting them to an implantable pulse generator usually placed in the buttock. However, before a permanent system is implanted, patients typically undergo a trial period of 3 to 10 days, during which time stimulation is provided by percutaneous electrodes to determine their overall efficacy.[57]

Placement of Percutaneous Electrodes

To place percutaneous electrodes, the patient is positioned in a comfortable prone position on a fluoroscopy table with a pillow underneath the abdomen. This position creates some kyphosis, which may facilitate electrode insertion.

A fundamental consideration in choosing the level of entry is that several centimeters of the lead have to lie in the epidural space to ensure maximal stability of the electrode and minimize unwanted migration. To ensure this, insertion must take place at least two spine segments below the desired target. For cervical placement one must bear in mind the cervical cord enlargement and insert the electrode below the T1-T2 level when possible. Insertion is performed under fluoroscopy; this equipment must be ready to function in both the anteroposterior and lateral planes at the time of needle insertion. A Tuohy needle is inserted with as shallow an angle as possible to minimize the risk of electrode breakage and a paramedian approach to avoid friction with the spinous process.

Although tactile feedback is important in locating the epidural space, it should not be the sole source of information. The most common method is feeling a loss of resistance while injecting fluid with a low-friction glass syringe; however, injecting a small amount of air may be superior because fluid injected in the epidural space may later be aspirated through the needle and give the false impression of being in the subarachnoid space. After multiple passes at one spine level have been performed, the loss-of-resistance method may lose its reliability. Therefore inserting a Seldinger wire through the needle can provide invaluable information about the degree of penetration into the spinal canal. If the needle tip is in the interspinous ligament and has not penetrated the ligamentum flavum, the wire cannot be advanced. The wire can be advanced only if the needle tip is in the paraspinal muscles or within the spinal canal. The pattern of advancement and the location of the wire under fluoroscopic imaging can further clarify its position.

If more than one electrode is inserted, it is wise to insert the other needles before inserting the electrodes since subsequent needle insertion might shear an already implanted electrode. Moreover, it is often possible to insert two electrodes simultaneously and advance them synchronously in the epidural space while maintaining their relative position and spacing.

Once the electrode is in the spinal canal, one has to be certain that it is positioned in the epidural space and not within the subarachnoid space. Although this may seem obvious, it may require multiple attempts at needle placement. This is particularly true if the dura has been previously pierced and CSF has escaped and pooled in the dorsal epidural space. One major difference is that in the subarachnoid space much less resistance is encountered when moving the electrode, particularly for lateral movements. The wire seems to be "floating" and undergoes large shifts of direction in the subarachnoid space; whereas in the epidural space movements are more discrete and obtained only with specific manipulations. Nevertheless, unfortunately the same type of wire/ electrode movement can be experienced epidurally if the dural sac

has collapsed significantly secondary to CSF loss. In such instances electrical stimulation clarifies the position; a subarachnoid placement elicits responses at much lower thresholds than an epidural placement.

When the epidural space is satisfactorily identified, the electrode is inserted gently under fluoroscopic guidance in the anteroposterior view. Once it has been inserted through the tip of the needle, the electrode must be removed without damage to the insulation surrounding the electrical contacts. If the electrode does not slide without minimal resistance, the needle and the electrode should be removed together. Every time the electrode is withdrawn through the needle, it should be inspected for minute breaks in the insulation, which would necessitate its disposal. Alternatively, a sleeve can be inserted over the guidewire in the epidural space. The guidewire is then removed, and the electrode is inserted through the sleeve. This obviates the risk of shearing the electrode during manipulation.

During placement the electrode may curve around the dural sac to the ventral epidural space. In the anteroposterior projection this might be indistinguishable from a proper midline dorsal location. A gentle lateral curve of the electrode shortly after its entry in the epidural space should raise the suspicion that it is actually lying ventrally. Absolute confirmation of the ventral location arises from stimulation generating violent motor contractions or observation in the lateral plane. An x-ray film should always be obtained to document electrode level and position. Care must be taken to identify either the bottom most visualized rib as the twelfth rib or to use the sacrum to count the number of lumbar vertebra to document the level of implant.

Once in place, the electrode must be secured to the interspinous ligament to minimize dislodgment. An important measure is to secure the wire as loops at the electrode insertion site to relieve the strain and reduce migration during bending. Applying suture directly to the leads has been shown to be safe since it does not cause substantial physical damage or any electrical impairment.[58] Nevertheless, manufacturers still do not recommend tying directly to the lead and continue to recommend the use of anchors to secure leads. When anchors are used to secure the electrode, one must remember to secure the anchor to both the electrode and the fascia.

Placement of Paddle Electrodes

Paddle electrodes require a surgical procedure for implantation under direct vision.[59] The patient may be placed in one of two basic positions: prone or semilateral. The prone position allows a more intuitive understanding of the spatial relations, which is more familiar to surgeons. At the same time, it can be difficult to obtain adequate sedation and maintain the airway in this position. In the semilateral position the surgeon has access to the spine and the flank, abdomen, or buttock for the implant of the pulse generator. The patient is asked to place himself or herself in the most comfortable position. If the pain is predominantly on one side, the patient is asked to lie on the less affected side. In this position airway management is safer than in the prone position, and the anesthesiologist is more comfortable in keeping the patient deeply sedated. For cervical placement the neck is slightly flexed but not excessively rotated laterally because extreme rotation substantially increases the difficulty of electrode placement. In general the variable degree of rotation with the patient in the semilateral position makes it more difficult to determine the location of the midline, which may be a significant problem in the cervical area.

A laminotomy is performed approximately one level below the intended level to allow the plate electrode to rest at the planned target for stimulation. Localization is performed with fluoroscopy or with a plain x-ray film, using metallic markers placed on the skin at the level of the planned incision. In a thin patient the incision is about 1 inch in length; and even in large individuals the incision seldom exceeds 2 inches because three to four levels can be accessed by extending the dissection and stretching the skin edges with a Gelpi retractor. Subperiosteal dissection is performed to expose the upper half of the inferior spinous process and the entire superior spinous process. Parts of the superior spinous process are then incrementally removed to expose the interposing ligamentum flavum. In the lower thoracic and upper lumbar area this usually requires the removal of the inferior third of the spinous process. However, in the midthoracic area the acute angle and significant overlapping of the spinous processes necessitates the removal of the whole spinous process. Following removal of the ligamentum flavum, the electrode is inserted into the dorsal epidural space; and its position is confirmed with fluoroscopy and by functional testing.

Such testing previously consisted of waking the patient and determining efficacy of stimulation from patient responses. This has gradually been replaced with intraoperative stimulation with electromyography (EMG) stimulation coupled with somatosensory evoked potential (SSEP) testing, which helps detect proper positioning of the electrode. EMG stimulation is performed with a signal consisting of a greater than 310 microseconds pulse width at a frequency of 5 Hz; the amplitude is gradually increased until EMG signal changes are detected. Alternatively, awake testing is commonly performed with 50-Hz stimulation. As one would expect, bilateral extremity stimulation suggests midline placement, and early root onset implies too lateral of a placement. In addition, stimulation of the dorsal columns results in a greater area of coverage with paresthesia—the percentage of body surface covered is inversely proportional to the distance between two electrodes.[60] To achieve this, most of the current has to be directed to an area within 2 to 3 mm on each side of the physiological midline. It is important to note that the physiological midline may differ from its anatomic counterpart by up to 2 mm[1]; in such instances one should rely on the former since it has a higher clinical correlation. With this feedback, the implant should be placed midline in cases of axial symptomatology or with a bias to one side for patients with unilateral pain. By correlating paddle position to the prior position of trial electrodes and testing motor stimulation responses, one can effectively find the proper location for implantation without waking the patient.

As with percutaneous leads, it is important to secure the leads with a strain relief loop with a diameter no less than 2.5 cm to minimize lead migration with movement. This loop can be sutured directly to the paraspinal muscles before closing the fascial layer.

Implantable Pulse Generator Placement

The IPG should be placed in an area where the unit will have enough overlying soft tissue but also not be pressing against bone, usually the abdomen or buttock. To find the appropriate area of implantation in the latter, three boney prominences are used as landmarks. The posterior superior iliac crest marks the medial border; the greater trochanter of the femur and the apex of the iliac crest define the lateral border. The IPG is implanted approximately 2 to 3 cm deep in the lateral aspect of this triangle (**Fig. 5-9**).

Postlaminectomy Syndrome/Failed Back Surgery Syndrome

In the treatment of postlaminectomy syndrome, a great challenge has been to obtain stimulation in the low back. Even with direct stimulation to the low back, the pattern of paresthesia is often

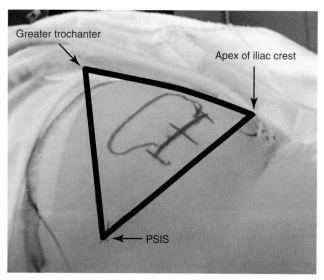

Fig. 5-9 Landmarks for battery placement.

replaced in time by an unpleasant segmental band of stimulation from the thoracic roots, which negates the benefits of the procedure. Previous pioneering work by Jay Law[61,62] has shown that stimulation in the low back can be obtained only if one uses multiple arrays of closely spaced bipoles at T9-T10. North and associates[63] have challenged the concept of the superiority of centered dual electrodes by showing that one single quadripolar electrode in midline has the ability to stimulate the axial low back. These were acute observations, and no data exist as to the long-term behavior of single vs. dual electrodes. The advent of the tripole electrodes and the ability to steer current has made it more plausible to aim for low-back paresthesia. This technology, which consists of a cathode flanked by lateral anodes, also theoretically increases the discomfort threshold.[46]

Angina

The most appropriate electrode location for the treatment of angina pectoris is most likely the lower cervical and upper thoracic region, although some have reported successful higher cervical placements.[64] In terms of its daily use, most patients use a low-intensity stimulation for several hours per day for prophylactic purposes.[65]

Brachial Plexitis/Neurogenic Thoracic Outlet Syndrome

With the currently available systems, stimulation of all areas is often not feasible with a single electrode. Stimulation of the shoulder and entire upper extremity requires an electrode placement in the upper cervical area; whereas stimulation in the axilla and upper chest wall area is typically achieved only with an electrode in the lower cervical/upper thoracic area. Only on rare occasions does an upper cervical placement reach all of the aforementioned areas. Therefore typically two electrodes are necessary to obtain appropriate coverage. In addition, a two-channel stimulating device might be indicated because the setting for the upper cervical region may be different from that required to optimally stimulate the axilla and anterior chest area.

One specific challenge with these patients is in the extreme hyperesthesia present in the brachial plexus region and the trapezius, which often extends to even larger areas of the posterior thorax. Any surgical manipulations in these areas of hypersensitivity must be avoided at all cost. Tunneling of the implanted wires must be planned carefully and must be at a substantial distance from the hypersensitive area. Lack of adherence to these principles often results in excruciating pain and intolerance to the implanted system.

Patient Management/Evaluation

Careful follow-up of the patients is necessary for successful long-term satisfaction. Equipment-related problems can arise at any time after implantation. Such problems include discomfort at the pulse generator/radio receiver site, electrode breakage or migration, and infection. Titration of the electrical parameters and careful follow-up of the patients is just as important as a technically correct surgical implant procedure. This process can be time consuming. The use of computer-assisted and patient interactive programming is showing great promise;[66,67] the ability to download several programs into the pulse generator/receiver, which can later be recalled by the patient at the push of a button, has greatly facilitated the management of the implanted stimulation systems.

There are three very important electrical parameters: the perception threshold, the discomfort threshold, and the usage range. The perception threshold is the voltage where the patient begins to perceive paresthesia;[68] the discomfort threshold is the voltage where the patient perceives the stimulation as uncomfortable, either because the paresthesias are too strong or because it elicits motor contractions; and the usage range is the difference between these two parameters. As previously indicated, the perception threshold is the lowest in the cervical area and highest in the midthoracic area because of the increasing thickness of CSF dorsal to the spinal cord in the midthoracic spine. For this reason electrode placement in the midthoracic spine favors more selective activation of the segmentary sensory system and seldom results in satisfactory long-term stimulation of the dorsal columns. The distance between electrode and nerve fibers is also affected by patient posture[69] and thus may require use of different programs throughout the day for such variations. This can be cumbersome, and no technology yet exists that is capable of adapting to these changes.

Once the optimal combination and stimulation voltage have been established, other electrical parameters must also be assessed to optimize the stimulation. The rate of stimulation is very important. Although most patients choose rates between 20 and 100 Hz, there is a high individual variability, and several different rates must be attempted before settling on the optimal one. Some evidence exists that patients with specific neuropathic pain syndromes may respond better to higher stimulation rates (>250 Hz).[66] The other parameter of pulse width provides a finer adjustment for the current intensity; and other features such as cycling, ramping, and biphasic pulses should be explored to promote the most effective delivery of stimulation. It is not unusual for optimal stimulation parameters not to be fully established for several weeks following implantation.

Outcomes Evidence

In selected patients SCS can produce at least 50% pain relief in 50% to 60% of the implanted patients; and with the proper follow-up care these results can be maintained over several years.

Postlaminectomy Syndrome/Failed Back Surgery Syndrome

Longitudinal studies by North and associates[70] evaluated 50 patients with postsurgical lumbar arachnoid or epidural fibrosis without surgically remediable lesions. In this group of patients SCS was superior to repeated surgical interventions on the lumbar spine for back and leg pain and superior to dorsal ganglionectomy for leg pain. Specifically a reduction in pain by at least 50% and patient satisfaction were obtained in 53% of patients at 2.2 years. These results are consistent with a 1995 systematic review of 41 studies,[71] in which approximately 50% to 60% of patients with failed back surgery syndrome (FBSS) had greater than 50% pain relief from SCS. Similarly, Burchiel and associates[72] conducted a prospective multicenter study in 1996 with 1-year follow-up and also reported 55% successful stimulation; but unfortunately medication usage and work status were not significantly changed. In 2007 a small retrospective series also demonstrated patient satisfaction of 73.5% with reduction in visual analog scale (VAS) scores and amount of additional medication required.[73]

North, Kidd, and Piantadosi[74] also conducted a prospective study randomizing patients with FBSS to repeat back surgery or SCS surgery; but allowing patients to cross over after 6 months. Although 10 of 15 patients crossed over from back surgery to SCS, only two of 12 patients crossed over from SCS to back surgery. North and colleagues[47] also compared the difference between paddle and percutaneous electrodes. Although laminectomy electrode placement is more invasive than percutaneous placement, it yielded significantly better clinical results in patients with FBSS at up to 3-year follow-up.

The PROCESS trial, published in 2008, involved randomizing 100 patients with FBSS to medical management alone or to SCS in addition to medical management.[75] In this 2-year study, the authors found that patients randomized to SCS demonstrated >50% leg pain relief, improved quality of life, and greater functional capacity more frequently (37%) than those randomized to medical management alone (2%). However, once again no difference was noted in the amount of opioid use between the two groups.

In a recent prospective cohort study of workers' compensation recipients who underwent SCS for FBSS, no significant difference was detected with regard to pain, function, medication use, and work time loss after 6 months of follow-up.[76] This study emphasizes the importance of patient screening to increase chances of a favorable outcome since those who underwent SCS in this study had low average mental health scores, poor baseline functioning, and axial back pain in addition to radicular leg pain.[77]

Complex Regional Pain Syndrome

In 1989 Barolat, Schwartzman, and Woo[78] reported reduction of pain in 10 of 13 patients implanted. No patients in that series were made pain free, but all 10 reported a definitive difference when the stimulation was stopped. In 1997 Kumar, Nath, and Toth[79] presented a median follow-up of 41 months on 12 patients with permanently implanted leads. Eight patients reported near complete resolution of their symptoms, and four also maintained good relief.

Kemler and associates[80] reported 23 cases with 78% of the patients reporting improvement. In 2000 this group published another series of 54 patients who underwent randomization to SCS with physical therapy or to physical therapy alone.[81] Using an intent-to-treat analysis, in the SCS-randomized group 67% of patients experienced significant pain relief, which persisted at 6 months. Specifically 2.4 cm decrease in VAS for pain was noted in the SCS group; compared to 0.2 cm increase in the group undergoing physical therapy alone. At the same time, no functional improvement was observed in either group. However, in subsequent publications Kemler and associates[82] noted that the effects of SCS that were maintained at 2-year follow-up, diminished over time for these patients such that, at 5-year follow-up, results were no longer statistically significant in favor of SCS. Nevertheless an as-treated analysis revealed near statistical significance for pain relief (p = 0.06) and statistically significant improvement in global perceived effect. When interviewed, 95% of patients with an implant reported that they would repeat treatment for the same result.[83]

Oakley and Weiner[84] reported a prospective study of 19 patients with CRPS implanted with SCS systems. Of the 10 patients about whom detailed long-term efficacy data were available, three reported full relief from their pain, and seven reported partial relief.

Three additional prospective studies without matched controls have been reported (total of 50 subjects).[59,84,85] Two of the studies reported success rates with an 84% overall success rate. The third study by Calvillo and colleagues[85] reported a significant improvement in pain scores (VAS) and a >50% reduction in narcotic use by 44% of subjects. In eight retrospective studies the overall success rate was 84% (192 patients).[86]

Chronic Critical Limb Ischemia (CCLI) and Pain

After the work by Cook and Weinstein,[26] in 1981 Meglio and associates[87] reported pain relief and ulcer healing in a patient with advanced peripheral arterial insufficiency. In 1988 Jacobs and colleagues[88] published clinical evidence that SCS improved the microcirculation as measured by capillary microscopy.

An early trial was performed by Klomp and associates,[89] who randomized 120 patients with critical painful limb ischemia to receive medical therapy alone or SCS in conjunction with medical therapy. At a mean follow-up of 19 months there was no significant difference in pain score improvement between the two groups. Yet Jivegard and colleagues[90] found benefits of SCS when they studied 51 patients who were randomized to receive either oral medication alone or SCS with oral medication. This group reported a significant improvement in pain scores of the SCS-treated group over the non-SCS group (p < 0.01). Similarly, a prospective randomized trial by Guarnera, Furgiuele, and Camilli[91] demonstrated superior pain control and increased ulcer healing of SCS (72%) compared to distal arterial reconstruction (40%).

Four prospective studies without matched controls reveal an overall success rate of 78% (n = 271); and an analysis of seven retrospective studies found an overall success rate of 76% (n = 308).[86] A review of the European literature demonstrates that 70% to 80% of patients achieved significant (>75%) pain relief. Moreover, pain relief with SCS was found to have more persistent effects than medical treatment alone. Cochrane reviewers have found evidence to favor SCS over conservative treatment to improve limb salvage and achieve pain relief in those unfit for surgery or who have persistent distal ischemia and pain despite revascularization.[92,93]

Angina

Vulink and colleagues[94] conducted a prospective study on quality of life changes in patients with refractory angina pectoris implanted with SCS. They found that both the pain and the health aspects of quality of life improved significantly after 3 months of SCS. Further, social, mental, and physical aspects of quality of life were found improved after 1 year of SCS.

Hautvast and associates[95] implanted SCS in patients with stable angina pectoris and randomized them. One group remained inactivated, and the other group was instructed to use the stimulator three times per day for 1 hour and with any angina attack. At 6 weeks the treatment group had increased exercise duration and time to angina and decreased angina attacks and sublingual nitrate consumption. Also observed was a decrease in ischemic episodes on electrocardiogram (ECG), with a decrease in observed ST

segment depressions on exercise ECG. There was an increase in perceived quality of life and decrease in pain. It was shown that a placebo effect from surgery in the treatment group was unlikely because all patients had implantation surgery at baseline.

In another prospective study of 104 patients who underwent SCS implantation for refractory angina pectoris there was a significant decrease in angina episodes at rest, angina episodes with activity, and total angina episodes.[96] Five additional studies are reported to be prospective but without matched controls.[94,97-100] Each of these also revealed significant benefit from SCS. The benefit indices ranged from reduction in angina attacks, decreased nitrate consumption, decrease in New York Heart Association (NYHA) grade, and improvement in Nottingham Health Profile (NHP) grade.

A recent randomized controlled study in patients already implanted with SCS for angina, demonstrated improvement in functional status and symptoms in treatment arms with conventional or subthreshold stimulation in comparison to a low-output placebo treatment arm.[101] This is the first blinded study in which stimulation below the sensory threshold for paresthesia has demonstrated therapeutic efficacy while eliminating the possibility of a placebo effect.

To compare SCS to coronary artery bypass graft (CABG), Mannheimer and associates[64] randomized 104 patients accepted for CABG to receive either CABG (n = 51) or SCS (n = 53) in the electrical stimulation versus coronary artery bypass surgery in severe angina pectoris (ESBY) study. This study demonstrated that patients randomized to SCS showed a greater than 30% improvement in Nottingham Health Profile (NHP) scores when compared with their baseline. This difference was significant and comparable to that shown by patients randomized to CABG[102] and were consistent on follow-up after 4 years. More important, the 5-year mortality of 27.9% in the ESBY study was similar between those receiving SCS and those who received CABG, with no difference in the percentage of cardiac deaths. In addition, whereas cardiac events were similar across the groups, significantly more cerebrovascular events were observed in the CABG group. Both groups experienced a significant and similar reduction in the number of angina attacks and the consumption of nitrates. Ultimately SCS appears to be equivalent to CABG in terms of symptom relief and may be an alternative to patients with increased surgical risk.

The concern of whether or not stimulation can conceal an acute myocardial infarction was directly addressed by Andersen, Hole, and Oxhoj.[103] They reported on 3 out of 45 patients treated with SCS for angina pain who survived a myocardial infarction (MI). All three patients noticed the pain to be different and unrelieved with SCS, and all patients correctly guessed that the pain was caused by a myocardial infarction. Therefore it was believed that SCS does not seem to conceal an acute MI.[104] Instead, SCS is believed to reduce the severity of angina attacks but not be able to suppress the conduction and perception of cardiac pain signals that act as indicators of cardiac distress.[105] Similarly, Murray and associates[106] have shown that SCS for refractory angina is effective in preventing hospital admissions without masking the ischemic symptoms or leading to silent infarction.

Abdominal/Visceral Pain Syndromes

Several early studies have since demonstrated the benefit of SCS in abdominal visceral disease. There was an initial hesitancy toward the application of SCS for visceral and somatic pain secondary to the belief that nociceptive pain could not be modulated via stimulation. However, Ceballos and colleagues[107] demonstrated reduction in pain scores and decrease in narcotic use in a patient treated for mesenteric ischemia with stimulation at T6. Similarly, Krames and Mousad[108] described a patient treated for irritable bowel syndrome who was developing escalating pain and diarrhea. After a stimulator was placed at T8, there was a subjective decrease in pain from 9/10 to 2/10 with only two diarrhea episodes and significant reduction in pain medications in the first 6 months. Even though the patient's pain recurred after 10 months, the significant reduction in the amount of diarrhea at that time persisted.

Kha, Raza, and Khan[109] reported the largest series of nine patients with refractory abdominal pain. Five of the nine patients had nonalcoholic pancreatitis, three had a presumed abdominal wall neuroma from frequent abdominal surgery, and another had postsplenectomy pain after trauma. All patients had a significant improvement in VAS scores and decreased narcotic use with placement of the leads at the T5-T7 level at 6- to 8-month follow-up.

Tiede and associates[110] reported on multiple abdominal surgeries and failed conservative measures. Each patient had an element of postprandial abdominal pain associated with nausea and vomiting. In both patients the leads were placed at the T2 level with significant improvement in pain, decreased narcotic use, and increased functioning such as return to work.

More recent studies have looked at the treatment of visceral pelvic pain specifically with SCS applied to the dorsal columns. Kapural and colleagues[111] reported on the value of neurostimulation for chronic visceral pelvic pain in six female patients with long-standing pelvic pain secondary to endometriosis, multiple surgical explorations, and dyspareunia. At an average follow-up of 30 months, they found a significant decrease in the VAS score with an average of more than 50% pain relief, accompanied with a decrease in opiate use.

Additional case reports have also demonstrated benefit of SCS for treatment of intractable abdominal or other etiologies, including familial Mediterranean fever and Bannayan-Riley-Ruvalcaba syndrome.[112,113]

Risk and Complication Avoidance

With the proper expertise, permanent complications are rare.[88] The most serious complication, which is shared with any type of spine surgery, is paralysis or severe neurological deficits, which are more likely during the dissection of epidural adhesions. Fortunately the number of cases of neurological injury involves far less than 1% of implants. An epidural hematoma is another rare but serious complication that can result from venous plexus damage on electrode insertion.

Electrode migration is not an uncommon problem and may require a reoperation to recapture adequate paresthesia. This phenomenon tends to occur most commonly in the first few days since it takes approximately 3 to 4 weeks for scar tissue to form around the plate electrode. In a retrospective review performed in 2006, lead migration was found to be slightly more common with plate electrodes (11.4%) than with percutaneous electrodes (9.8%); and this complication was also found to occur sooner in the former.[114] Close attention to programming is essential since a change in voltage requirements or sudden loss in previously captured paresthesia may hint at this problem. The incidence of electrode migration has varied significantly in the literature but is more accurately between 1% and 15%.

As technology continues to improve, hardware-related complications continue to decrease. Overall complications with the equipment include a 1% to 4% incidence of unspecified hardware failure or <2% incidence of battery failure. There is also a 1% to 8% incidence of lead breakage, which is common in the cervical spine and with plate electrodes.[114] An x-ray film may not reveal the

break—particularly if the break is limited to a small number of filaments—and high impedance is the only indication of this diagnosis. Most hardware-related problems are simply corrected with replacement.

Infection of the implanted hardware has occurred with a 3% to 5% rate. Infection usually affects the IPG or the cabling connecting to the electrode; very seldom does infection spread to the epidural space. Patients typically present with persistent tenderness over the implanted hardware, which can be difficult to differentiate from their baseline pain. The ultimate treatment is complete removal of the hardware followed by a prolonged course of intravenous antibiotics. Even when the infection is limited to the IPG, removal of that component alone leaves the patient at risk for spread of infection to the electrode.

A CSF leak may occur in less than 1% of implants. The clinical presentation consists of spinal headaches and fluid accumulation at the pulse generator site. These patients can be treated initially with bed rest for a few days and a tight abdominal binder over the pulse generator site for 2 to 3 weeks. If symptoms persist, a blood patch or surgical exploration may be required. When the CSF leak threatens the incision, surgical intervention is imperative.

Persistent pain at the implant site has been seen in about 5% of patients with CRPS. Recalcitrant CSF leakage has been encountered in a few patients, requiring multiple surgical revisions. Breakage or malfunction of the implanted hardware, particularly the electrodes and the subcutaneous extension cables, has been encountered in about 10% of the implanted systems. Disruption of the programmed settings can be minimized with appropriate patient education. For example, patients should be informed to turn off the device before going through an antitheft device in a retail store and to avoid strong magnetic fields, including magnetic resonance imaging (MRI) scanners. Painful stimulation, necessitating either repositioning or removal of the electrode, has also been reported in a number of cases.

Conclusions

SCS has been performed for over 30 years, and slow but steady progress with this technology has been made. As the equipment and stimulation parameters are improved, selection criteria have been better defined, and applications are slowly being expanded. More important, experience in the technique and equipment has increased the reliability and safety of SCS. Like all the modalities performed for chronic pain management, its results are generally favorable. Nonetheless, it is important to remember that the goal of neurostimulation is to reduce pain rather than to completely eliminate it. SCS has been shown to have approximately 50% improvement in pain relief that persists over years of follow-up, which is superior to many other invasive modalities. For this reason SCS has earned a well-established role in contemporary chronic pain management.

References

1. Oakley JC et al: transverse tripolar spinal cord stimulation: results of an international multicenter study. *Neuromodulation* 9(3):192-203, 2006.
2. Barolat G, Sharan A: Spinal cord stimulation for chronic pain management. *Arch Med Res* 31:258-262, 2000.
3. North RB et al: Spinal cord stimulation for chronic, intractable pain: superiority of "multi-channel" devices. *Pain* 44(2):119-130, 1991.
4. Barolat G et al: Mapping of sensory responses to epidural stimulation of the intraspinal neural structures in man. *J Neurosurg* 78:233-239, 1993.

5. Hayek SM, Veizi IE, Stanton-Hicks M: Four-limb neurostimulation with neuroelectrodes placed in the lower cervical epidural space. *Anesthesiology* 110(3):681-684, 2009.

6. Melzack R, Wall PD: Pain mechanisms: a new theory. *Science* 150:971-979, 1965.

7. Coburn B: Electrical stimulation of the spinal cord: two-dimensional finite element analysis with particular reference to epidural electrodes. *Med Biol Eng Comput* 18:573-584 1980.

8. Coburn B: A theoretical study of epidural electrical stimulation of the spinal cord–Part II: Effects on long myelinated fibers. *IEEE Trans Biomed Eng* 32:978-986, 1985.

9. Coburn B, Sin WK: A theoretical study of epidural electrical stimulation of the spinal cord–Part I: Finite element analysis of stimulus fields. *IEEE Trans Biomed Eng* 32:971-977, 1985.

10. Holsheimer J et al: Significance of the spinal cord position in spinal cord stimulation. *Acta Neurochir Suppl* 64:119-124, 1995.

11. Holsheimer J, Struijk JJL: How do geometric factors influence epidural spinal cord stimulation? A quantitative analysis by computer modeling. *Stereotact Funct Neurosurg* 56:234-249, 1991.

12. Holsheimer J, Wesselink WA: Effect of anode-cathode configuration on paresthesia coverage in spinal cord stimulation. *Neurosurgery* 41:654-659 (discussion 659-660), 1997.

13. Schlaier JR et al: Effects of spinal cord stimulation on cortical excitability in patients with chronic neuropathic pain: a pilot study. *Eur J Pain* 11(8):863-868, 2007.

14. Foreman RD et al: Effects of dorsal column stimulation on primate spinothalamic tract neurons. *J Neurophysiol* 39:534-546, 1976.

15. Linderoth B et al: Dorsal column stimulation induces release of serotonin and substance P in the cat dorsal horn. *Neurosurgery* 31:289-296 (discussion 296-297), 1992.

16. Linderoth B, Stiller CO, Gunasekera L et al. Gamma-aminobutyric acid is released in the dorsal horn by electrical spinal cord stimulation: an in vivo microdialysis study in the rat. *Neurosurgery* 34:484-488 (discussion 488-489), 1994.

17. Brandwin MAK, Kewman DG: MMPI indicators of treatment response to spinal epidural stimulation in patients with chronic pain and patients with movement disorders. *Psychological Rep* 51(3 Pt 2):1059-1064, 1982.

18. Kupers RC et al: Spinal cord stimulation: a nation-wide survey on the incidence, indication, and therapeutic efficacy by health insurer. *Pain* 56:211-216, 1994.

19. Nielson KD, Adams JE, Hosobuchi Y: Experience with dorsal column stimulation for relief of chronic intractable pain: 1968-1973. *Surg Neurol* 4(1):148-152, 1975.

20. Monsalve V, de Andres JA, Valia JC: Application of a psychological decision algorithm for the selection of patients susceptible to implantation of neuromodulation systems for the treatment of chronic pain. a proposal. *Neuromodulation* 3(4):191-200, 2000.

21. Olson KA et al: Psychological variables associated with outcome of spinal cord stimulation trials. *Neuromodulation* 1(1):6-13, 1998.

22. Burchiel KJ et al: Prognostic factors of spinal cord stimulation for chronic back and leg pain. *Neurosurgery* 36(6):1101-1110, 1995.

23. Ruchinskas R, O'Grady T: Psychological variables predict decisions regarding implantation of a spinal cord stimulator. *Neuromodulation* 3(4):183-189, 2000.

24. Daniel MSL et al: Psychological factors and outcome of electrode implantation for chronic pain. *Neurosurgery* 17(5):773-777, 1985.

25. Cook AW, Weinstein SP: Chronic dorsal column stimulation in multiple sclerosis; preliminary report. *N Y State J Med* 73:2868-2872, 1973.

26. Cook AW et al: Vascular disease of extremities: electric stimulation of spinal cord and posterior roots. *NY State J Med* 76:366-368, 1976.

27. Benyamin R, Kramer J, Vallejo R: A case of spinal cord stimulation in Raynaud's Phenomenon: can subthreshold sensory stimulation have an effect? *Pain Physician* 10(3):473-478, 2007.

28. de Vos CC et al: Effect and safety of spinal cord stimulation for treatment of chronic pain caused by diabetic neuropathy. *J Diabetes Complications* 23(1):40-45, 2009. Epub Apr 16, 2008.

29. Augustinsson LE: Spinal cord electrical stimulation in severe angina pectoris: surgical technique, intraoperative physiology, complications, and side effects. *Pacing Clin Electrophysiol* 12:693-694, 1989.

30. de Jongste MJ et al: Effects of spinal cord stimulation on myocardial ischaemia during daily life in patients with severe coronary artery disease. A prospective ambulatory electrocardiographic study. *Br Heart J* 71:413-418, 1994.

31. de Jongste MJ et al: Efficacy of spinal cord stimulation as adjuvant therapy for intractable angina pectoris: a prospective, randomized clinical study: Working Group on Neurocardiology. *J Am Coll Cardiol* 23:1592-1597, 1994.

32. Mannheimer C et al: Epidural spinal electrical stimulation in severe angina pectoris. *Br Heart J* 59:56-61, 1988.

33. Sanderson JE et al: Epidural spinal electrical stimulation for severe angina: a study of its effects on symptoms, exercise tolerance and degree of ischaemia. *Eur Heart J* 13:628-633, 1992.

34. Hautvast RW et al: Effect of spinal cord stimulation on myocardial blood flow assessed by positron emission tomography in patients with refractory angina pectoris. *Am J Cardiol* 77:462-467, 1996.

35. Meller ST, Gebhart GF: A critical review of the afferent pathways and the potential chemical mediators involved in cardiac pain. *Neuroscience* 48:501-524, 1992.

36. Thamer V et al: Pain and myocardial ischemia: the role of sympathetic activation. *Basic Res Cardiol* 85(suppl 1):253-266, 1990.

37. Linderoth B, Fedorcsak I, Meyerson BA: Is vasodilatation following dorsal column stimulation mediated by antidromic activation of small diameter afferents? *Acta Neurochir Suppl (Wien)* 46:99-101, 1989.

38. Brindley GS et al: Sacral anterior root stimulators for bladder control in paraplegia: the first 50 cases. *J Neurol Neurosurg Psych* 49:1104-1114, 1986.

39. Brindley GS, Rushton DN: Long term follow-up of patients with sacral anterior root stimulator implants. *Paraplegia* 28:469-475, 1990.

40. Van Kerrebroeck PEV et al: Results of the treatment of neurogenic bladder dysfunction in spinal cord injury by sacral posterior root rhizotomy and anterior sacral root stimulation. *J Urol* 155:1378-1381, 1996.

41. Van Kerrebroeck PCV et al: Urodynamic evaluation before and after intradural posterior sacral rhizotomies and implantation of the Finetech-Brindley anterior sacral root stimulator. *Urodinamica* 1:7, 1992.

42. O'Flynn KJ et al: The effect of sacral rhizotomy on lower urinary tract function in spinal injury patients. *Eur Urol* 18:8, 1990.

43. Vallès M et al: Effect of sacral anterior root stimulator on bowel dysfunction in patients with spinal cord injury. *Dis colon rectum* 52(5):986-992, 2009.

44. Krainick JU, Thoden U, Riechert T: Pain reduction in amputees by long-term spinal cord stimulation: long-term follow-up study over 5 years. *J Neurosurg* 52:346-350, 1980.

45. Waltz JM: Computerized percutaneous multi-level spinal cord stimulation in motor disorders. *Appl Neurophysiol* 45:73-92, 1982.

46. Sharan A: *Selective dorsal column activation with three column electrode arrays using percutaneous and paddle leads*, Washington, DC, 2007, AANS.

47. North R et al: Spinal cord stimulation electrode design: a prospective randomized comparison of percutaneous and insulated paddle electrodes. *Fourth International Congress of the INS*, 1998, p 211.

48. Holsheimer J et al: Clinical evaluation of paresthesia steering with a new system for spinal cord stimulation. *Neurosurgery* 42:541-547 (discussion 7-9), 1998.

49. Hornberger J et al: Rechargeable spinal cord stimulation versus non-rechargeable system for patients with failed back surgery syndrome: a cost-consequences analysis. *Clin J Pain* 24(3):244-252, 2008.

50. Van Buyten JP et al: The restore rechargeable, implantable neuro-stimulator: handling and clinical results of a multicenter study. *Clin J Pain* 24(4):325-334, 2008.

51. Shealy CN, Cady RK: Historical perspective of pain management. In Weiner RS, editor: *Pain management: a practical guide for clinicians*, ed 5, Florida, 1998, St Lucie Press, pp 7-15.

52. Shealy CN, Mortimer JT, Reswick JB: Electrical inhibition of pain by stimulation of the dorsal columns: preliminary clinical report. *Anesth Analg* 46:489-491, 1967.

53. Hoppenstein R: A device for measuring intracranial pressure. *Lancet* 1:90-91, 1965.

54. Larson SJ et al: A comparison between anterior and posterior spinal implant systems. *Surg Neurol* 4:180-186, 1975.

55. Lazorthes Y, Verdie JC, Arbus L: Anterior and posterior medullary analgesic stimulation, using a percutaneous implantation technic. *Acta Neurochir (Wien)* 40:277-223, 1978.

56. Dooley DM: *Percutaneous electrical stimulation of the spinal cord*, Bal Harbour, Fla, 1975, Associations of Neurology Surgeons.

57. Cepeda MS et al: An N-of-1 trial as an aid to decision-making prior to implanting a permanent spinal cord stimulator. *Pain Med* 9(2):235-239, 2008.

58. Kreis PG, Fishman SM, Chau K: Impact to spinal cord stimulator lead integrity with direct suture loop ties. *Pain Med* 10(3):495-500, 2009.

59. Ebel H et al: Augmentative treatment of chronic deafferentation pain syndromes after peripheral nerve lesions. *Minimally Invasive Neurosurg* 43:44-50, 2000.

60. Barolat G, Zeme S, Ketcik B: Multifactorial analysis of epidural spinal cord stimulation. *Stereotact Funct Neurosurg* 56:77-103, 1991.

61. Law JD: Targeting a spinal stimulator to treat the "failed back surgery syndrome". *Appl Neurophysiol* 50:437-438, 1987.

62. Law JD: Spinal stimulation in the "failed back surgery syndrome": comparison of technical criteria for palliating pain in the leg vs. in the low back. *Acta Neurochir* 117:95, 1992.

63. North R et al: Spinal cord stimulation for axial low back pain: single versus dual percutaneous electrodes, *Fourth International Congress of the INS*, 1998, p 212.

64. Mannheimer C et al: Electrical stimulation versus coronary artery bypass surgery in severe angina pectoris: the ESBY study. *Circulation* 97:1157-1163, 1998.

65. Norrsell H et al: Effects of spinal cord stimulation and coronary artery bypass grafting on myocardial ischemia and heart rate variability: further results from the ESBY study. *Cardiology* 94:12-18. 2000.

66. Alò K et al: Computer assisted and patient interactive programming of dual octrode spinal cord stimulation in the treatment of chronic pain. *Neuromodulation* 1:30-45, 1998.

67. North R et al: Patient-interactive microprocessor-controlled neurological stimulation system. *Neuromodulation* 1:185-193, 1998.

68. He J et al: Perception threshold and electrode position for spinal cord stimulation. *Pain* 59:55-63, 1994.

69. Abejón D et al: Effect of posture on spinal cord stimulation in patients with chronic pain syndromes: analysis of energy requirements in different patient postures. *Rev Esp Anestesiol Reanim* 56(5):292-298, 2009.

70. North RB et al: Failed back surgery syndrome: 5-year follow-up after spinal cord stimulator implantation. *Neurosurgery* 28:692-699, 1991.

71. Turner JA, Loeser JD, Bell KG: Spinal cord stimulation for chronic low back pain: a systematic literature synthesis. *Neurosurgery* 37:1088-1095 (discussion 1095-1096), 1995.

72. Burchiel KJ et al: Prospective, multicenter study of spinal cord stimulation for relief of chronic back and extremity pain. *Spine* 21:2786-2794, 1996.

73. De Andrés J et al: Patient satisfaction with spinal cord stimulation for failed back surgery syndrome. *Rev Esp Anestesiol Reanim* 54(1):17-22, 2007.

74. North RB, Kidd DH, Piantadosi S: Spinal cord stimulation versus reoperation for failed back surgery syndrome: a prospective, randomized study design. *Acta Neurochir Suppl* 64:106-108, 1995.

75. Kumar K et al: The effects of spinal cord stimulation in neuropathic pain are sustained: a 24-month follow-up of the prospective randomized controlled multicenter trial of the effectiveness of spinal cord stimulation. *Neurosurgery* 63(4):762-770, 2008.

76. Turner JA et al: Spinal cord stimulation for failed back surgery syndrome: outcomes in a workers' compensation setting. *Pain* 148(1):14-25, 2010.

77. Wasan AD: Spinal cord stimulation in a workers' compensation population: how difficult it can be to interpret a clinical trial. *Pain* 148(1):3-4, 2010.

78. Barolat G, Schwartzman R, Woo R: Epidural spinal cord stimulation in the management of reflex sympathetic dystrophy. *Stereotact Funct Neurosurg* 53:29-39, 1989.

79. Kumar K, Nath RK, Toth C: Spinal cord stimulation is effective in the management of reflex sympathetic dystrophy. *Neurosurgery* 40:503-508 (discussion 508-509), 1997.

80. Kemler MA et al: Electrical spinal cord stimulation in reflex sympathetic dystrophy: retrospective analysis of 23 patients. *J Neurosurg* 90:79-83, 1999.

81. Kemler MA et al: Spinal cord stimulation in patients with chronic reflex sympathetic dystrophy. *N Engl J Med* 343:618-624, 2000.

82. Kemler MA et al: Spinal cord stimulation for chronic reflex sympathetic dystrophy—five-year follow-up. *N Engl J Med* 354:2394-2396, 2006.

83. Kemler MA et al: Effect of spinal cord stimulation for chronic complex regional pain syndrome Type I: five-year final follow-up of patients in a randomized controlled trial. *J Neurosurg* 108(2):292-298, 2008.

84. Oakley J, Weiner, RL: Spinal cord stimulation for complex regional pain syndrome: a prospective study of 19 patients at two center. *Neuromodulation* 2:47-50, 1999.

85. Calvillo O et al: Neuroaugmentation in the treatment of complex regional pain syndrome of the upper extremity. *Acta Orthop Belg* 64:57-63, 1998.

86. Cameron T: Safety and efficacy of spinal cord stimulation for the treatment of chronic pain: a 20-year literature review. *J Neurosurg* 100:254-267, 2004.

87. Meglio M et al: Pain control and improvement of peripheral blood flow following epidural spinal cord stimulation: case report. *J Neurosurgery* 54:821-823, 1981.

88. Jacobs MJ et al: Epidural spinal cord electrical stimulation improves microvascular blood flow in severe limb ischemia. *Ann Surg* 207:179-183, 1988.

89. Klomp HM et al: Spinal-cord stimulation in critical limb ischaemia: a randomised trial: ESES Study Group. *Lancet* 353:1040-1044, 1999.

90. Jivegard LE et al: Effects of spinal cord stimulation (SCS) in patients with inoperable severe lower limb ischaemia: a prospective randomised controlled study. *Eur J Vasc Endovasc Surg* 9:421-425, 1995.

91. Guarnera G, Furgiuele S, Camilli S: Spinal cord electric stimulation vs. femoro-distal bypass in critical ischemia of the legs: preliminary results in a randomized prospective study. *Minerva Cardioangiol* 42:223-227, 1994.

92. Ubbink DT, Vermeulen H: Spinal cord stimulation for non-reconstructable chronic critical leg ischaemia (update of Cochrane Database Syst Rev. 2003;(3):CD004001; PMID: 12917998) *Cochrane Database Systematic Rev* CD004001, 2005.

93. Pedrini L, Magnon F: Spinal cord stimulation for lower limb ischemic pain treatment. *Interactive Cardiovasc Thorac Surg* 6:495-500, 2007.

94. Vulink N et al: The effects of spinal cord stimulation on quality of life in patients with therapeutically chronic refractory angina pectoris. *Neuromodulation* 2:33-34, 1999.

95. Hautvast RW et al: Spinal cord stimulation in chronic intractable angina pectoris: a randomized, controlled efficacy study [see comment]. *Am Heart J* 136:1114-1120, 1998.

96. Di Pede F et al: Immediate and long-term clinical outcome after spinal cord stimulation for refractory stable angina pectoris. *Am J Cardiol* 91:951-955, 2003.

97. Andersen C: Complications in spinal cord stimulation for treatment of angina pectoris: differences in unipolar and multipolar percutaneous inserted electrodes. *Acta Cardiol* 52:325-333, 1997.

98. Bagger JP, Jensen BS, Johannsen G: Long-term outcome of spinal cord electrical stimulation in patients with refractory chest pain. *Clin Cardiol* 21:286-288, 1998.

99. Eliasson T et al: Safety aspects of spinal cord stimulation in severe angina pectoris. *Coron Artery Dis* 5:845-850, 1994.

100. Sanderson JE et al: Spinal electrical stimulation for intractable angina–long-term clinical outcome and safety. *Eur Heart J* 15:810-814, 1994.

101. Eddicks S et al: Thoracic spinal cord stimulation improves functional status and relieves symptoms in patients with refractory angina pectoris: the first placebo-controlled randomised study. *Heart* 93:585-590, 1997.

102. Ekre O et al: Long-term effects of spinal cord stimulation and coronary artery bypass grafting on quality of life and survival in the ESBY study (see comment). *Eur Heart J* 23:1938-1945, 2002.

103. Andersen C, Hole P, Oxhoj H: Will SCS treatment for angina pectoris pain conceal myocardial infraction? Abstracts of the First Meeting of the International Neuromodulation Society. Rome, 1992.

104. Andersen C, Hole P, Oxhoj H: Does pain relief with spinal cord stimulation for angina conceal myocardial infarction? *Br Heart J* 71:419-421, 1994.

105. Hautvast R: *Cardiac nociception in rats-neuronal pathways and the influence of dermal stimulation on conveyance to the central nervous system*, Netherlands, 1997, Kader, Groningen.

106. Murray S et al: Spinal cord stimulation significantly decreases the need for acute hospital admission for chest pain in patients with refractory angina pectoris. *Heart* 82:89-92, 1999.

107. Ceballos A et al: Spinal cord stimulation: a possible therapeutic alternative for chronic mesenteric ischaemia. *Pain* 87:99-101, 2000.

108. Krames E, Mousad DG: Spinal cord stimulation reverses pain and diarrheal episodes of irritable bowel syndrome: a case report. *Neuromodulation* 7:82-88, 2004.

109. Khan Y, Raza S, Khan, E: Application of spinal cord stimulation for the treatment of abdominal visceral pain syndromes: case reports. *Neuromodulation* 8:14-27, 2005.

110. Tiede JM et al: The use of spinal cord stimulation in refractory abdominal visceral pain: case reports and literature review. *Pain Pract* 6:197-202, 2006.

111. Kapural L et al. Spinal cord stimulation is an effective treatment for the chronic intractable visceral pelvic pain. *Pain Med* 7:440-443, 2006.

112. Kapur S, Mutagi H, Raphael J: Spinal cord stimulation for relief of abdominal pain in two patients with familial Mediterranean fever. *Br J Anaesth* 97:866-868, 2006.

113. Yakovlev AE, Resch BE: Treatment of intractable abdominal pain patient with Bannayan-Riley-Ruvalcaba syndrome using spinal cord stimulation. *WMJ* 108(6):323-326, 2009.

114. Rosenow JM et al: Failure modes of spinal cord stimulation hardware. *J Neurosurg Spine* 5(3):183-190, 2006.

6 Spinal Cord Stimulation: Implantation Techniques

Richard L. Rauck, Sean Nagel, James L. North, and Andre G. Machado

CHAPTER OVERVIEW

Chapter Synopsis: Spinal cord stimulation is a valuable tool for managing patients with chronic pain of spinal origin, complex regional pain syndrome, as well as other chronic pain syndromes. Patients who are considered good candidates typically undergo a trial period of SCS before permanent implantation is considered. The techniques for implantation with percutaneous leads or paddle leads are reviewed in this chapter. Percutaneously placed cylindrical leads are commonly used for trialing as well as for permanent implantation. The procedure for permanent implantation of a cylindrical lead is less invasive than required to implant a plate lead and good outcomes can be accomplished. However, surgically implanted plate/paddle leads are less likely to migrate, less susceptible to positional effects, and often result in better clinical outcomes compared to percutaneous leads. In candidates for SCS, these potential benefits should be weighed against the more invasive surgery required for implantation.

Important Points:
- Spinal cord stimulation trialing techniques vary among implanters.
- Use of biplanar fluoroscopy is critical to safe and successful lead placement.
- No studies exist to validate a particular trialing technique over another, although advantages and disadvantages of each approach exist.
- Trialing varies by duration, number of leads used, type of leads, entry point, and technique.
- Either percutaneous cylindrical leads or surgically placed plate leads are used for permanent implantation.
- Plate leads are less likely to migrate and are less susceptible to position but require a more invasive surgery for implantation.
- The generator pocket should be deep enough to avoid erosion but superficial enough for interrogation and recharging.
- It may be advantageous to minimize extensions, and tension on the leads should be avoided.

Clinical Pearls:
- Careful planning is essential to successful outcomes when utilizing SCS systems. Planning includes appropriate patient selection; trialing technique; lead type and location; and generator type and location.
- Trialing and implant techniques vary among practitioners. Each technique carries unique advantages and disadvantages. Techniques should be carefully selected by practitioners based on their experience and individual patient characteristics.
- Optimal lead placement seeks to achieve non-painful paresthesias in the areas of pain. This typically occurs in the posterior epidural space, near midline, at a spinal level common for a particular pain distribution.
- Lead anchoring must be carried out meticulously to minimize migration. This involves redundant suturing techniques and utilization of optimal fascia.
- Fluoroscopic imaging in both AP and lateral views should be utilized frequently to ensure patient safety and device stability during placement.
- Generator location selection should be individualized based on each patient's anatomy and the stimulator position.

Clinical Pitfalls:
- Practitioners who choose to implant SCS systems should be prepared to manage the potential complications; this includes SCS repositioning, revision, and explantation.
- Lead damage can occur both during placement and post-placement. To minimize future damage, one must appreciate the lead location relative to the supraspinous and interspinous ligaments.
- Physiological trespass in the neuraxial space can have devastating consequences. Meticulous care should be taken at all times regarding surgical and aseptic technique.
- Lead migration and signal interruption can manifest following poor anchoring techniques, insufficient lead length, and excessive use of extensions.
- Inappropriate generator location or depth can lead to tissue erosion, patient discomfort, and difficulty with interrogation and charging.

Introduction

Neuromodulation achieves analgesia without producing destruction of nerves. Attempts to alter pain perception in the cerebral cortex by neuromodulation can take place via the peripheral nervous or the central nervous system. Neuromodulation within the central nervous system occurs at the spinal cord level or within the brain. All of these sites have been used to decrease the perception of pain and produce analgesia.

The recent clinical focus of neuromodulation techniques in chronic pain medicine center on two main areas: electrical (nondrug) stimulation and intrathecal drug delivery. This chapter looks at electrical stimulation as a neuromodulatory way of producing pain relief in patients suffering from chronic pain syndromes. Specifically, the chapter focuses on percutaneous and surgical techniques of spinal cord stimulation (SCS).

Patient Selection

Several factors are considered when selecting patients for SCS. The type (neuropathic vs. nociceptive) and location (radicular vs. axial) of pain are considered key components in the selection process. However, it is equally important to consider physical characteristics of the patient when deciding if he or she is an appropriate candidate for SCS. This consideration is also important for implanters who only perform percutaneous techniques to a decision about potentially referring the patient for surgical or paddle lead placement.

Patient selection for SCS is reviewed in detail elsewhere in this book. The ideal candidates for percutaneous leads are younger patients who do not have significant degenerative spine disease or pronounced scoliosis and/or kyphosis. The patients depicted in **Figs. 6-1** and **6-2** have significant scoliosis and were considered potentially difficult percutaneous placements. Approaching from the convex side of the scoliotic curve, the trials proceeded uneventfully as did the subsequent permanent percutaneously placed epidural leads.

It can prove difficult to place and anchor percutaneous leads to appropriate fascial tissue in morbidly obese patients. Percutaneously placed trial leads can often be maintained in the obese patient for 1 to 2 weeks without incident.

Migration of percutaneously placed spinal cord stimulator leads has been reported in many studies.[1-3] The reported incidence

ranges from 5% to 23% in different series.[1-4] Proper patient selection should help to minimize the likelihood of subsequent migration. As with morbidly obese patients, very thin patients may prove more technically challenging for the percutaneous implanter. This may include finding appropriate space for the generator and anchors and fixation of the leads.

Trialing

Trialing methods for SCS vary from one implanter to the next. No consensus exists for duration of trials, percutaneous or surgically implanted leads, or number of leads used for the trial (commonly, one or two leads).

Most implanters trial from 48 hours to 10 days. The overwhelmingly and single most important goal of a spinal cord stimulator trial attempts to determine the likelihood of a patient achieving

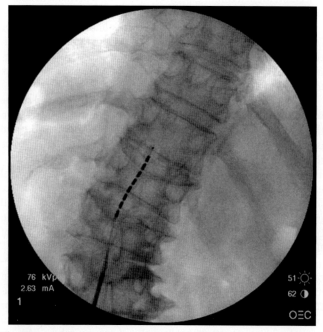

Fig. 6-1 Scoliotic patient undergoing trial spinal cord stimulator lead placement. Note position of needle on convex side of scoliosis. This approach facilitates successful lead placement.

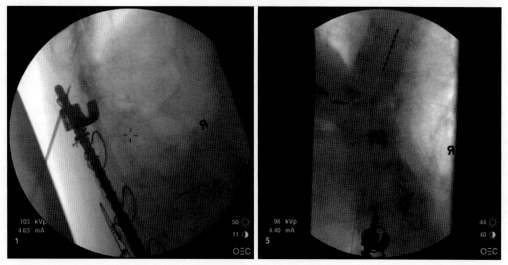

Fig. 6-2 Scoliotic patient with hardware in place from previous surgery. Note approach is from convex side of scoliotic curve.

clinically meaningful long-term pain relief from the device. No studies have determined the length of time needed for a trial to answer this question.

How much pain relief is necessary before considering a trial successful for subsequent permanent implant? The literature often reports 50% pain relief as an outcome for judging a successful trial.[5-6] No good studies have looked at whether a criterion of 50% pain relief during a trial period predicts long-term success with SCS. It is quite possible that some patients with less than 50% relief may find acceptable relief long term and/or significant improvement in activities of daily living and increased functional abilities. It is known that some patients who report 50% or greater pain relief during a trial do not sustain relief long term and eventually become therapy failures.

Pain relief estimated at 50% often does not correlate with 50% reduction as measured by a numeric pain rating scale (NPRS) (Rauck, unpublished data). It is unclear if implanters who use 50% as a cutoff for determining whether to implant a permanent system should use the patient's verbal response or an NPRS.

Percutaneously implanted spinal cord stimulator leads can be inserted less invasively than surgically implanted trial leads. Surgically implanted trial leads are commonly sutured to spinal elements. An unsuccessful trial requires a second surgical procedure to remove the leads.

Percutaneously implanted spinal cord stimulator leads can be tunneled and exteriorized. These leads commonly are anchored in the deep fascia tissue of the back at the time of insertion. If the trial is unsuccessful, a second surgical procedure is required to remove the anchors and lead(s).

Many percutaneous implanters place leads through a special epidural needle with no intention of leaving the lead in place for long-term use. The lead or leads are exteriorized and sutured in place against the skin. At the end of the trial the lead(s) can be removed in the office without a surgical procedure or use of fluoroscopy.

The effort to place surgically implanted trial leads or percutaneous leads that are anchored, tunneled, and exteriorized may present a bias for second-stage completion or implantation of the generator. Patients with marginal results during the trial may opt for permanent implantation rather than agreeing to a second surgical procedure for removal. The downside to removing the trial leads at the end of the trial is the risk that subsequently placed permanent lead(s) may not recreate paresthesias exactly as the trial. Patients may report that the permanent system does not perform as well as the trial.

The implanting physician must decide whether to use one or two leads during a trial. Cost, increased procedural time, and increased risk of complications mitigate against placing two leads for all trial purposes. However, placing only one spinal cord stimulator lead for the trial may prove inadequate for producing sufficient paresthesias and analgesia for the patient. Many implanters use two leads for all permanent implants; thus one can argue that two leads should be used at trial to mimic the long-term paresthesias one expects over time.

Risk of infection during spinal cord stimulator trial has been infrequent.[7-8] Meticulous sterile technique should be followed during the trial placement. Literature from other implantable trial catheters suggest that the risk of infection increases with the duration of the trial.[9] A recent study with intrathecal catheters (in which the risk of serious neuraxial infection would be expected to be greater than epidurally placed spinal cord stimulator leads) reported no infections until week 3 and thereafter an incidence of 16% for catheters placed longer than 2 weeks.[9]

Our policy (RR and JN) has been to implant one percutaneously placed lead for most of our spinal cord stimulator trials. During paresthesia mapping in the fluoroscopy suite, we place a second lead if we are unable to get adequate paresthesias in the area of pain as reported by the patient. This occurs occasionally in our practice.

We inform patients to expect the trial to last 1 week. Patients are followed closely by telephone to make sure that the trial is progressing smoothly. If paresthesias are inadequate, too light, or too strong, patients are brought back to the clinic for reprogramming. Occasionally trials are extended beyond 1 week if patients cannot adequately assess the results of the trial.

If the lead migrates or pulls out (very rare) before 1 week, the results of the trial are assessed and reviewed with the patient. If sufficient pain relief (>50%) is reported and the patient and implanter agree, the decision to go forward with a permanent implantation is often made. Similarly, if no or minimal pain relief has been obtained, no permanent implantation is performed. Occasionally the trial lead is replaced 1 to 2 weeks later if the patient cannot assess the effects of the trial at the time of lead migration.

Finally, after removal of the percutaneous trial lead, we wait 1 to 2 weeks before permanent implantation. This allows for any indolent infection from the trial to manifest before moving forward with a permanent implantation. It is always preferred to find a subcutaneous or other skin infection from the trial and eradicate it before placing the permanent implant.

Positioning the Spinal Cord Stimulator Lead

Ultimately the location of any spinal cord stimulator lead depends on individual patient characteristics. No single location produces the same paresthesias in all patients. The optimal time for finding the location that produces paresthesia in the patient's pain distribution is during trial lead placement. The implanter and the programmer coordinate efforts along with feedback from the patient to map paresthesias that cover the patient's complaints of pain. Nevertheless, it is important to mention that it is not always possible to reproduce the paresthesias reported during the trial by implanting the permanent leads in the same radiologically defined location. Often, the permanent lead is implanted in the vicinity of the area where the trial lead was placed.

Patients are most commonly positioned prone for both percutaneous trial and permanent lead placement. If necessary, clippers are preferred over shaving and should be used the day of surgery. Prophylactic intravenous antibiotics should be administered within 1 hour of the permanent implant unless there is a strong contraindication present. We also routinely administer intravenous antibiotics before the percutaneous trial implant, although all implanters do not agree on its efficacy.

After sterile surgical preparation (e.g., chlorhexidine), many implanters use an Ioban drape over the surgical site. Standard sterile surgical techniques are used. Needle entry for percutaneous placement depends in part on anticipated final placement of the lead(s). Common needle entry for the lower extremity and/or axial low back pain is the midlumbar region. Skin entry commonly is marked at L2-3, L3-4, or L4-5. Entry into the epidural space should be as flat as possible, dependent in part on the body habitus of the patient. Entry into the epidural space is either one or often two levels above skin insertion. A paramedian approach should be used to avoid both the forces of the supraspinous and interspinous ligaments and the tendency of the spinous process to fracture a lead placed through a midline approach. The percutaneous implanter should not hesitate to use a longer-than-standard epidural needle to ensure that the angle of approach to the epidural space is shallow (less than 45 degrees whenever possible). A lateral view should be taken to ensure that the lead has not migrated anteriorly in the epidural space or into the dura (**Fig. 6-3**).

Common lead placement for lower-extremity paresthesias vary from T9 to T12 (**Figs. 6-4** and **6-5**). Lead placement below T12 will not consistently stimulate posterior columns since the spinal cord often terminates at L1 or L2. Stimulation for axial back paresthesias commonly requires placement of the leads at T7 and/or T8. As

stated previously, final lead placement should always be individualized to the patient response during intraoperative mapping.

For upper-extremity paresthesias, leads are commonly placed from C2 to C7. Needle insertion should be in the thoracic region. A choice exists between the upper and lower thoracic region. The upper thoracic area is a stable and good site for needle placement. Skin location of T4 or T5 allows the needle to advance easily in a shallow orientation to the epidural space. The normal kyphotic nature of the upper thoracic spine can make insertion in this area technically difficult or nonintuitive to the novice implanter. On the skin the needle often appears perpendicular, whereas the fluoroscopic image (particularly the lateral image) verifies that the approach to the epidural space is shallow (**Fig. 6-6**). Although insertion at T3 or T2 is certainly achievable, this kyphotic tendency enhances the direction of the needle. Skill and practice in learning this technique are necessary before implementation. The lateral view on fluoroscopic imaging can be difficult to interpret (see **Fig. 6-6**). However, as described in the following paragraphs, there are significant advantages to using the lateral view as one advances the needle in this location. With practice, the implanter can learn to interpret and understand this approach in the lateral view. The major advantage of needle placement in this area is less threading or passing of the electrode lead in the epidural space.

Proponents of a lower thoracic needle placement with subsequent passage of the lead to cervical sites counter that the lower skin insertion site for the needle and lead obviates the need to tunnel the lead(s) from the upper thoracic space to the generator site (usually a flank or buttock location).

In our practice we use a lower thoracic approach when the patient is young or we expect threading or passing of the lead in the epidural space to proceed without difficulty. In the older patient or one with significant spine disease we commonly choose the upper thoracic space for needle entry. Passing the lead(s) long distances through the thoracic spine region in the presence of significant spondylolysis, facet arthropathy, spurs, thickened ligamentum flavum, or other degenerative diseases can be technically challenging and fraught with difficulty. The lead can bow when significant

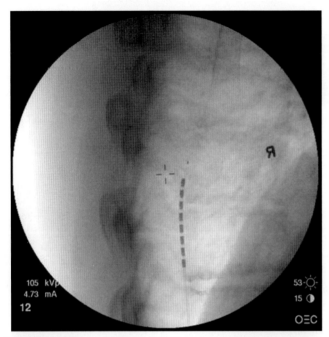

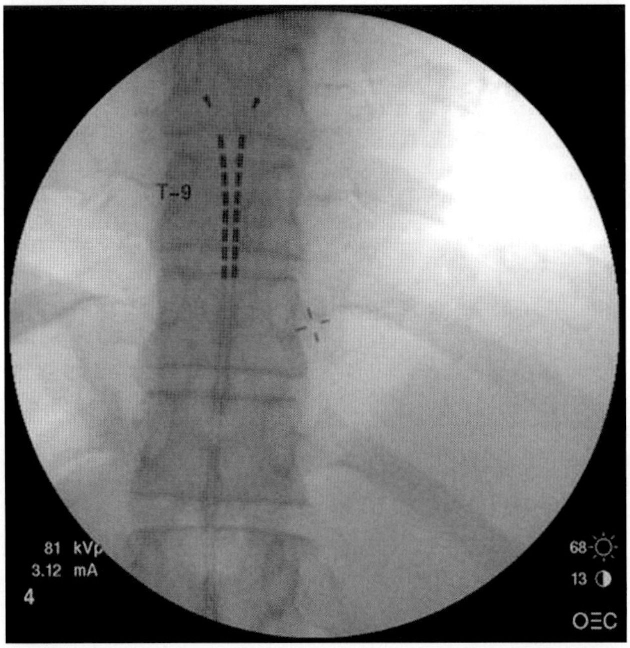

Fig. 6-3   Lateral view of spinal cord stimulator lead positioned erroneously in the anterior epidural space. Note that it is not possible to ascertain that a lead is anterior in the epidural space with a standard anteroposterior view.

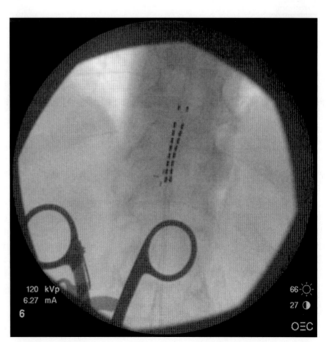

Fig. 6-4   Lead placement for typical spinal cord stimulation of lower extremities and axial back pain.

Fig. 6-5   Spinal cord lead placement for axial low back pain with leads positioned across vertebral body levels of T8-T9.

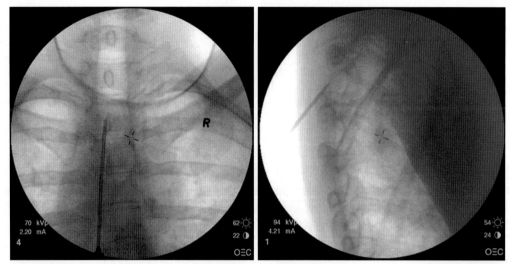

Fig. 6-6 Approach to epidural space in the upper thoracic region. Paramedian approach is used on anteroposterior view. Lateral view can be difficult to understand but becomes easier with repeated use.

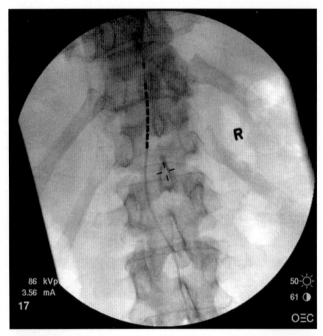

Fig. 6-7 Spinal cord stimulator that has bowed laterally. This lead can easily produce paresthesias on the nerve root and can migrate anteriorly in the epidural space.

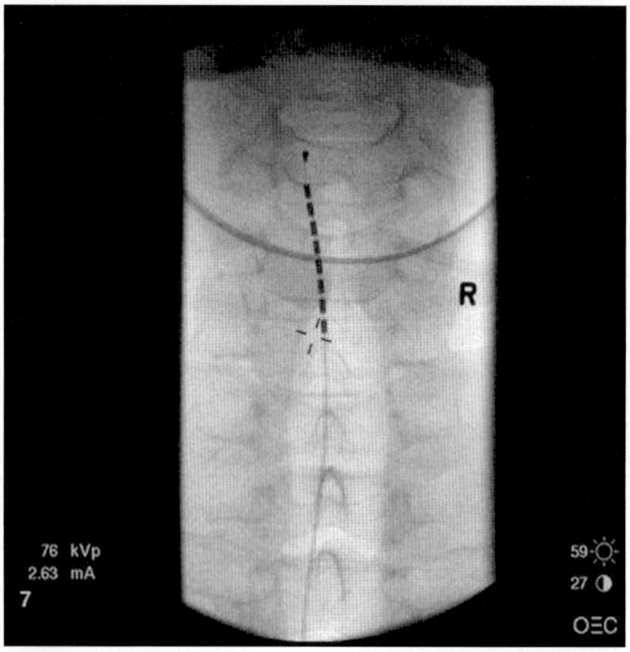

Fig. 6-8 Cervical trial lead positioned at C2 with lead extending laterally. This placement provides optimal chance of producing pain-relieving paresthesias in the neck.

obstructions are encountered, with painful paresthesias reported by the patient if the lead contacts a corresponding nerve root (**Fig. 6-7**).

In our experience it can be very difficult to obtain adequate paresthesias with SCS in patients who have significant neck pain. The best attempt at achieving paresthesia relies on placement of the electrode at C2 with an exaggerated lateral location as seen on the anteroposterior (AP) fluoroscopic image (**Fig. 6-8**). One alternative is to attempt a trial with a paddle lead placed retrograde over C1-C2, in a midline position. In the experience of the authors, this often allows for paresthesia coverage of the neck.

There have been case reports demonstrating four-limb paresthesias with leads placed in the lower cervical region.[10] Most patients considered candidates for SCS do not have pain in three to four extremities. However, this observation of four-limb stimu-

lation has been useful in the rare patient and may prevent placement of a second generator and two additional leads.

Lead placement for angina pectoris patients is commonly performed at C7 to T3 (**Fig. 6-9**). Needle insertion is usually in the lower thoracic level (T9 to 12). Two leads are commonly used and are positioned over both posterior columns. The leads should be placed close to the midline to avoid uncomfortable paresthesias of the chest wall.

A note should be made about the placement of two percutaneous leads. For trial purposes, the second needle is sometimes placed on the opposite side of the spine from the first needle or an interspace one level below the first needle. One should avoid placing the second needle above the first needle on the same side of the spine because the needle can potentially damage the lead coming from

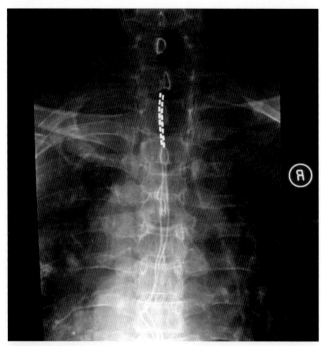

Fig. 6-9 Spinal cord stimulator leads placed in patient with refractory angina pectoris. Note leads are positioned between C7 and T2.

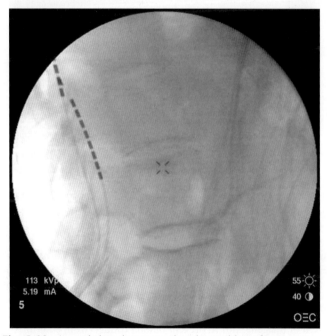

Fig. 6-10 Lateral view demonstrating the position of two 17-gauge Tuohy needles at the same vertebral level. Note that second needle is appropriately positioned beneath the first needle/lead to prevent possibility of the needle shearing or damaging the first lead.

the first needle (**Fig. 6-10**). It is possible to use the same interspace as the first needle, use a skin insertion site 1 to 2 cm below the first needle, and approach the space using the first needle as a guide.

For permanent implantation, two leads are commonly used. This often produces optimal paresthesia possibilities and also assists the programmer in maintaining adequate coverage if there is minor migration following surgery. Both leads can be inserted

through the same intervertebral space using the same paramedian approach from either the right or left side of the spine. In fact, it is our personal preference to insert both epidural needles at the same level and on the same side of the spine. The second epidural needle should always be inferior to the first needle. The second needle is positioned after the first percutaneous lead has been positioned. It is acceptable for the second needle to slide slightly medial or lateral relative to the first needle, depending on the location of the first needle and the desired location of the second lead. Lateral fluoroscopy greatly helps the implanter watch the second needle as it approaches the epidural space. The implanter can easily discern that the needle is staying inferior relative to the first needle as it approaches the epidural space. The first needle also serves as an excellent marker for where the posterior epidural space lies.

If there is difficulty placing the second needle, the opposite paramedian side or a lower epidural space can be used. It is very unusual to have to use an additional space; once the implanter becomes comfortable using the same interspace, the initial needle serves as an excellent landmark for depth and location of the posterior epidural space.

Subcutaneous Cut-Down and Lead Anchoring Techniques

Implanters vary during permanent implantation on when to perform the subcutaneous cut-down for anchoring the leads. Some implanters perform the cut-down before either needle placement. Others prefer to perform it after the initial needle is placed but before the second needle. Either method is acceptable and can result in satisfactory outcomes.

If the cut-down is performed after needle and lead placement, the needle should be left in place to protect the lead during cut-down. A self-retaining retractor aids exposure. Monopolar cautery should be avoided in the area of the epidural needles because the electrical current and heat from contact with the Bovie can be carried down the needle to the epidural space.

Once site preparation is complete, stylets and needles should be removed. Fluoroscopic guidance is used to ensure no change in position of the leads. Final lead arrangement can have several patterns. In addition, some electrode asymmetry can be considered acceptable in the majority of cases.

Meticulous anchoring of the leads is essential to prevent subsequent migration of the lead array. Anchoring devices are preferred by the authors as sutures placed directly around the leads may facilitate lead deterioration, failure, and possibly fracture. Non-absorbable sutures placed into deep fascial planes help hold the anchor in place. Multiple sutures around some of the anchoring devices help to minimize subsequent migration (**Fig. 6-11**). When using an anchoring sleeve, it should be positioned forward on the lead such that the distal end is abutting or directed into the deep fascial tissue. Placement of the anchor in this fashion minimizes the chance of the lead migrating out of the epidural space and into the space between the fascial tissue and the anchoring sleeve. It is a good idea to take frequent fluoroscopic images during the anchoring process to ensure that no lead migration occurs. A final fluoroscopic image in both the AP and lateral views at the end of this process ensures that there has been no migration.

Lateral Fluoroscopic Imaging

Fluoroscopic imaging is used to aid in placement of the epidural needle and subsequent passage of the spinal cord stimulator lead into the posterior epidural space. Standard fluoroscopic machines

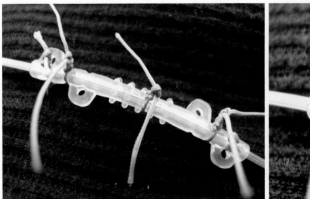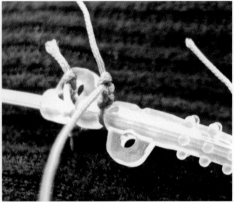

Fig. 6-11 Suturing technique of anchor. Note constriction of anchor around the lead using a sturdy suture.

are limited to two-dimensional views. AP views inform the implanter if the needle or lead is too medial or lateral. AP views cannot tell the depth of the needle. Lateral fluoroscopic views cannot help with left/right orientation of the needle but can help visualize the depth of the needle.

Some implanters use AP fluoroscopic guidance exclusively during placement of the epidural needle, relying on the feel of the lamina and a loss of resistance technique to guide them into the epidural space. In the authors' technique, the needle is placed firmly into fascial tissue using the AP view. The AP view is used initially to ascertain left/right direction and orientation. Once it is evident that the needle is headed in the correct direction, the fluoroscopic machine is rotated to the lateral view for final approach to the epidural space. Careful attention is made not to change the left/right orientation during lateral imaging. Whether the lead is in the lumbar, lower thoracic, or upper thoracic space, our preference is to position the fluoroscopic machine in the lateral view as the needle approaches the epidural space. (This is also our approach for cervical epidurals without SCS and all other approaches to the epidural space.) It takes skill and practice to interpret the location of the posterior epidural space, particularly in the upper thoracic area, but with experience it can be done consistently and reliably.

Further, the lateral fluoroscopic view shows where the lumbar lamina is and where access to the epidural space can be gained (**Fig. 6-12**). If the implanter learns the anatomy and understands the images, it becomes possible to predict if the approach of the needle will gain access to the epidural space or require redirection to avoid the protective lamina.

Generator Site Location and Preparation

The generators, particularly for rechargeable systems, have greatly diminished in size over the past several years. This allows additional options for placement of the generator. Generators can be placed in the posterior hip area/buttock area, the flank (single incision), midaxillary line over the inferior ribs, or subclavian area (for upper-extremity leads and upper-thoracic needle placement). Abdominal placement of the pulse generators is also possible and it has been suggested that it may reduce the risk of lead migration, although this is not a consensus among implanters.

The most common site for generator placement has been in the posterior hip area. The goal is to place the generator above where the patient sits but below the belt line. This can sometimes be problematic and the generators may coincide with the belt line. Incisions are usually made horizontally. The depth of the pocket is commonly 1 to 3 cm, and recommendations vary among the

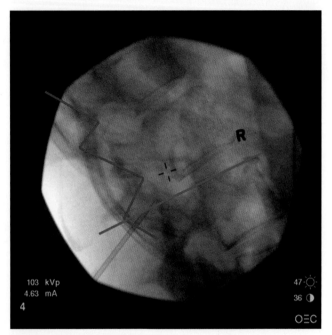

Fig. 6-12 Lateral fluoroscopic imaging showing anatomic relationships to entry site for epidural space. Red lines (shadows of pedicles and lamina) are analogous to stairs with entry on "risers" of steps. Blue line is superior endplate of vertebral body.

suppliers for actual depth of generator placement. Ideally the generator is placed deep enough to avoid subsequent discomfort or erosion but superficial enough for recharging and interrogation of the system with subsequent programming.

Adequate hemostasis in the pocket is important before placement of the generator to prevent blood products from entering the portals between the generator and the leads. The leads or extension wires are tunneled between the electrode and anchor site and the pocket site using a tunneler. Some implanters prefer to leave a tensioning loop in the back incision to minimize the potential for the leads migrating when the patient moves.

The electrical contact sites on the lead should be inspected for blood or tissue products and cleaned with a wet, then dry, sponge before insertion into the generator. After connecting to the generator, excess lead is coiled and maintained under or around the generator. Connecting cables may be needed to reach the IPG site. This should be considered against the possibility that each additional connector adds risk for disconnecting or for electrical interface problems.

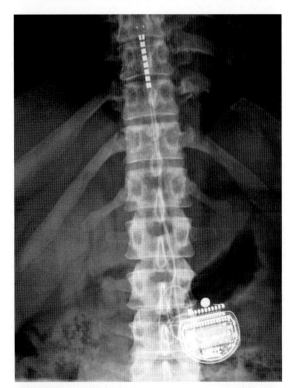

Fig. 6-13   Final placement of bilateral spinal cord stimulator leads with pocket and generator placed in right flank/paramedian locations.

The integrity of the system should be checked before closure. The generator is sutured into the pocket to prevent its migration, flipping over, or twiddling by the patient. A final AP and lateral fluoroscopic image is obtained to demonstrate no migration during the process.

An alternative location for the generator is in the flank. This location allows for placement of the generator lateral to where the leads are anchored in lumbar epidural insertions. Large generators are not well tolerated in this area. However, small (rechargeable) generators work very well in a lateral flank location. **Fig. 6-13** shows final lead placement with generator positioned in the flank. Flank locations make it unnecessary to have two incisions. This should reduce the risk of skin or superficial infections. In addition, no tunneling is necessary between leads and pocket site. The implanter must make the pocket large enough so the generator stays off the midline area. Patients do not tolerate pockets migrating over the spinal processes. Besides anchoring the generator to fascial tissue, an additional two or three retaining sutures to close the pocket site help keep the generator from migrating.

A few implanters and patients prefer the pocket in the abdominal region, in the midaxillary line, or more anteriorly over the inferior ribs. These are acceptable sites but may require the use of longer leads or connected extensions. It also can be problematic to perform the entire procedure in the prone position and may require re-preparation and re-draping of the patient for pocket incision and generator placement.

Revisions

Complications of SCS placement are reviewed elsewhere in this book. However, it should be noted that all implanters will experience a need to revise SCS systems. This may be replacing a

generator, moving a generator to a different site, replacing or repositioning a migrated lead, or removing an infected system.

The steps to perform a permanent, percutaneously placed SCS system can be relatively straightforward. Managing SCS systems after placement can prove challenging in some cases. Anyone who chooses to do permanent SCS implantations should be prepared to deal with the complications and perform the necessary maintenance and revisions to provide long-term satisfaction and favorable outcomes.

Summary

Percutaneously placed SCS leads can be performed for both trial conditions and permanent implants. The procedure for permanent implantations is less invasive than surgically placed leads. Long-term favorable outcomes can be expected with many patients and physicians who choose this route of implantation.

Paddle/Plate Leads

Cylindrical leads, inserted percutaneously through a Touhy needle or through superficial incisions as discussed in previous paragraphs, are a less invasive option. Incisions are small and typically do not breach the fascia. The advantages of this technical option include limited postoperative pain, discomfort, and length of stay. Most patients can be discharged on the same day as the procedure. Implantation of percutaneous leads is routinely done under local anesthesia with or without intravenous sedation. This minimizes anesthesia-related risk, particularly in the elderly and in those with multiple co-morbidities. However, the design limitations inherent in a cylindrical lead may limit stimulation efficacy. The tips of percutaneous leads are frequently placed several segments rostral to the spinal entry level and then anchored at the point of entry. Although technique modifications[11] and improved anchoring devices may limit longitudinal lead migration, lateral lead migration, not always easily identifiable in x-ray films, remains a concern. Furthermore, cylindrical leads are prone to positional effects with changes in activity or posture. This often limits efficacy and practical clinical value in patients who are (or want to be) more active and in those who continue to work.

Plate leads are a valuable alternative to cylindrical leads. Unlike cylindrical leads, plate leads have contacts that are insulated on one side. The contacts are flat and therefore cover a greater surface area. The expanded electrode-tissue interface maximizes efficiency and requires lower stimulation amplitude to generate a similar therapeutic response.[12] In 2005, North and associates[12] reported a prospective study comparing 12 patients implanted with cylindrical leads to 12 patients implanted with plate leads for the management of failed back surgery syndrome. Patients with plate leads had significantly better clinical results than those with cylindrical leads at 1.9 months follow-up.[2] Similarly in a retrospective study Villavicencio and colleagues[13] reported that patients implanted with paddle leads also had improved pain control. Lead migration and positional effects observed with cylindrical leads are minimized with the flat or semicurved lead body design of the plate lead. Depending on the model, the lead body can be anchored to spinal elements, or extensions from the lead body can be anchored to the muscle or fascia during wound closure. These anchoring options provide stabilization points that are closer to the electrical contacts than with cylindrical leads. The risk for lead migration is reduced, although migration can still occur in some cases, particularly at the nonanchored distal tip of the lead.

Plate Lead Specifications

Hardware selection often depends on the surgeon's experience. To date there is no direct comparative study demonstrating clinical superiority of devices from one manufacturer over another. Plate lead electrode configuration varies from a single column of four to sixteen electrode contacts divided into three columns. The postimplantation programming options increase with the number of contacts. The contact array length and width specifications range from approximately 30 to 55 mm and 2.5 to 8 mm, respectively. The thickness of the lead bodies ranges from 1.5 to 2 mm. Length and width of the lead bodies range from approximately 40 to 75 mm and 4 to 13 mm, respectively. The differences in lead body dimensions may not be insignificant for some patients. The potential for causing critical spinal canal narrowing and cord injury can be magnified by lead size and shape. Manufacturer warnings have been added to the product labeling.

Implantation Technique

The technique for implantation of a paddle lead is sometimes straightforward for the experienced surgeon. However, revision surgery is often challenging. Imaging of the spine can be helpful to assess the size of the canal and evaluate the degree of degenerative disease or post-surgical changes that may influence the type of lead selected and implant strategy. As for other posterior thoracic or cervical spinal procedures, there is always a concern for spinal cord injury, dural tears, or other complications.[3,14-16] In this chapter we focus on the thoracic implantation of plate leads in two common scenarios: (1) implantation of the plate lead following a temporary test with a percutaneous cylindrical lead, and (2) implantation of a plate lead after removing chronically implanted SCS cylindrical leads.

Implantation of a New Plate Spinal Cord Stimulator Lead
Plate leads can be selected as the first choice for chronic implantation of a SCS system. This decision often follows a test period of SCS with externalized cylindrical leads. If the placement of the test leads is without complication, placement of the permanent system can follow shortly after. Adhesions in the epidural space tend to be minimal after a percutaneous trial and usually do not pose a significant challenge for permanent implantation.

The procedure can be performed under general anesthesia or sedation, with or without regional anesthesia.[17-20] If the implant is done under sedation, intraoperative testing of the pattern of paresthesia coverage can be verified during the procedure, in a fashion similar to that of implantation of percutaneous leads.[18,20] The plate leads can be adjusted until the induced paresthesias cover all or the majority of the area of chronic pain. Implantation under general anesthesia is often preferred. Reasons include patient choice and concerns for deep sedation in the prone position. Although this option precludes intraoperative testing, implantation of the plate lead can often be successfully accomplished with intraoperative radiographic verification by placing the lead in the topographical region that was adequate for stimulation during the test period. Intraoperative neurophysiological monitoring is often used as for other spine procedures. If, after surgery, paresthesias cannot be created in the areas of chronic pain, revision of the lead may be required to accomplish this goal. The posterior elements of the spine are exposed with standard surgical exposure techniques. The length of the incision may vary with the patient's body habitus, and usually it is not necessary to extend the dissection as laterally as for spinal instrumentation. Depending on the lead type and planned level of implantation, a unilateral partial laminectomy or

laminotomy of the inferior margin of a lamina, sparing the spinous process and supraspinal ligament, is performed. For some lead models and for midline implantation, the exposure may be extended to include a midline partial laminectomy or laminotomy to clear an opening that allows for safe passage. Under most circumstances the tip of the paddle lead is advanced into the canal until the length of the lead is just beyond the laminotomy (**Fig. 6-14**).

If the opening of bone and ligamentum flavum is insufficient, resistance at the edges can direct the lead along unintended trajectories in the spinal canal or against the dural sac and cord. To protect the thecal sac and spinal cord from the paddle lead tip, the inferior spinous process may be removed to accommodate a shallower approach. As for cylindrical leads, implantation of the plate lead is usually planned for a median or paramedian position to optimize stimulation of the spinal cord while limiting spread of stimulation to the nerve roots laterally. The partial laminectomy or laminotomy is planned below the level intended for the tip of the lead. If a relatively short lead is used and the plan is to place the tip at the level of the top of a thoracic vertebral body, the opening can be created on the inferior margin of the corresponding lamina. However, depending on the length of the lead and the site for planned implantation, the laminectomy or laminotomy is created one or more levels below the intended vertebral body level for tip placement. The lead is inserted and aimed at the midline or paramedian position that favors the side of the pain. The location can be verified with intraoperative x-ray films and/or fluoroscopy.

Epidural adhesions, osteophytes, or thickening of the ligamentum flavum can cause resistance when the lead is passed. The nerve roots or the dural sac may also block lead advancement. In these situations it is often necessary to remove the lead and attempt reimplantation until a satisfactory trajectory into the canal and

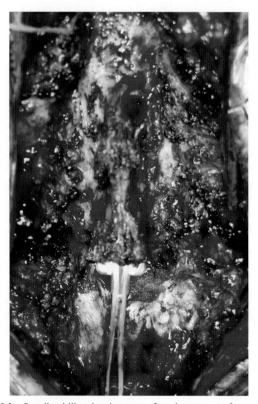

Fig. 6-14 Small midline laminotomy for placement of a paddle lead. Note that only the bottom of the lead is seen while most of the body is sublaminar. The bottom of the lead was sutured to the ligamentum flavum for anchoring

final location are seen. The dural guide is a useful instrument to facilitate dissection. Some plate lead kits include a tool for dissection of epidural adhesions. When resistance is identified, fluoroscopy can be helpful to identify what level and structure may be causing the resistance. For example, if the lead is directed laterally, resistance may be related to a nerve root, and repeated attempts may result in damage to the root or dural tear. In addition, forcing the lead beyond resistance could push it toward the sac and result in tear or cord injury. Complications from dissection of the sublaminar epidural space and lead placement are not limited to direct injury to the cord and roots during dissection alone. Hematoma formation,[21] inadvertent dural tear with leakage of cerebrospinal fluid, and pseudomeningocele formation are infrequent but recognized complications for this type of operation.

The lead can be anchored directly to the ligamentum flavum. Anchoring to the dura can be attempted, but the suture through the dura may create fluid leakage. Some leads have a portion of the body configured for suture anchoring. If the lead is not anchored directly to the spinal elements, the extensions from the lead body can be anchored to the soft tissues during closure. Some anchors provided with the SCS leads or in separate packages are designed for this purpose. Different anchoring techniques and anchoring devices can be used. Bench data have suggested that the position and type of anchor may influence the stress on the lead and promote hardware failure,[14] although these findings have not yet been validated clinically. Implantation of the implantable pulse generator (IPG) and connection to the lead directly or via extension wires is performed in a similar fashion as described for cylindrical leads.

Implantation of a Spinal Cord Stimulator Plate Lead After Removal of Cylindrical Leads

Patients experiencing limited benefits or complications associated with cylindrical lead implantation such as migration, positional effects, or hardware failure are often referred for revision of the SCS system and implantation of a paddle lead replacing the cylindrical leads. If cylindrical lead migration or limited benefits are observed early, before extensive scar formation, replacement with a plate lead is less complicated. The complexity and risk of the operation increases over time as scar formation around the cylindrical leads thickens. Computed tomography myelograms may be of value to assess the lead location and canal dimensions when revision surgery is planned. Magnetic resonance imaging is not possible in patients implanted with current SCS systems. Surgical exposure is essentially the same as for a new lead; however, caution (or avoidance) must be used with Bovie electrocautery in a patient already implanted with a neurostimulation system. The cylindrical leads are removed from their entry and anchoring site. The laminectomy is planned in accordance with the intended level of implantation of the lead. The scar buildup around the previously implanted leads may be obvious in the epidural space (**Fig. 6-15**). Dural guides and implantation tools for clearing the sublaminar space can be used to dissect epidural scar. If significant resistance is noted with passing the lead and the epidural scar is resistant to dissection, another laminotomy may be opened one or two levels cranially to facilitate dissection of the epidural scar and adhesions. In some cases a full laminectomy is needed. This should be weighed against the risk of a late deformity. However, if at least a "bridge" of lamina can be preserved, it can assist in stabilizing the lead and preventing dorsal migration away from the dura (**Fig. 6-16**).

Test Period With a Plate Lead

Externalized trials of SCS are typically performed with cylindrical leads, but externalized trials with a plate lead can be an option for

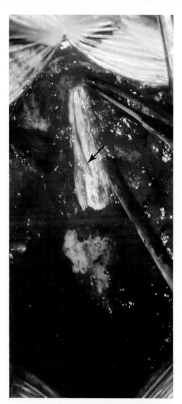

Fig. 6-15   Laminectomy in a patient who had previous spinal cord stimulation implanted with percutaneous leads. Note the thick cylindrical scar bands in the epidural space (*arrow*) corresponding to the tracts of encapsulation around the percutaneous leads.

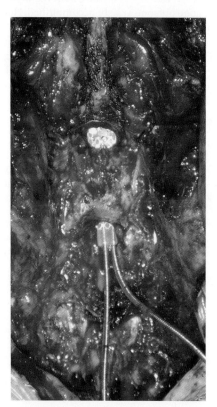

Fig. 6-16   Implantation of a paddle lead via a small midline laminotomy. Note that a second midline laminotomy was opened cranially to the initial (bottom) laminotomy to allow for dissecting epidural scar and adhesions that prevented adequate placement of the lead through a single opening.

some patients. Cylindrical leads can be challenging to advance in patients with extensive epidural adhesions or scar from previous operations. In addition, cylindrical lead migration can occur shortly after implantation, limiting the validity of the trial. This choice is weighed, taking into consideration the more invasive operation needed for placement of the paddle lead for a trial. During the test period the plate lead is connected either directly to the external pulse generator or via externalized extensions. In the latter option the goal is to preserve the plate lead for permanent implantation. The extensions can be tunneled to a point distant (i.e., laterally at the flank) to the laminectomy incision, whereas the connectors between the plate lead and the externalized extension can be placed at the level of the laminectomy incision. To internalize the SCS system at the end of a successful testing period, the laminectomy incision is reopened superficially, and the extensions are cut distal to the connectors. The extensions are then pulled through the externalized area away from the midline surgical incision. Although any externalized procedure carries in principle a higher risk of infection, this approach minimizes the chance of contamination of the plate lead and its extensions. In the experience of these authors, infection is uncommon when externalized extensions are used. An externalized trial with a plate lead is also an option in patients that completed a test period with cylindrical leads but report equivocal results because of suboptimal coverage, positional effects, or other limitations.

Summary

Percutaneously placed cylindrical leads are used for trialing and permanent implantation. The procedure for permanent implantation of a cylindrical lead is less invasive than required to implant a plate lead and good outcomes can be accomplished. However, surgically implanted plate/paddle leads may be less likely to migrate, less susceptible to positional effects, and may result in better clinical outcomes in some patients when compared to percutaneous leads. In candidates for SCS, these potential benefits should be weighed against the more invasive surgery required for implantation.

References

1. Barolat G: Spinal cord stimulation for chronic pain management. *Arch Med Res* 31:258-262, 2000.
2. North RB et al: Spinal cord stimulation electrodes design: a prospective, randomized controlled trial comparing percutaneous with laminectomy electrodes: part II-clinical outcomes. *Neurosurgery* 57: 990-996, 2005.
3. Cameron T: Safety and efficacy of spinal cord stimulation for the treatment of chronic pain: a 20-year literature review. *J Neurosurg* 100:254-267, 2004.
4. Kumar K et al: Spinal cord stimulation versus conventional medical management: a multicenter randomized controlled trial of patients with failed back surgery syndrome. *Pain* 132:179-188, 2007.
5. Kapural L et al: Spinal cord stimulation for chronic visceral pain. *Pain Med* 11:347-355, 2010.
6. Jang HD et al: Analysis of failed spinal cord stimulation trials in the treatment of intractable chronic pain. *J Korean Neuro* 43:85-89, 2008.
7. Rauchwerger JJ et al: Epidural abscess due to spinal cord stimulation trial. *Pain Pract* 8:324-328, 2008.
8. Kumar K, Wilson JR: Factors affecting spinal cord stimulation outcome in chronic benign pain with suggestions to improve success rate. *Acta Neurochir* 97(suppl):91-99, 2007.
9. Wallace MJ et al: Intrathecal ziconotide for severe chronic pain: safety and tolerability results of an open-label, long-term trial. *Anesth Analg* 106:628-637, 2008.
10. Hayek S, Veizi ID, Stanton-Hicks M: Four-limb neurostimulation with neuroelectrodes placed in the lower cervical spine. *Anesthesiology* 110:681-684, 2009.
11. Renard VM, North RB: Prevention of percutaneous electrode migration in spinal cord stimulation by a modification of the standard implantation technique. *J Neurosurg Spine* 4(4):300-303, 2006.
12. North RB et al: Spinal cord stimulation electrode design: prospective, randomized, controlled trial comparing percutaneous and laminectomy electrodes-part I: technical outcomes. *Neurosurgery* 51(2):381-389, 2002.
13. Villavicencio AT et al: Laminectomy versus percutaneous electrode placement for spinal cord stimulation. *Neurosurgery* 46:399-406, 2000.
14. Kumar K et al: Complications of spinal cord stimulation, suggestions to improve outcome and financial impact, *J Neurosurg* 5:191-203, 2006.
15. Turner JA et al: Spinal cord stimulation for patients with failed back surgery syndrome or complex regional pain syndrome: a systematic review of effectiveness and complications. *Pain* 108:137-147, 2004.
16. Taub A, Collins WF, Venes J: Partial, reversible, functional spinal cord transection: a complication of dorsal column stimulation for the relief of pain. *Arch Neurol* 30:107-108, 1974.
17. Vangeneugden J: Implantation of surgical electrodes for spinal cord stimulation: classical midline laminotomy technique versus minimal invasive unilateral technique combined with spinal anaesthesia. *Acta Neurochir* 97(suppl):111-114, 2007.
18. Beems T, van Dongen RT: Use of a tubular retractor system as a minimally invasive technique for epidural plate electrode placement under local anesthesia for spinal cord stimulation: technical note. *Neurosurgery* 58:ONS-E177; discussion ONS-E177, 2006.
19. Garcia-Perez ML et al: Epidural anesthesia for laminectomy lead placement in spinal cord stimulation. *Anesth Analg* 105:1458-1461, 2007.
20. Lind G et al: Implantation of laminotomy electrodes for spinal cord stimulation in spinal anesthesia with intraoperative dorsal column activation. *Neurosurgery* 53:1150-1153; discussion 1153-1154, 2003.
21. Franzini A et al: Huge epidural hematoma after surgery for spinal cord stimulation. *Acta Neurochir (Wien)* 147:565-567; discussion 567, 2005.

7 Spinal Cord Stimulation: Parameter Selection and Equipment Choices

Claudio Andres Feler

CHAPTER OVERVIEW

Chapter Synopsis: In principle, electrical spinal cord stimulation (SCS) can be delivered by the simplest of electrodes applied directly to the back, but today's implanted devices are far more complex. In efforts to maximize the benefits of SCS, designers of medical devices have constructed ever more complicated electrode arrays. For clinicians wisdom seems to come from experience when it comes to selecting the device and other details of SCS implantation. This chapter addresses the many technical considerations driven by clinical and basic science research and the underlying neurophysiology. A common electrophysiological goal of SCS is to stimulate A-beta fibers that innervate the painful region, thereby switching the pain "gate" to allow nonpainful signals to overwhelm neuropathic pain. Stimulation of sympathetic fibers resulting from SCS also has beneficial effects in multiple indications. Optimal implantation of the proper device can improve the chances of success in these aims. The electrode array itself is the first consideration in selecting a patient's individual course of treatment with SCS. Other factors to consider include power requirements, the optimal power source (rechargeable vs. battery), and placement of the power source in the body. Finally the stimulation pattern used at the electrode can produce varying results and should also be individualized.

Important Points: Contemporary neurostimulators allow changes in amplitude or voltage, frequency, and pulse width; they likely provide different electrophysiological effects at the level of the cord fibers, potentially increasing throughput in some settings while diminishing (blocking) spinal cord transmission in others.

Clinical Pearls: Changing parameters such as frequency may salvage a potentially bad outcome.

Clinical Pitfalls: Reliance on parameters does not relieve the implanter from properly selecting a patient, selecting a device, and completing a properly done implant.

Parameter Selection

The selection of targets for stimulation and the attendant selection of devices is in many respects easy and at the same time complicated, largely because of the massive amounts of anecdotal information and biases. These points of selection should be determined by desired impact on the nervous system and intent of paresthetic overlap on pain. Even more clouded is the selection of parameters of stimulation, wherein device selection may produce limitations and little has been published to support clinical perspectives. Claims among manufacturers of clinical advantage for one reason or another have been based on absent or at best poor science. Experienced users who have developed a keen eye for the characteristics of "responders" in their own hands further mystify new users of the technology as they announce, "this is it!" but fail to acknowledge other treatment perspectives as potentially valid. Yet there are reasonable guidelines for the selection of devices and their parameters that are both sensible and anatomically and physiologically specific.

Although spinal cord stimulation at its simplest requires only that a cathode be placed in position over cord with a closely spaced or distant anode to complete the circuit, many other factors may enter into play to change the stimulation experience for the patient. The intrinsic anatomy and physiology of a given patient is something that must be understood and considered.[1] The selection of a device and its parameters for stimulation is impactful in

patients. Most obvious among decisions of device selection is that of the lead or leads comprising the functional array. Array geometry and lead design have been demonstrated to be powerful in fiber selection for stimulation.[2-4] In particular, much of the recent lead development has been in designing arrays and leads to exclude stimulation of certain fibers, specifically the segmental fibers, in an effort to be better able to stimulate those desired within the cord.[5] The primary example of this is the ability to stimulate the back area rather than the dorsal roots representing the lower quadrants of the abdomen. Other topographic areas of desired stimulation have necessitated the use of alternate targets, such as the sacral nerve roots in patients with pelvic pain disorders.[6,7]

Much has been said and written about arrays. However, the parameters of stimulation have had relatively little attention.[8] Parameters of stimulation include the frequency or number of pulses per second expressed in Hertz (Hz); pulse width (PW), the duration of each pulse expressed in microseconds; and the amplitude or voltage, representing the power output from the generator. Another factor with potential impact on the experience of the patient is the waveform of each pulse. Although stimulation is done through ramped currents, they are essentially square waves; but the recovery phase of each pulse varies. However, the impact of this variance is less quantifiable because waveforms vary from company to company and may also vary within a given company's family of devices. Other factors such as constant current vs. constant voltage

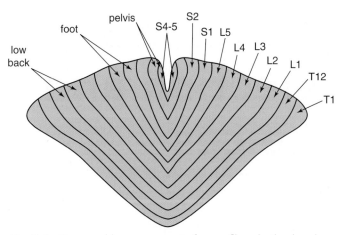

Fig. 7-1 Topographic arrangement of nerve fibers in the dorsal column. (Adapted from Feirabend HKP et al: Morphometry of human superficial dorsal and dorsolateral column fibres: significance to spinal cord stimulation, *Brain* 125(5):1137-1149, 2002.)

variances make objective comparisons between one waveform and the next difficult.

The anatomy and physiology relevant to stimulation of spinal cord structures is relatively straightforward. The *sine qua non* of a properly selected and implanted device for spinal cord stimulation (SCS) is comfortable paresthetic overlap on the pain segment. Although this teaching is correct, it may not be necessary to achieve this overlap in all cases, as follows.

To produce paresthesia, Aβ fibers should be stimulated. These lie in the dorsal columns of the spinal cord and have a somatotopic arrangement with the most caudal segments arranged medially, whereas the more cephalad fibers present laterally (**Fig. 7-1**). Activation of nerve fibers depends on current density, pulse frequency, and specific fiber sensitivity to stimulation. Current density at a target is a function of power output, frequency, and distance to the target. Fiber characteristics that are most impactful to depolarization are size and resting membrane potential and curvature to or from the field.[9] All other things being equal, larger fibers depolarize more readily than smaller fibers. Notably within the spinal cord, different tracts have varying sensitivities to current than others. Because the descending sympathetic tracts (intermediolateral fasciculus) are relatively sensitive to stimulation, it is reasonable to consider that pain relief secondary to stimulation may be related to direct inhibition of these pathways rather than large-fiber afferent activation. It is known that efficacious stimulation in patients treated for angina pectoris may be delivered below sensory perceptual threshold.[10] Similarly, consideration for the use of stimulation below sensory threshold must be given in those patients who suffer from other conditions in which modulation of the sympathetic nervous system plays a part. Examples of this include complex regional pain syndrome (CRPS) 1 with predominant sympathetically maintained pain (SMP) and Raynaud disease. Some have theorized that attention to the patient's response to sympathetic blocks may predict the outcome from stimulation below sensory perception. This theory has not yet been proven in clinical practice.

Frequency is the parameter that has been easiest to study. Case studies report benefit in many patients achieved by using "high frequencies" to treat when "normal frequencies" have failed.[8] Anecdotal experience shows that most patients prefer frequencies of stimulation of 50 Hz ± 10 Hz. This perception has been supported by Gordon and associates.[11] In some patients with CRPS 1, frequencies have been required that exceed 250 Hz to achieve and

or maintain satisfactory outcome. The physiological impact of stimulations as high as 1200 Hz is not well understood. It is conceivable that high-frequency stimulation functions by blocking transmission, perhaps by keeping neurons in their relative refractory period. This would be a frequency-dependent mechanism, as opposed to increasing signal throughput at more conventional frequency ranges (100 ± 50 Hz). The need in some patients for high-frequency stimulation, which is not necessarily predictable based on a trial of stimulation, presents a potential problem if a properly selected generator has not been implanted. Fortunately most current-generation rechargeable generators and some conventional batteries and radiofrequency units are capable of producing high-frequency rates. The obvious disadvantage of conventional batteries in a high-frequency setting is that of early depletion. It would be advisable to consider rechargeable power sources or transcutaneous induction generators that are capable of high-frequency stimulation in patients who suffer with pain from CRPS 1.

Equipment Choices

Matching a device to a patient should always begin with consideration of the best lead array to produce the desired result. In my opinion, the use of percutaneous leads for both trial and permanent implants is an excellent option for treating patients with lower-extremity pain and thoracic radicular pain and angina. In making the decision regarding lead selection for a permanent device, consideration must be given to the topography of pain and the durability of the patient's implant. Durability is the ability to comfortably stimulate the intended target predictably and repeatedly for the duration of the pain (i.e., the lifetime of the patient). This requires proper device selection, implant methods, and technique and reliability of the equipment. When possible, patients should benefit from additional freedom with the use of these devices, as opposed to increased limitations in activities. A case in point is placing a permanent device in a patient who is found to have high power requirements during the trial, yet implanting them with a percutaneous instead of a paddle system. It is predictable that such a patient will have to lie in the supine position to achieve satisfactory paresthesia after the maturation of the scar increases the impedance to stimulation. This will increase the confinement of the patient. Although more effort may be required to implant paddle leads, they are more efficient than percutaneous leads. They allow a patient to use his or her stimulator with longer intercharge intervals; or, if a conventional battery has been used, to benefit from greater battery life. A commonly treated target that requires higher power output is the low back area. This target is commonly treated as part of a lower extremity pain problem but may need to be considered independently because of its resistance to satisfactory stimulation when using percutaneous leads.

Migration and positional stimulation is problematic in the cervical spine; thus it is advantageous to use retrograde paddle leads under C1-C2 in these cases (**Fig. 7-2**).[12] The use of paddle leads below the disc space of C2 should be avoided if possible because of concern for both acute and subacute acquired spinal stenosis and resultant paresis or plegia. Preoperative evaluation with magnetic resonance imaging or myelography is essential to the proper evaluation of the cervical canal both before placing a paddle lead and before placing a percutaneous lead (**Fig. 7-3**). In certain cases percutaneous implantation in the cervical spine may be beneficial for another reason. The patient may prefer stimulation carefully limited to his or her pain area but physiologically may also need a centrally placed lead to help with his or her underlying pathophysiology (**Figs. 7-4** and **7-5**).

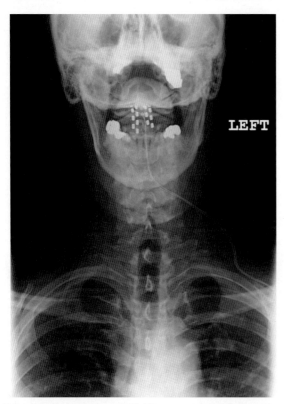

Fig. 7-2 Bilateral implant of C1-C2 retrograde leads for treatment of upper-extremity pain. Lead stability is good without significant risk of neurologic deficit.

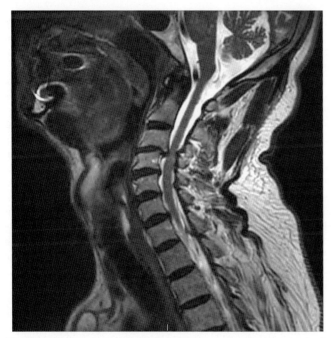

Fig. 7-3 Magnetic resonance imaging demonstrating focal spinal stenosis at C3-C4 with obliteration of the subarachnoid space. Placing a lead through the area of stenosis is likely to produce neurological deficit.

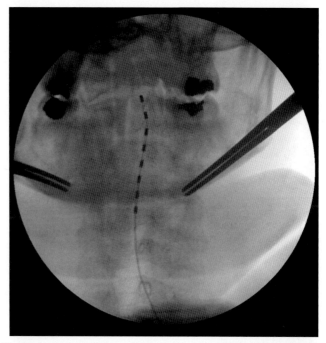

Fig. 7-4 An initially placed paramedian lead produces paresthesia overlap that is global. The patient wants more focused stimulation.

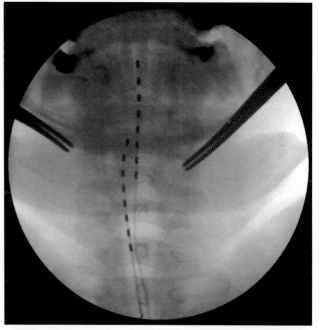

Fig. 7-5 A second lead is added over the nerve roots to provide a focused, specific current deployed over the nerve roots. The paramedian lead is left in place for stimulation below paresthetic perception to aid in reducing the sympathetic throughput.

Strategies to improve coverage of the back include multilead methods such as tripolar lead configurations (**Fig. 7-6**). This helps the implanter produce low back coverage by truncating the field between the dorsal rootlets and hyperpolarizing the nerve roots, thus reducing radicular stimulation. Although these arrays may be created with percutaneous leads, maintaining proper alignment of three independent percutaneous catheters can be quite challenging (**Fig. 7-7**). In contrast, creating the same array with a tripolar paddle lead is straightforward, with the caveat that the lead must be placed so it properly straddles the midline. Recently a five-column lead has become available that offers the user the ability to selectively stimulate dermatomes in the low back and lower extremities through the use of small textured contacts that allow

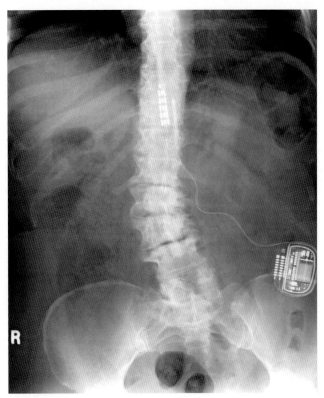

Fig. 7-6 Tripolar paddle lead with 16 contacts implanted to treat back and leg pain.

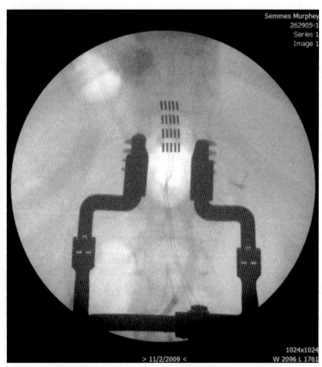

Fig. 7-8 Five-column lead. There are 16 active electrodes in the closely spaced array. This creates narrowly truncated fields that penetrate well and are very specific, allowing discreet evoked paresthesias. (Penta, St. Jude Medical, Plano, TX.)

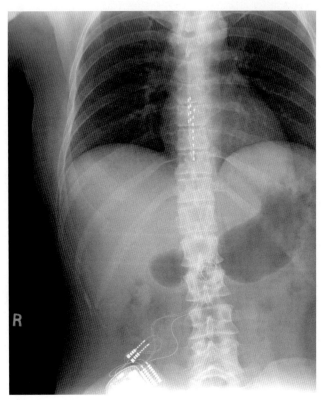

Fig. 7-7 Tripolar array implanted with percutaneous leads. There has been interval relative motion between the columns, potentially making the array less useful.

both aggressive field truncation and anodal hyperpolarization (**Fig. 7-8**).[2] In spite of the sophistication of these paddle leads, without question the percutaneous array has the edge in treating distant multifocal pain topographies (**Fig. 7-9**).

The history of generators available for SCS is relevant to the topic of parameters because not all generators have historically been capable of the same parametric variance. Frequencies in particular have varied substantially from device to device. Some generators have been limited to frequencies less than 130 Hz, excluding the possibility of high-frequency stimulation as an option in patients who are not responding favorably to permanent implants (**Table 7-1**). One would assume that frequency limitations are related to the use of conventional batteries and that high frequencies would be available with rechargeable devices, but neither of these assumptions is correct. Furthermore, frequency capability changes with the addition of programs or stim sets (depending on the manufacturer's terminology). An implanter should know the capabilities of the devices that they implant so they may provide the most appropriate care for their patients.

Beyond the issue of specific generator capabilities is the question of patient compliance. Some patients may not be able to manage a rechargeable system because of diminished mental faculties. Older patients may not need the life expectancy of a rechargeable generator. These newer devices are more costly, but they last longer than conventional batteries. In some markets price drives this selection.

Patient Management/Evaluation

It would seem empirically true that prediction of a patient's need for high frequency stimulation would be reliable based on that given patient's trial of SCS. However, this is not the case. During the trial, patients usually do not have their stimulation optimized, and trials are rarely long enough for a patient to truly understand the limitations of conventional frequencies in their pain modulation. Optimization and realization take time. On the basis of the literature, it is reasonable to use a high-frequency system in patients who are being treated for CRPS 1. These patients in particular may need this system capability. Not having

the opportunity to stimulate at high frequency may result in a suboptimal or nonexistent response to stimulation. There are less data regarding CRPS 2 patients. Bennett and associates[8] report the use of frequencies greater than 250 Hz but do not identify the treatment population physiologically. It is not unreasonable to hypothesize that some of these patients might have CRPS 2. While SCS as

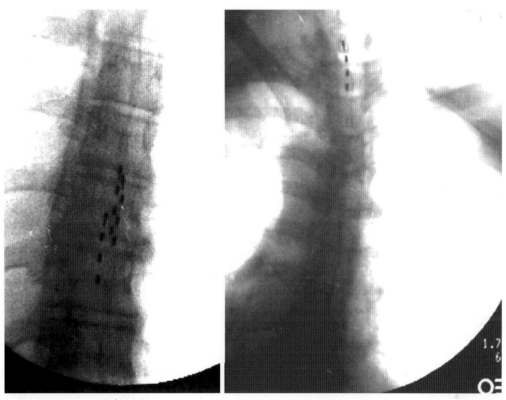

Fig. 7-9 A patient referred with low-back and lower-extremity pain in a postlaminectomy setting was found on history to have angina. Each portion of the array treats a separate target.

Table 7-1: Comparative Generator Data

Small Rechargeable IPGs

	Precision	RestoreULTRA	Eon Mini
Company	Boston Scientific	Medtronic	St. Jude Medical
IPG engine	Constant current	Constant voltage	Constant current
Amplitude	0-12.7 mA	0-10.5 V	0-25.5 mA
Maximum amplitude with single cathode at 524 ohms	12.7 mA	21.8 mA	24.7 mA
Pulse width	20-1000 µs	60-1000 µs	50-500 µs
Frequency	2-1200 Hz	2-1200 Hz	2-1200 Hz
Maximum sustainable frequency	1200 Hz for 1 stim set 130 Hz for 2 stim sets 80 Hz for 4 stim sets	1200 Hz for 1 stim set 600 Hz for 2 stim sets 300 Hz for 4 stim sets	1200 Hz for 1 stim set 600 Hz for 2 stim sets 300 Hz for 4 stim sets 200 Hz for 6 stim sets 150 Hz for 8 stim sets
Programs and stim sets	4 programs 4 stim sets each	8 programs 16 total stim sets	24 programs 8 stim sets each
Recommended maximum implant depth	2 cm	1 cm	2.5 cm
Device life approval	5 yr, open-ended	9 yr, end-of-life	10 yr, open-ended

Continued

Table 7-1: Comparative Generator Data—Cont'd

High-capacity IPGs

	N/A	RestoreADVANCED	Eon
Company	Boston Scientific	Medtronic	St. Jude Medical
Battery capacity	None available	300 mA/hr	325 mA/hr
IPG engine		Constant voltage	Constant current
Amplitude		0-10.5 V	0-25.5 mA
Maximum amplitude with single cathode at 524 ohms		21.8 mA	24.7 mA
Pulse width		60-450 µs	50-500 µs
Frequency		2-130 Hz	2-1200 Hz
Maximum sustainable frequency		130 Hz for 1 stim set 130 Hz for 2 stim sets 65 Hz for 4 stim sets	1200 Hz for 1 stim set 600 Hz for 2 stim sets 300 Hz for 4 stim sets 200 Hz for 6 stim sets 150 Hz for 8 stim sets
Recommended implant depth		Up to 1 cm	Up to 2.5 cm
Battery life approval		9 year, end-of-life	10 years, open-ended

Primary Cell IPGs

	N/A	PrimeADVANCED	EonC
Company	Boston Scientific	Medtronic	St. Jude Medical
Volume	None available	39 cc	49 cc
Battery capacity		6.9 Ahr	8.9 Ahr
IPG engine		Constant voltage	Constant current
Amplitude		0-10.5 V	0-25.5 mA
Pulse width		60-450 µs	50-500 µs
Frequency		2-130 Hz	2-1200 Hz
Maximum sustainable frequency		130 Hz for 1 stim set 130 Hz for 2 stim sets 65 Hz for 4 stim sets	1200 Hz for 1 stim set 600 Hz for 2 stim sets 300 Hz for 4 stim sets 200 Hz for 6 stim sets 150 Hz for 8 stim sets
Programs and stim sets		8 programs 16 total stim sets	24 programs 8 stim sets each
Recommended implant depth		Up to 4 cm	Up to 4 cm
Longevity at average settings		4 years	7 years
Approval settings		Medium settings	High settings

IPG, implantable pulse generator.

a modality to help patients with mechanical back pain is not well supported,[13] consideration must be given to a trial of high-frequency stimulation in these patients to potentially block C-fiber transmission rather than the more conventional mechanistic concept of large-fiber activation to reduce throughput at the level of the gate.

Summary

As suggested previously, before selection of an SCS system, proper understanding of a patient's physiology and topography of pain is essential. Furthermore, it is relevant to know the patient's anatomic idiosyncrasies, if present. The latter helps to avoid complication. Consideration should be given to using generators with rechargeable power sources and both conventional and high-frequency capabilities to improve the opportunity for a patient's satisfactory long-term benefit. Although in some environments cost may drive selection, rechargeable longevity should more than make up for the difference in initial costs.

Electrode selection and placement are more complicated, in part because of the superficial similarities and subtle, but important differences in platforms among companies. Implanter experience is undeniably important in the process, especially when there is enough experience that the implanter's eye for evaluating each patient is based on his or her refined personal outcomes. Nonetheless, careful lead placement that allows for specific paresthesia overlap on the patient's pain, in which the paresthesia perception begins within the area of pain, is most likely to provide satisfactory long-term stimulation.

As research and development and our knowledge regarding stimulation continue to evolve, paradigms in stimulation change. There has been much evolution, especially in the past 15 years. It will be interesting to see whether the future evolution of stimulation will simplify or complicate matters further.

References

1. Barolat G: Epidural spinal cord stimulation: anatomical and electrical properties of the intraspinal structures relevant to spinal cord stimulation and clinical correlations. *Neuromodulation* 1:63-71, 1998.
2. Feler C, Garber J: Selective dermatome activation using a novel five-column spinal cord stimulation paddle lead: a case series, *NANS* poster presentation, 2009.
3. Struijk JJ, Holsheimer J, Boom HBK: Excitation of dorsal root fibers in spinal cord stimulation: a theoretical study. *IEEE Trans Biomed Eng* 40:632-639, 1993.
4. Struijk JJ et al: Theoretical performance and clinical evaluation of transverse tripolar spinal cord stimulation. *IEEE Trans Rehab Eng* 6:277-285, 1998.
5. Smith S: Stimulation coverage of transverse tripole programming using the Lamitrode Tripole 16c surgical lead: preliminary evaluation from one clinic in a prospective, multi-centered, post-market study, *NANS 2007*.
6. Feler C et al: Recent advances: sacral nerve root stimulation using a retrograde method of lead insertion for the treatment of pelvic pain due to interstitial cystitis. *Neuromodulation* 2:211-216, 1999.
7. Feler C, Whitworth LA, Fernandez J: Sacral neuromodulation for chronic pain conditions. *Anesth Clin North Am* 21:785-791, 2003.
8. Bennett DS et al: Spinal cord stimulation for complex regional pain syndrome I (RSD): a retrospective multicenter experience from 1995 to 1998 of 101 patients. *Neuromodulation* 2:202-210, 1999.
9. Holsheimer J, Struijk JJ, Tas NR: Effects of electrode geometry and combination on nerve fibre selectivity in spinal cord stimulation. *Med Biol Eng Comput* 33(5):676-682, 1995.
10. Wesselink W, Holsheimer J, Boom H: Analysis of current density related parameters in spinal cord stimulation. *IEEE Trans Rehab Eng* 6(2):200-220, 1998.
11. Gordon A et al: Challenges to setting spinal cord stimulator parameters during intraoperative testing: factors affecting coverage of low back and leg pain. *Neuromodulation* 7(10):133-141, 2007.
12. Whitworth LA, Feler CA: C1-C2 Sublaminar insertion of paddle leads for the management of chronic painful conditions of the upper extremity. *Neuromodulation* 6(3):153-157, 2003.
13. Barolat G et al: Epidural spinal cord stimulation with a multiple electrode paddle lead is effective in treating intractable low back pain. *Neuromodulation* 4(2):59-66, 2001.

8 Spinal Cord Stimulation as a Treatment of Failed Back Surgery Syndrome

Richard B. North

CHAPTER OVERVIEW

Chapter Synopsis: Failed back surgery syndrome (FBSS) is the term used for chronic neuropathic pain that persists or reoccurs after a surgical procedure on the lumbosacral spine. FBSS patients comprise the largest population of recipients for spinal cord stimulation (SCS) in the United States, but patient selection is a key factor in successful SCS treatment, which is generally defined as a significant reduction in pain. This chapter reviews the research data that contribute to our understanding of how SCS works to alleviate pain and discusses the techniques used for SCS treatment. The basic science literature shows that SCS modifies activity of wide dynamic range (WDR) neurons and the release of many different neurotransmitters. Imaging data should be used to assess the patient's presurgical spinal anatomy for patient selection and to ensure proper electrode implantation. Selection of the proper device, placement location, and stimulation pattern are also key factors in optimizing SCS success. The SCS screening trial is the best indicator of a patient's potential to respond favorably to treatment.

Important Points:
- SCS is a minimally invasive, reversible, cost-effective treatment that can reduce the pain associated with FBSS in carefully selected patients.
- A screening trial mimics the therapeutic effect of SCS and thus predicts the results of system implantation.
- Modern SCS systems provide a myriad of programming options. Rechargeable batteries can reduce patient risk associated with battery replacement and improve cost-effectiveness.

Clinical Pearls:
- An examination of recent imaging studies (an MRI or CT myelogram) before a patient undergoes any SCS procedure will provide information about the depth of dorsal cerebrospinal fluid and the position of the spinal cord and allow the surgeon to optimize electrode selection, placement, and adjustment.
- Applying silicone elastomer adhesive during electrode anchoring can prevent longitudinal electrode migration. (This is not necessary or possible with some anchors and techniques, and alternatives are under development.) During system implantation, decrease mechanical stress by avoiding unnecessary bends of small radius and superfluous connectors and by not crossing a mobile joint or body segment with subcutaneous lead wire or extension cable.

Clinical Pitfalls:
- SCS success requires the right patient, the right equipment, and the right technique. Failure in any of these will increase the possibility of treatment failure.

Introduction

Failed back surgery syndrome (FBSS) is the name given to the chronic pain syndrome that occurs when a surgical procedure involving the lumbosacral spine culminates in persistent or recurrent pain.

By 1985, investigators recognized that FBSS is an important public health problem affecting 25,000 to 50,000 new patients each year.[1] Many causes have been implicated for the development of FBSS, including inappropriate patient selection criteria for lumbosacral surgical procedures, shortfalls in the surgeon's diagnostic or technical skills (operation not indicated, wrong site, incomplete decompression, and/or fusion),[2] and inadequacies in available surgical techniques.

In the United States, FBSS is the primary indication for spinal cord stimulation (SCS), even though SCS is not the primary therapy for FBSS. SCS is a modern application of the ancient use of electricity to treat pain (in ancient times healers used current generated by electrical fish).

Electrical stimulation with implanted devices followed the 1965 publication of Melzack and Wall's gate control theory of pain[3] and the development of cardiac pacemaker technology. Today SCS is delivered with sophisticated techniques that take advantage of multichannel pulse generators powered by rechargeable batteries.

By reducing the level of pain associated with FBSS, SCS can allow patients to decrease or eliminate use of pain medication, improve their physical functioning and ability to engage in the activities of daily life, enhance their quality of life, and return to work. The success of SCS, however, depends in large part on the physician's ability to (1) select appropriate candidates, (2) use the right equipment to treat a specific pain condition, and (3) implant and adjust the equipment in an optimum manner.

Establishing Diagnosis

Diagnosing FBSS seems fairly straightforward in patients suffering from persistent or recurrent pain following a surgical procedure on the lumbosacral spine. However, because FBSS has many possible etiologies, identification of the syndrome is merely the first step in meeting its treatment challenges.

The assessment of an FBSS patient should be multifaceted and should follow the same procedure used for any chronic pain syndrome. Review of the patient's history and operative record (which should be sought routinely) helps to establish the underlying diagnosis. The presence of any issues of secondary gain, psychological or behavioral problems, or co-morbid pain conditions is of interest. A thorough pertinent physical examination helps to corroborate the diagnosis. A validated numeric rating or visual analog scale (VAS) can help to determine the intensity of the pain and follow the patient's progress.[4] Imaging studies provide valuable information that will guide treatment. Abnormalities revealed by imaging studies and the physical examination should be consistent with the patient's pain. The patient might demonstrate nonorganic responses (Waddell signs) during the physical examination,[5] but organic findings should predominate.

Specific prognostic factors have been identified for patients with FBSS concerning the likelihood that they might benefit from SCS. For example, the extent to which the patient's pain is radicular is important (relieving axial low back pain with SCS is technically more difficult than relieving radicular pain).[6,7] Technological advances, however, continue to permit clinicians to improve outcomes and extend the circumstances in which SCS is indicated for FBBS.

Anatomy

FBSS often occurs because a surgeon has assumed that a patient's pain was caused by an anatomical abnormality that could be corrected with a surgical procedure. The same or similar anatomical abnormalities, however, might occur in asymptomatic individuals.[8] Indeed, in consecutive patients with FBSS, Long and associates[2] reported that most did not meet standard indications for their first surgical procedure. Treatment of FBSS with a repeat surgical procedure remains indicated, however, if a patient has a large disc fragment or severe stenosis compressing a nerve or nerves and causing a significant neurologic deficit or if there is gross spinal instability.

Computer modeling of the electrical fields produced by SCS in the spinal cord[9,10] revealed current and voltage distributions consistent with those found in studies of cadavers and primate spinal cords. The modeling studies have predicted that bipolar stimulation with closely spaced electrical contacts separated by 6 to 8 mm or less would be the best way to target longitudinal midline fibers and that the electrical field between two cathodes bracketing the physiological midline does not sum constructively in the midline.[11] Modeling has also predicted advantages for three or more columns of contacts with lateral anodes.[12] Clinical experience has confirmed that correct positioning and spacing of SCS electrodes is essential for pain relief.[13] The longitudinal position of an electrode largely determines the segmental effects of stimulation; and rather than being beneficial, positioning electrodes more cephalad than the target area commonly elicits unwanted local segmental effects.[14]

Electrical impulses are more easily conducted through cerebrospinal fluid (CSF) than through any other tissue in the spinal canal. Because the depth of cerebrospinal fluid differs at various locations in the spine, thresholds and recruitment patterns vary; because CSF depth changes as an individual shifts between supine and prone positions, patients usually report that the perceived intensity of stimulation-induced sensation (paresthesia) changes when they change their posture.

Basic Science

Neuropathic pain, which often produces a radiating, burning sensation, results from nerve or nervous system damage. Activation of peripheral nerve fibers in pathological conditions can more easily activate wide dynamic range (WDR) neurons in the superficial laminae of the corresponding dorsal horn, resulting in hyperalgesia (extreme sensitivity to pain) and/or allodynia (pain from normally nonpainful stimuli).

In experimental studies SCS suppressed long-term potentiation of WDR neurons by reducing the C-fiber response[15] and also changed the concentration of several neurotransmitters and their metabolites in CSF, including serotonin and substance P,[16] glycine, adenosine, and noradrenaline.[17,18] Supraspinal microdialysis in conscious rats revealed that SCS causes γ-aminobutyric acid (GABA) release in periaqueductal grey matter.[19] SCS also induces GABA release in the dorsal horn[20] (activation of the GABA-B receptor might be responsible for the therapeutic effect of SCS) and decreases the release of glutamate and aspartate.[21] It is likely that SCS has additional, complicated effects on as-yet-unidentified neural transmitters and modulators. SCS is not thought to affect opioid receptor-mediated analgesia because naloxone does not inhibit SCS efficacy.[22]

In patients undergoing successful SCS treatment to reduce otherwise intractable neuropathic leg pain, positron emission tomography (PET) studies suggest that SCS also modulates supraspinal neurons.[23] In these patients SCS increased cerebral blood flow significantly in the thalamus contralateral to the painful leg and in the associated bilateral parietal area, and this was associated with changes in pain threshold. SCS also activated the anterior cingulate cortex and prefrontal areas, which control the emotional response to pain.

Imaging

Imaging studies undertaken to establish the diagnosis of FBSS provide information about the patient's postsurgical anatomy and whether or not the anatomic goals of the surgical procedure were met. This might explain the failure of the surgical procedure to relieve pain; however, established nerve injury can lead to persistent pain, even after technically successful surgery (**Table 8-1**). Radiographic imaging studies should reveal abnormalities concordant with the patient's current pain complaints (see **Table 8-1**).

Imaging is also used to guide SCS treatment (see **Table 8-1**). For example, imaging the thoracic spine provides valuable information about the placement of thoracic electrodes. Imaging should take place before the procedure to rule out any pathological condition that might contribute to the patient's pain or confound (or increase the risk of) electrode placement (e.g., stenosis). Fluoroscopic imaging during the procedure helps guide placement of the electrode and documents the final electrode position. Imaging is also used to diagnose the cause of a complication such as suspected electrode migration or fracture.

Guidelines

Many guidelines are published for medical therapies, invoking principles of evidence-based medicine (EBM). Ironically, to date little evidence exists that EBM or guidelines have improved patient care. We have published a set of practice parameters as a reference

Table 8-1: Uses of Imaging Technology in Spinal Cord Stimulation Treatment

Type	Timing	Purpose
MRI or CT myelogram of lumbar spine	Before SCS screening trial	Establish diagnosis of FBSS. Reveal postsurgical anatomy. Were goals of surgery met? Are abnormalities consistent with current pain complaint?
MRI or CT myelogram of thoracic spine	Before SCS screening trial	Rule out pathology contributing to symptoms. Rule out pathology that would compromise electrode placement. Aid in planning electrode placement.
Fluoroscopy	During SCS procedure	Guide electrode placement.
Fluoroscopy or x-ray	After SCS procedure	Document electrode placement.
X-ray	Diagnosis of cause of complication	Electrode migration or fracture is possible.

CT, Computed tomography; *FBSS,* failed back surgery syndrome; *MRI,* magnetic resonance imaging; *SCS,* spinal cord stimulation.

for referring physicians, clinicians offering SCS treatment, and patients.[24]

Indications/Contraindications

To be eligible for SCS, FBSS patients must have pain that is refractory to more conservative care. The definition of "more conservative" is not precise; for example, it is a matter of opinion whether opioid therapy is more or less "conservative" than SCS, and some patients are referred for SCS to avoid opioids. Neuropathic pain is generally more responsive to SCS than is nociceptive pain; distinguishing these is not always straightforward (e.g., FBSS), and a therapeutic trial of SCS might be the most practical approach to determining eligibility. Likewise, radicular pain is generally more responsive than axial low back pain; again, individual cases might be most practically approached by simply offering an SCS trial.

Relative contraindications to SCS include unresolved issues of secondary gain (e.g., an outstanding lawsuit or compensation claim), a major untreated psychiatric co-morbidity, and/or inappropriate medication use. The presence of a demand cardiac pacemaker requires electrocardiogram (ECG) monitoring and/or changing the pacemaker mode to a fixed rate.[25]

Absolute contraindications include uncorrected coagulopathy, untreated sepsis, a patient's inability to cooperate or to control the device, and/or a projected need for the patient to undergo magnetic resonance imaging (MRI).

SCS is problematic if the patient has a separate, co-morbid chronic pain syndrome. As noted previously, before receiving SCS treatment some FBSS patients require a repeat surgical procedure to correct a serious anatomical defect.

Equipment

Equipment needed for the SCS screening trial (see following paragraphs) includes an electrode that will be connected to an external pulse generator and external programming equipment. A complete

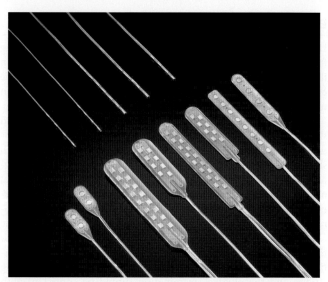

Fig. 8-1   Spinal cord stimulation electrodes are arrays with multiple contacts. Some require laminectomy; others are inserted percutaneously through a modified Tuohy needle.

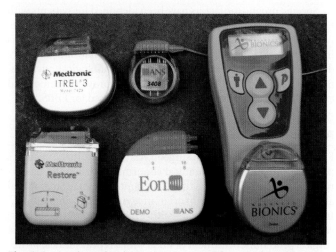

Fig. 8-2   Implanted pulse generators used for spinal cord stimulation support multiple contacts, which may be programmed noninvasively as anodes and cathodes. Some are powered by implanted batteries (visible here); older versions accept or require power from an external device.

SCS system for chronic use requires at least one electrode (**Fig. 8-1**) with an extension cable and an implantable pulse generator (IPG) (**Fig. 8-2**).

Two types of SCS electrodes are available: percutaneous catheter electrodes and plate/paddle electrodes (also known as laminectomy, surgical, or insulated electrodes). Percutaneous electrodes can be inserted with a minimally invasive procedure using a Tuohy needle. When performed under fluoroscopy, percutaneous placement facilitates longitudinal mapping of multiple levels for optimal positioning of the electrode.

Placement of plate/paddle electrodes requires surgical exposure of the epidural space. Plate/paddle electrodes have dorsal insulation to protect against excess posterior stimulation, and they offer better performance than do percutaneous electrodes in FBSS patients.[26,27] They are available in one-, two-, three-, and five-column configurations. Compared with percutaneous electrodes, plate/paddle electrodes require only half the battery power.[28] They require open (albeit minimal) exposure; this limits longitudinal mapping. They are more difficult to revise, remove, or replace, once encapsulated in scar tissue; however, this makes them inherently more resistant to migration.

Each type of electrode has multiple electrical contacts that can be configured in a multitude of ways (various combinations of anode/cathode/off/on). The SCS programming options are so numerous that it is impossible to test every combination (e.g., a four-contact electrode has 50 functional bipolar combinations of anodes and cathodes, an eight-contact electrode has 6050). Computerized methods are useful in finding and recording options for an individual patient.[29] Typical stimulation parameters are set at 60 Hz frequency (pulse repetition rate) with 0.2- to 1-msec pulse width. Amplitude should be adjusted to the minimum level, on a scale from perceptual to discomfort (or motor) threshold that elicits adequate coverage of the area(s) of pain by paresthesia.

The longitudinal position of the electrode determines which segment of the body will experience paresthesia, and bipolar (or tripolar) stimulation has the greatest selectivity for longitudinal midline fibers.[13] FBSS patients with associated axial low back pain require low thoracic electrode placement and sometimes need complex electrode arrays.

As shown in **Fig. 8-2**, the stimulator energy sources in use are: (1) radiofrequency-coupled passive implants that have a long life but require an external antenna, which can cause skin irritation and fluctuations in stimulation amplitude; (2) primary cell IPGs that require replacement at the end of battery life; and (3) IPGs with rechargeable batteries. Patients can turn IPGs on and off and use either an external magnet to make limited adjustments in amplitude or a remote transmitter capable of complicated adjustments.

Technique

This following discussion of the placement of an SCS system should not be confused with installation instructions. This information is meant to give the reader an idea of what is involved in the procedure rather than to bestow permission to undertake SCS implantation. Any specialist who wishes to offer SCS must have appropriate training, which must be supervised by an experienced implanter. The SCS procedure is straightforward, but positive results require facility and complete understanding of sophisticated details. Therefore, the following should be considered a general description.

The technical goal of SCS for FBSS is to cover the area of pain with a tingling sensation known as *paresthesia* (**Table 8-2**). Pain/paresthesia overlap is necessary (but not sufficient) to achieve pain relief. The paresthesia must be comfortable, and the stimulation must not cause a motor reaction. If pain/paresthesia overlap only occurs with uncomfortable stimulation (i.e., outside of the [often narrow] "usage range" between perception of paresthesia and discomfort or motor effects), treatment is compromised. In addition, the perception of extraneous stimulation paresthesia outside the area(s) of pain should be minimized.

Paresthesia can be directed to one location or another by changing stimulation parameters (pulse amplitude, width, and repetition rate) and specific contact combinations (anode/cathode/off).

Screening Trial

SCS candidates typically undergo a 3- to 10-day screening trial after insertion of a temporary percutaneous catheter electrode (or in special circumstances, implantation of a plate/paddle electrode) connected to an external pulse generator. This screening trial provides information about the potential technical and clinical success of SCS.

Table 8-2: Positive Outcomes of Spinal Cord Stimulation Treatment

Desired outcome	Goal	Requirements
Technical	Overlap pain with comfortable paresthesia Minimize extraneous paresthesia No motor effects	Well-trained implanter Correct longitudinal, left-right, and dorsal-ventral position of electrode Correct stimulation parameters (pulse amplitude, width, and repetition rate) Correct contact combination (anode/cathode/off) Appropriate use of plate/paddle electrode
Clinical	≈50% relief of baseline pain	Well-trained implanter Proper patient selection Use of appropriate equipment Equipment implanted and adjusted optimally
Potential benefits	Decrease or eliminate pain medication Improve physical functioning and ability to engage in activities of daily life Enhance quality of life Return to work Improve emotional state	Factors beyond successful spinal cord stimulation therapy

Because the patient must be able to describe pain/paresthesia overlap, placement of a percutaneous catheter electrode is best done under local anesthesia. The electrode is inserted under fluoroscopy with a Tuohy needle that is advanced cephalad at a shallow angle from 1 to 2 segments (depending on the patient's girth) below the target interlaminar space. (If additional interlaminar space is needed, the degree of spinal flexion can be increased.) Loss of resistance to a Seldinger guidewire confirms entry into the epidural space (use of injected air or saline might interfere with steering and with test stimulation).

While advancing the electrode incrementally along the radiographic midline, use of bipolar stimulation with adjacent contacts reveals the physiological midline at each level. The electrode can be repositioned as needed to achieve symmetry and paresthesia/pain overlap.

Mapping the epidural space longitudinally during the screening trial reveals the optimal placement for the permanent implant (assuming that the patient passes the screening trial) and helps the clinician determine the best type of electrode and generator for the patient. When the electrode is optimally positioned, the Tuohy needle is withdrawn, and the lead is sutured to skin.

If the patient had prior surgery that precludes percutaneous access, the screening trial is conducted with a surgical plate/paddle electrode that remains in place for chronic use if the patient passes the screening trial. A percutaneous temporary extension cable connects the electrode to an external generator.

A patient who is satisfied with SCS treatment and achieves at least 50% pain relief despite everyday provocative activity, with the use of stable or reduced analgesics, can proceed to full system implantation.

In our practice we remove percutaneous electrodes used during the screening trial. It is possible to implant a temporary percutaneous electrode so it can be adapted to permanent use, but (as is the case for paddle electrodes implanted via minilaminectomy) doing this for a trial has disadvantages: the need for an incision, anchoring, or sutures; requires operating room resources; and, even if the trial is unsuccessful, a second procedure in an operating room is required just to remove the electrode. Incisional pain might confound interpretation of the effects of the SCS trial on pain. Use of a temporary extension cable can only increase the risk of infection.

Percutaneous Catheter Electrode Implantation

To implant a percutaneous electrode for chronic use, insert the electrode as described previously. Make an incision longitudinally around the Tuohy needle to the dorsal fascia and put two self-retaining retractors in position. Then make two sutures with No. 0 nonabsorbable material (e.g., Tevdek) through the supraspinous ligament caudal to the needle.

After removing the needle, pass the anchoring sleeve/strain relief through the dorsal fascia and tie it with one suture before injecting a small amount (<0.1 mL) of silicone elastomer adhesive between the inner surface of the sleeve and the outer surface of the lead. This virtually eliminates electrode migration.[30] Add ligatures around the anchor as appropriate and secure the sleeve flat against the dorsal fascia with the most caudal anchoring suture. Finally, confirm the position of the electrode under fluoroscopy.

Surgical Plate/Paddle Electrode Implantation

Implantation of a surgical plate/paddle electrode and subcutaneous tunneling requires intravenous sedation with intermittent boluses or a propofol drip. Under fluoroscopy center a 1- to 2-inch incision on the target area, just below the intended position of the most caudal electrode contact. Infiltrate the paravertebral muscles with local anesthetic and dissect them subperiosteally before performing a minilaminectomy of sufficient size to allow insertion of the electrode at a shallow angle. Insert the electrode cephalad beneath intact lamina. Conduct test stimulation to confirm symmetry and pain/paresthesia overlap. Finally, anchor the lead wire to supraspinous ligament, incorporating sleeve/strain relief and adhesive as described previously.

Pulse Generator Implantation

Common pulse generator implantation sites are the lateral abdomen and lower chest wall, the infraclavicular area (for cervical electrodes), and the upper buttocks below the belt line. (Compared with abdominal placement, implantation in the upper buttocks increases stress on the system with normal patient flexion or extension.)

The incision and pocket should be made in a location that makes it possible to close the wound adjacent to (not directly over) the implant. The skin thickness over the pocket should be sufficient to maintain integrity and patient comfort without compromising power transfer or telemetry; 1 cm is typically appropriate.

The proximal lead and/or extension from the electrode(s) is connected to the generator via a subcutaneous tunnel. It is best to avoid use of connectors (which introduce stress and can cause discomfort). Placing loops of excess wire in the pocket beneath the generator relieves strain. All incisions should be closed in layers.

Patient Management/Evaluation

After a routine postoperative examination and SCS programming adjustment, the patient should return for suture or staple removal and any needed additional adjustments on postoperative day 7 to 14. Routine follow-up visits should taper from monthly to annually, with additional visits scheduled as needed to ensure safe and effective operation of the stimulator.

SCS patients should disable the system before entering an electromagnetic field produced by antitheft devices, a metal detector, or any other security-scanning device. They should also avoid scuba diving more than 10 m deep or entering hyperbaric chambers with an absolute pressure above 2.0 atm. They should not engage in any activity that might place excessive stress on the implanted system.

Special precautions are required for an SCS patient to undergo certain medical tests such as cardiac monitoring, radiation therapy with the IPG in the active field, radiofrequency ablation, and electrocautery. Ultrasound over the device and diathermy anywhere are contraindicated, as is MRI, although the latter is under study.

If SCS pain relief disappears, it is important to determine first if the system is operating correctly. Sometimes fibrosis around implanted electrodes increases impedance and interferes with treatment; this generally can be overcome through reprogramming. A minority of SCS patients experience clinical failure, which is the unexplained loss of pain relief despite a functioning system that continues to provide appropriate pain/paresthesia overlap. When this occurs, SCS can sometimes be potentiated with adjuvant medication.[31]

Successful treatment of infection usually requires removal of the entire SCS system. A new system can be placed after the infection clears. Therefore, not only is infection costly, but the patient loses the SCS pain control during the treatment period. Clinicians and patients should take appropriate measures to avoid infection.

Outcomes Evidence

Patient-rated pain relief is the usual primary outcome criterion for SCS and for pain treatments in general, with success commonly defined as a minimum 50% relief (see **Table 8-2**). Secondary outcome measures include ability to conduct activities of daily living, work status, medication requirements, neurological function, and patient satisfaction with the procedure. To reduce bias in SCS studies, collection of follow-up data by a disinterested third party is desirable. Since SCS elicits paresthesia, blinding is not feasible; thus any randomized controlled trial (RCT) of SCS loses points on rating scales commonly used in EBM.

Two decades ago we compared retrospective data in FBSS patients who underwent reoperation[32] with those who received SCS and found that SCS patients enjoyed reduced morbidity and pain and improved neurological function, quality of life, and ability to engage in activities of daily living.[6,33]

In the first RCT of SCS vs. reoperation in FBSS patients,[34] 45 subjects (90% of those who received insurance authorization for study participation) were available for a mean follow-up of 3 years. SCS success was 9 of 19, whereas reoperation success was 3 of 26. Only 5 of the 24 subjects randomized to SCS crossed to reoperation, whereas 14 of the 26 randomized to reoperation crossed to SCS. No patient who crossed from SCS to reoperation achieved success with reoperation, but 6 of the 14 who crossed from reoperation to SCS achieved success with SCS. Success was defined as at least 50% pain relief and patient satisfaction with treatment.

An international multicenter RCT (the PROCESS study)[35] randomized 100 subjects with FBSS to conventional medical management (CMM) or SCS plus CMM. By 6 months the subjects randomized to SCS achieved significantly greater pain relief and improved functional capacity and health-related quality of life than did those randomized to CMM. The investigators followed the 42 subjects randomized to SCS who actually received SCS for 24 months and found significantly improved leg pain relief, functional capacity, and quality of life compared with baseline scores.[36] At the time the randomized group reached 24 months' follow-up, 72 patients had received SCS as a final treatment, through either randomization or cross over. Of these, 34 (47%) achieved the primary outcome (more than or equal to 50% pain relief) vs. 1 of 15 patients who received only CMM.

The initial cost of an SCS system is high. Nevertheless, several cost-effectiveness analyses have demonstrated that SCS treatment lowers the total cost of health care for patients with neuropathic pain compared with alternative treatments. In a cost study based on data from the first 40/42 (of 50) patients enrolled in the RCT of SCS vs. reoperation,[34] every analysis (intention-to-treat, treated-as-intended with cross over counted as failure of randomized treatment, and final treatment) showed that SCS achieved economic dominance by being more effective and less expensive than reoperation.[37]

In 2008 the National Institute for Health and Clinical Excellence (NICE) in the United Kingdom conducted a systematic review and technology assessment of the use of SCS.[38] The model, which compared the cost of treating FBSS with SCS vs. CMM and reoperation and assumed an IPG battery life of 4 years, predicted that SCS would produce additional quality-adjusted life years at a cost the United Kingdom health service would be willing to pay.

Despite the fact that the rechargeable IPG systems cost more initially than the primary cell systems, the rechargeable systems should improve the cost-effectiveness of SCS by reducing the cost and potential morbidity associated with replacing IPGs because of battery depletion.

Technical Aspects of Spinal Cord Stimulation

Beginning in 1986 we developed and used a patient-interactive computer program to allow patients to find the parameter settings that would optimize pain/paresthesia overlap and battery life and as a means of conducting blinded RCTs comparing electrode designs.[39] In one study, we compared results with a four-contact percutaneous electrode vs. a four-contact surgical plate/paddle electrode and found that the plate/paddle electrode provided the best pain/paresthesia coverage, low back coverage, and battery longevity.[28] At mean follow-up of 1.9 years, compared with patients with percutaneous electrodes, twice as many patients with plate/paddle electrodes reported a successful outcome (at least 50% sustained relief of pain and patient satisfaction) and a reduction or elimination of pain medication.[26] A statistically significant advantage for the plate/paddle electrode disappeared, however, at longer follow-up in our small sample of 24 patients.

To determine if use of two percutaneous electrodes bracketing the physiological midline would enhance paresthesia coverage of the low back, we tested parallel percutaneous electrodes bracketing the midline (for chronic use) vs. a single percutaneous electrode placed on the midline for temporary use during the screening trial.[40] The single electrode provided the best pain/paresthesia overlap at the lowest amplitude requirement. Nevertheless, 53% of the patients reported success at 2.3-year mean follow-up with the parallel percutaneous electrodes.

Next we compared results of treating axial low back pain using a four-contact percutaneous electrode with those obtained using a surgical plate/paddle electrode with two parallel rows of eight contacts (16 total).[41] The percutaneous electrode provided marginally better pain/paresthesia overlap with significantly improved symmetry using significantly lower voltage. Compared with the surgical plate/paddle electrode, however, the percutaneous electrode required a slightly higher scaled amplitude to cover the low back and produced significantly increased extraneous coverage.

Our findings indicate that an electrode array comprising dual columns of contacts bracketing the midline presents disadvantages that might be overcome if a third column is placed on the midline. Indeed, a computer model developed at the University of Twente predicts the effect of such electrode configurations on the stimulation of dorsal column and root fibers.[42] Both a longitudinal tripole electrode and a transverse tripole (each with a central cathode) reportedly have advantages in selectively recruiting the presumed stimulation target neurons.[12]

Reducing Risks and Avoiding Complications

The risks and complications associated with SCS can be characterized as biological, procedural, and equipment-related. Sometimes routine system maintenance (e.g., replacing a depleted battery or adjusting stimulation parameters) is mistakenly referred to as a complication.

SCS implantation can lead to spinal cord or nerve injury, dural puncture causing CSF leakage, hematoma, or infection (**Table 8-3**). To avoid spinal cord or nerve injury, it is helpful to obtain an MRI or computed tomography (CT) myelogram of the target area before placing an electrode. To avoid dural puncture, the patient should be conscious during the procedure; and, if possible, electrodes should not be placed in scarred areas. A standard preoperative coagulation profile should be undertaken to help avoid hematoma, and the patient should be monitored overnight. Standard precautions should be taken to avoid infection.

Table 8-3: Reducing the Risk of Spinal Cord Stimulation Complications	
Potential Adverse Outcomes	**Risk Reduction**
Spinal cord or nerve injury	Image (MRI, CT myelogram) target area before electrode placement. Patient is conscious during procedure.
Dural puncture (CSF leak)	Avoid placing electrodes in area with scarring. Patient is conscious during procedure.
Hematoma	Perform preoperative review of coagulation history. Monitor patient overnight.
Infection	Prophylactic antibiotics Standard sterile precautions
Generator failure	Train patient in proper system use. Consider IPGs with rechargeable batteries.
Lead fatigue fracture	Avoid unnecessary extension cables and connectors. Position service loops to relieve strain. Avoid crossing mobile body segments.
Electrode migration	"Glue" lead anchor to lead.
Disturbance from exposure to electromagnetic field	Educate patient to avoid exposure.

CSF, Cerebrospinal fluid; *CT*, computed tomography; *IPG*, implantable pulse generator; *MRI*, magnetic resonance imaging.

Equipment-related complications include generator failure, electrode fatigue fracture, electrode migration, and disturbance from exposure to an electromagnetic field (see **Table 8-3**). Generators can fail, but the incidence of battery failure can be reduced by helping the patient learn to use the system properly and by implanting rechargeable batteries. Lead fatigue failure can be reduced by minimizing the use of connectors, positioning service loops to relieve strain, avoiding crossing mobile body segments, and placing the generator in the patient's flank or lateral abdomen. Fixing the electrode in place properly virtually eliminates migration.[30]

Conclusion

The multiplicity of the factors that affect chronic pain, even in syndromes less complex than FBSS, makes it difficult to construct and conduct rigorous studies to determine appropriate therapies and patient selection criteria. The cross-over randomized trial comparing SCS with reoperation is likely as rigorous as possible and shows clear benefits for SCS in its carefully selected patient population. The available literature on cost-effectiveness provides evidence that, despite its initial cost, SCS pays for itself within a few years.

FBSS patients will likely be best served when clinicians and investigators begin to identify, study, and treat subcategories of FBSS (i.e., to redefine the syndrome). This is likely the necessary first step toward identifying the most appropriate medical, surgical, and neuromodulation therapy for the various subtypes of FBSS. In the meantime, the paucity of available literature despite the large number of people who suffer from FBSS indicates that, until we learn to prevent FBSS, more research on its treatment needs to be conducted and published. In the present state of the art, SCS has proved to be superior to alternative treatments for FBSS in properly selected patients, and SCS technology continues to improve.

References

1. Heithoff KB, Burton CV: CT evaluation of the failed back surgery syndrome. *Orthop Clin North Am* 16:417-444, 1985.
2. Long DM et al: Clinical features of the failed-back syndrome. *J Neurosurg* 69:61-71, 1988.
3. Melzack R, Wall PD: Pain mechanisms: a new theory. *Science* 150:971-978, 1965.
4. Jensen MP, Karoly P, Braver S: The measurement of clinical pain intensity: a comparison of six methods. *Pain* 27:117-126, 1986.
5. Waddell G et al: Nonorganic physical signs in low back pain. *Spine* 5:117-125, 1980.
6. North RB et al: Spinal cord stimulation for chronic, intractable pain: experience over two decades. *Neurosurgery* 32:384-394, 1993.
7. Burchiel KJ et al: Prospective, multicenter study of spinal cord stimulation for relief of chronic back and extremity pain. *Spine* 21:2786-2794, 1996.
8. Tong HC et al: Magnetic resonance imaging of the lumbar spine in asymptomatic older adults. *J Back Musculoskeletal Rehab* 19:67-72, 2006.
9. Coburn B, Sin W: A theoretical study of epidural electrical stimulation of the spinal cord. I. Finite element analysis of stimulus fields. *IEEE Trans Biomed Eng* 32:971-977, 1985.
10. Holsheimer J, Strujik JJ, Rijkhoff NJM: Contact combinations in epidural spinal cord stimulation: a comparison by computer modeling. *Stereotact Funct Neurosurg* 56:220-233, 1991.
11. Holsheimer J, Wesselink WA: Effect of anode-cathode configuration on paresthesia coverage in spinal cord stimulation. *Neurosurgery* 41:654-659, 1997.
12. Struijk JJ et al: Theoretical performance and clinical evaluation of transverse tripolar spinal cord stimulation. *IEEE Trans Rehabil Eng* 6:277-285, 1998.
13. Barolat G et al: Mapping of sensory responses to epidural stimulation of the intraspinal neural structures in man. *J Neurosurg* 78:233-239, 1993.
14. Law J: Spinal stimulation: Statistical superiority of monophasic stimulation of narrowly separated bipoles having rostral cathodes. *Appl Neurophysiol* 46:129-137, 1983.
15. Wallin J et al: Spinal cord stimulation inhibits long-term potentiation of spinal wide dynamic range neurons. *Brain Res* 973:39-43, 2003.
16. Linderoth B et al: Dorsal column stimulation induces release of serotonin and substance P in the cat dorsal horn. *Neurosurgery* 31:289-296, 1992.
17. Meyerson BA, Brodin E, Linderoth B: Possible neurohumoral mechanisms in CNS stimulation for pain suppression. *Appl Neurophysiol* 48:175-180, 1985.
18. Cui JG et al: Adenosine receptor activation suppresses tactile hypersensitivity and potentiates spinal cord stimulation in mononeuropathic rats. *Neurosci Lett* 223:173-176, 1997.
19. Linderoth B et al: An animal model for the study of brain transmitter release in response to spinal cord stimulation in the awake, freely moving rat: Preliminary results from the periaqueductal grey matter. *Acta Neurochir(Wien)* 58(suppl):156-160, 1993.
20. Stiller CO et al: Release of gamma-aminobutyric acid in the dorsal horn and suppression of tactile allodynia by spinal cord stimulation in mononeuropathic rats. *Neurosurgery* 39:367-374, 1996.
21. Cui JG et al: Spinal cord stimulation attenuates augmented dorsal horn release of excitatory amino acids in mononeuropathy via a GABAergic mechanism. *Pain* 73:87-95, 1997.
22. Freeman TB, Campbell JN, Long DM: Naloxone does not affect pain relief induced by electrical stimulation in man. *Pain* 17:189-195, 1983.
23. Kishima H et al: Modulation of neuronal activity after spinal cord stimulation for neuropathic pain; H(2)15O PET study. *Neuroimage* 49:2564-2569, 2010.
24. North RB, Shipley J: Practice parameters for the use of spinal cord stimulation in the treatment of neuropathic pain. *Pain Med* 8(S4):S200-S275, 2007.
25. Ekre O et al: Feasibility of spinal cord stimulation in angina pectoris in patients with chronic pacemaker treatment for cardiac arrhythmias. *Pacing Clin Electrophysiol* 26:2134-2141, 2003.
26. North RB et al: Spinal cord stimulation electrode design: s prospective, randomized, controlled trial comparing percutaneous with laminectomy electrodes. Part II. Clinical outcomes. *Neurosurgery* 57:990-995, 2005.
27. Villavicencio AT et al: Laminectomy versus percutaneous electrode placement for spinal cord stimulation. *Neurosurgery* 46:399-405, 2000.
28. North RB et al: Spinal cord stimulation electrode design: a prospective, randomized, controlled trial comparing percutaneous and laminectomy electrodes. Part I. Technical outcomes. *Neurosurgery* 51:381-389, 2002.
29. North RB et al: Patient-interactive, computer-controlled neurological stimulation system: clinical efficacy in spinal cord stimulator adjustment. *J Neurosurg* 76:967-972, 1992.
30. Renard VM, North RB: Prevention of percutaneous electrode migration in spinal cord stimulation by a modification of the standard implantation technique. *J Neurosurg Spine* 4:300-303, 2006.
31. Lind G et al: Baclofen-enhanced spinal cord stimulation and intrathecal baclofen alone for neuropathic pain: long-term outcome of a pilot study. *Eur J Pain* 12:132-136, 2008.
32. North RB et al: Failed back surgery syndrome: five-year follow-up in 102 patients undergoing repeated operation. *Neurosurgery* 28:685-691, 1991.
33. North RB et al: Failed back surgery syndrome: Five-year follow-up after spinal cord stimulator implantation. *Neurosurgery* 28:692-699, 1991.
34. North RB et al: Spinal cord stimulation versus repeated lumbosacral spine surgery for chronic pain: a randomized, controlled trial. *Neurosurgery* 56:98-106, 2005.
35. Kumar K et al: Spinal cord stimulation versus conventional medical management for neuropathic pain: a multicenter randomized

controlled trial in patients with failed back surgery syndrome. *Pain* 132:179-188, 2007.

36. Kumar K et al: The effects of spinal cord stimulation in neuropathic pain are sustained: a 24-month follow-up of the prospective randomized controlled multicenter trial of the effectiveness of spinal cord stimulation. *Neurosurgery* 63:762-768, 2008.

37. North RB et al: Spinal cord stimulation versus reoperation for failed back surgery syndrome: a cost effectiveness and cost utility analysis based on a randomized, controlled trial. *Neurosurgery* 61:361-369, 2007.

38. National Institute for Health and Clinical Excellence (NICE). Spinal cord stimulation for chronic pain of neuropathic or ischemic origin, London, 2008, NICE Technology Appraisal Guidance, National Institute for Health and Clinical Excellence, accessed from http://www.nice.org.uk/nicemedia/live/12082/42367/42367.pdf July 8, 2010.

39. Fowler K, North R: *Patient-interactive PC interface to implanted, multichannel stimulators, Proceedings of 39th Annual Conference on Engineering in Medicine and Biology*, Baltimore, Md, 1986, Biomedical Engineering Society, p 380.

40. North RB et al: Spinal cord stimulation for axial low back pain: a prospective, controlled trial comparing dual with single percutaneous electrodes. *Spine* 30:1412-1418, 2005.

41. North RB et al: Spinal cord stimulation for axial low back pain: a prospective, controlled trial comparing 16-contact insulated electrode arrays with 4-contact percutaneous electrodes. *Neuromodulation* 9:56-67, 2006.

42. Holsheimer J, Struijk JJ, Tas NR: Effects of electrode geometry and combination on nerve fibre selectivity in spinal cord stimulation. *Med Biol Eng Comput* 33;676-682, 1995.

9 Neurostimulation in Complex Regional Pain Syndrome

I. Elias Veizi, Joshua P. Prager, and Salim M. Hayek

CHAPTER OVERVIEW

Chapter Synopsis: This chapter deals with electrical stimulation of the spinal cord (SCS) in patients with complex regional pain syndrome (CRPS). This broad diagnosis refers to chronic regional pain with variable neuropathic and inflammatory features that usually occurs following injury or surgery and whereby pain is out of proportion with the expected nociceptive response. CRPS usually results in decreased function of the affected limb and occasional disability. Sympathetic nerve activity may make an important contribution to the pain of CRPS, and the condition likely includes an inflammatory response as well as a neuropathic component. Central sensitization results from persistent hyperalgesic signals from the periphery, which can cause pain to worsen and spread beyond the initially affected region. CRPS type II requires underlying nerve damage and was once referred to as *causalgia*, whereas type I CRPS was once called *reflex sympathetic dystrophy* (RSD) and there is no obvious evidence of direct nerve injury. Women are affected far more often by CRPS, usually at postmenopausal age, suggesting a hormonal contribution to the syndrome. Therapies for CRPS include physical therapy as a mainstay and sympathetic nerve blocks, pharmacological intervention, and psychological interventions aimed at facilitating rehabilitation. SCS is generally considered for intractable CRPS. Hypotheses to explain its effects include the usual "gating" of signals from nociceptors, increasing blood flow, and releasing vasoactive substances from antidromic activation of sympathetic nerves. Some studies suggest that early treatment with SCS can reverse CRPS entirely; thus perhaps it should be considered as an initial rather than a final attempt at treatment. However, there are not enough data to make such a recommendation. Although not always effective, SCS appears to be the only treatment that provides long-term (two-year) pain relief in CRPS patients.

Important Points:

- CRPS is a regional pain disorder of uncertain etiology with likely inflammatory and neuropathic components.
- Diagnosis is based purely on clinical criteria, which are being refined.
- Management centers on functional rehabilitation. Psychiatric and pain medicine interventions are often critical to management and facilitation of functional restoration.
- One randomized controlled trial showed that SCS is effective in long-term pain relief (2 years) in refractory CRPS patients.
- Retrospective data and case series suggest potential effectiveness of peripheral nerve stimulation and motor cortex stimulation.
- Before offering neurostimulation to patients with CRPS, less invasive options are usually tried, and patients need to have careful psychological screening and preferably an interdisciplinary committee recommendation for neuromodulation.
- It is critical to stress to patients that neurostimulation is only one component of the management of CRPS and that it may only offer the patient a window of improved pain control to facilitate rehabilitation.
- Although expensive upfront, SCS is cost-effective in the management of refractory pain in CRPS patients.
- Recent technological improvements in SCS devices may result in lower complication rates than those that have been reported in the literature to date.
- Further randomized controlled studies on the role of neurostimulation in CRPS are needed.

Clinical Pearls:

- Diagnosis of the syndrome using the available IASP criteria is the first step in clinical management.
- SCS may be part of a treatment plan that focuses on rehabilitation through desensitization and active functional improvement strategies.
- Careful psychological screening is necessary to avoid failure of therapy due to unrelated issues.
- Chronicity of the syndrome might influence the outcome of the SCS treatment.
- Meticulous surgical technique and careful placement of the SCS leads may improve outcomes and limit revisions.

Clinical Pitfalls:

- Spinal cord stimulation is not effective in all CRPS patients.
- The analgesic effects of spinal cord stimulation on pain intensity appear to decrease with time.
- Placement of a spinal cord stimulator device involves surgery along with the risks and benefits associated with it.
- Lead migration, unwanted stimulation, and discomfort at the generator site may lead to loss of analgesia and multiple revisions may be necessary. Surgical site infection is another complication that curbs effectiveness of the therapy early on.
- Placement of a spinal cord stimulation device may limit the patient from obtaining MRI imaging of the body.
- Though early implantation of SCS may alter symptom progression, no such evidence exists at this stage and risk-to-benefit ratio of SCS placement should be considered individually for every patient.

Introduction

Complex Regional Pain Syndrome History and Nomenclature

Complex regional pain syndrome (CRPS) is the newer nomenclature encompassing the clinical entities of reflex sympathetic dystrophy (RSD) and causalgia.[1] It is characterized by intractable pain usually affecting one or more extremities. Even though it was originally described over a hundred years ago, much debate lingers over the clinical and basic pathophysiological characteristics of this condition. Named as *causalgia* (from Greek, *kausos* [heat], *algos* [pain]), it was initially described in 1864 during the American Civil War by Silas Weir Mitchell from the observation of soldiers developing chronic pain following traumatic nerve injuries.[2] Since its original description, it has been given a number of different names such as algodystrophy, posttraumatic dystrophy, sympathetic-maintained pain syndrome, hand-shoulder syndrome, Sudeck atrophy, and other names. Early in the twentieth century Paul Sudeck[3] described a syndrome with predominantly trophic symptoms that developed following distal bone fractures not affecting directly peripheral nerves. Patients experiencing Sudeck syndrome obtained significant pain relief by sympathetic block, thus suggesting at the time a central role for the autonomic nervous system in the pathophysiology of the condition. An articulation of the belief in a central role of sympathetic system was the term *reflex sympathetic dystrophy (RSD)*, coined by Evans in 1946 to label all syndromes characterized by excessive chronic pain following injury, responsive to sympathetic blocks and as such driven by the sympathetic system.[4] As understanding of the condition evolved, it was clear that sympatholytic interventions and sympathetically maintained pain (SMP) were not specific to RSD but common in other neuropathic pain disorders. In addition, dystrophic changes were not always observed, and there was no evidence that the condition was a reflex. As such, a working group of the International Association for the Study of Pain (IASP) developed a consensus definition in 1994 and proposed a new terminology reflecting a more accurate description of the condition. The term *CRPS type I* replaces RSD; the term *CRPS type II*, which requires demonstrable peripheral nerve injury, replaces the term *causalgia*.[1] Various diagnostic tests have been proposed (without much success) to confirm the diagnosis of CRPS, including among others radiological studies, triple-phase bone scans, quantitative sensory testing, quantitative sudomotor axon reflex test (QSART), and limb thermography with or without sympathetic block. However, diagnosis of CRPS remains a clinical process relying mostly on history and potentially on physical examination. The current IASP diagnostic criteria define CRPS type I as a syndrome that usually develops following a trauma, fracture, surgery, or immobilization, with pain that is disproportionate to the inciting event in a regional/nondermatome pattern (not limited to the distribution of a single peripheral nerve or nerve root). CRPS II requires the same set of descriptive criteria; however, an identifiable nerve injury is required for diagnosis. Although these diagnostic criteria had a high sensitivity (98%), their specificity was poor (36%), resulting in a correct diagnosis in as few as 40% of patients.[5] The lack of an objective test that serves as a gold standard for diagnosis has led to extensive efforts to validate a set of bedside diagnostic criteria to improve the accuracy of CRPS diagnosis. The new proposed diagnostic criteria (**Box 9-1**) do not imply at all the pathogenesis of the disease; however, they supply a set of descriptive signs and symptoms that are adequately sensitive and specific in diagnosing CRPS[6] (**Table 9-1**). The same set of criteria would be applied with varied stringency, depending on the intent, and thus defined as research criteria or clinical diagnostic criteria. These newer criteria

---

Box 9-1: Revised International Association for the Study of Pain Diagnostic Criteria

A. Must have *continuing pain out of proportion* to the inciting event
B. Symptoms
   i. Sensory: Reports hyperesthesia or allodynia
   ii. Vasomotor: Reports skin temperature asymmetry or skin color changes
   iii. Sudomotor/edema: Edema and/or sweating changes
   iv. Motor/trophic: Decreased range of motion and/or motor dysfunction (weakness, tremor, dystonia) and/or trophic changes (hair, nails, skin)
C. Signs
   i. Sensory: Evidence of hyperalgesia or allodynia
   ii. Vasomotor: T° or skin color asymmetry
   iii. Sudomotor/edema: Evidence of edema and/or sweating changes and/or sweating asymmetry
   iv. Motor/trophic: Evidence of decreased range of motion and/or motor dysfunction (weakness, tremor, dystonia) and/or trophic changes (hair, nails, skin)
D. *No other diagnosis* to explain the signs and symptoms

Diagnosis of CRPS (Clinical) Requires:	Diagnosis of CRPS (Research) Requires:
Criteria A: **Fulfilled**	Criteria A: **Fulfilled**
Criteria B: At least **3 Symptoms out of 4** fulfilled	Criteria B: **4 Symptoms out of 4** fulfilled
Criteria C: At least **2 Signs out of 4** fulfilled	Criteria C: At least **2 Signs out of 4** fulfilled
Criteria D: **Fulfilled**	Criteria D: **Fulfilled**

From Harden et al: Proposed new diagnostic criteria for complex regional pain syndrome, *Pain Med* 8:326-331, 2007.
Clinical diagnostic criteria have a specificity of 69% and sensitivity of 85%. Research diagnostic criteria have a specificity of 94% and sensitivity of 70%.

Table 9-1: Criteria and Decision Rules Considered for Complex Regional Pain Syndrome Diagnosis

Criteria/Decision Rules for Proposed Criteria	Sensitivity	Specificity
2+ sign categories and 2+ symptom categories	0.94	0.36
2+ sign categories and 3+ symptom categories	0.85	0.69
2+ sign categories and 4 symptom categories	0.70	0.94
3+ sign categories and 2+ symptom categories	0.76	0.81
3+ sign categories and 3+ symptom categories	0.70	0.83
3+ sign categories and 4 symptom categories	0.86	0.75

From Harden et al: Proposed new diagnostic criteria for complex regional pain syndrome, *Pain Med* 8:326-331, 2007.

---

have not yet been ratified by the taxonomy committee of the IASP and will undergo further validation studies before full adoption.[5-8]

Patient Demographics and Risk Factors

There are only two population-based epidemiological studies of CRPS in the general population. One reported the population-based incidence rate in North America,[9] and the other in Europe (Netherlands).[10] The reported incidence rates are different; the U.S. study reporting an incidence of 5.6 per 100,000 person-years; the more recent European study reported a rate of 26.2. The inclusion criteria for both studies were different, which could be one of the factors accounting for varying results. CRPS affects females more than males at a ratio almost 4:1,[11] and the majority of CRPS cases in females occur in the postmenopausal stage of life, suggesting a potential hormonal etiological role in CRPS. The observed mean age of diagnosis in these studies of CRPS is 50 to 70 years old with a mean of 52.7 years old.[9,10,12] This age peak is higher than is generally expected and observed in some nonpopulation-based investigations.[13] Before the mid-1980s there were only scattered case reports of RSD in children. However, over the last 10 to 15 years it has become apparent that CRPS does occur in children, with a mean age of onset of about 12.5 years (range 3 to 18 years),[14] particularly following sports injuries.

No single causative factor has been found that explains the development of this complex disorder, but an inciting event often precedes the onset of CRPS. Initial observations correlated CRPS with wounds and crushing limb injuries. Fractures are the most common trigger, wrist fractures in particular.[15] Cast immobilization appears to be another condition associated with development of CRPS.[16] During cast immobilization increased pressure and early complaints of tightness are predictive risk factors for the onset of CRPS. On the other hand, CRPS cases developing as a consequence of remote processes such as stroke,[17] spinal cord injury, and myocardial infarction[18] have been reported. The risk for developing CRPS may depend on susceptibility to exaggerated responses, probably through genetic predisposition to basic pain-related mechanisms such as inflammation and sensitization. This has led to a search for gene polymorphisms that could predict development of CRPS. In a study from Herlyn and colleagues[19] a single nucleotide polymorphism within the α-adrenoceptor appears to be a risk factor for the development of CRPS I after distal radius fracture. Polymorphisms in the human leukocyte antigen (HLA) system have been studied, and loci from all three HLA classes reportedly have been associated with CRPS onset.[20] Studies on co-occurrence of disorders such as migraine, osteoporosis, menstrual cycle–related problems, and neuropathies with CRPS[21,22] can potentially give clues to shared etiologic factors and reveal risk factors.

Complex Regional Pain Syndrome Pathophysiology

The pathophysiology of CRPS is not fully understood; however, based on animal and human studies several hypothesized mechanisms appear to play an important role. In the acute (early) stage as described by Veldman and associates[13] CRPS presents with skin discoloration, edema, increased nail or hair growth, temperature difference, limited movement, or reported sweating. Traditional sequential staging of CRPS into acute inflammatory, subacute dystrophic, and chronic atrophic stages has been largely supplanted by classifying the condition based on limb appearance and warmth. Thus CRPS has been more recently subdivided into a "warm and a cold form."[13,23] The difference in temperature between affected and unaffected extremities has led to the use of thermography, albeit with low specificity for either diagnosis or prognosis.[24,25] Symptoms such as edema, trophic changes, sweating, and vasomotor-related changes have been considered signs of autonomic system dysregulation (sympathetic); pain responding favorably to sympathetic blocks is considered sympathetically maintained pain (SMP). However, the role of the sympathetic system in CRPS has been debated since the vasomotor instability

can be explained by other mechanisms[26-28] such as abnormal sensitivity of adrenergic receptors to normal sympathetic outflow.[29] Moreover, α-adrenoceptors appear to be overexpressed in hyperalgesic skin from CRPS-affected limbs.[30] The reverse hypothesis of diminished sympathetic stimulation has been postulated as an underlying cause of adrenergic receptor up-regulation and sensitization in CRPS patients.[31] A generally acknowledged view today is that SMP and sympathetic dysregulation can be important but not obligatory components of CRPS.

Aseptic neuroinflammation may be a mechanism that is active early in the establishment of CRPS.[32] Trauma-related events could lead to activation and sensitization of primary neuronal afferents to cytokines and neuropeptides released in the affected body region, mainly substance P (SP) and calcitonin gene-related peptide (CGRP).[32] Evidence of a neuroinflammatory process is also obvious from analysis of fluid derived from artificially produced blisters on CRPS-affected extremities. Analysis of blister fluid with a multiplex array testing for 25 different cytokines revealed a strong proinflammatory expression profile, with increased markers for activated monocytes and macrophages.[33] Recently neuropeptide Y and angiotensin-converting enzyme (ACE) have been also suggested as potential modulators of neuroinflammatory responses.[34] Despite the commonly found increase in proinflammatory cytokines in human studies, there is a lack of correlation between cytokine expression and severity and duration of CRPS, suggesting that neuroinflammation is only partly involved in the pathophysiology of CRPS.[35]

Pain and hyperalgesia are the predominant symptoms in CRPS. Persistent peripheral nociceptive input in CRPS results in spinal cord central sensitization with features of mechanical hyperalgesia and allodynia.[36,37] A hallmark of central sensitization is spreading of hyperalgesia, which goes far beyond the initial site of injury. This expansion of nociceptive receptive fields occurs as a result of neuroplasticity changes in the central nervous system (CNS) between the dorsal horn (DH) of the spinal cord and the somatosensory cortex. At the spinal level DH central pain-projecting neurons are pathologically activated by N-methyl-D-aspartate (NMDA) receptor–mediated processes, which leads to hyperexcitability and central sensitization.[38] Furthermore, changes in central representation of somatosensory input in the thalamus and cortex have been found by various studies.[39,40] This cortical reorganization correlates linearly with the amount of CRPS pain and is reversed following pain relief as confirmed by magnetoencephalography (MEG) studies.[40]

Recently the hypothesis of progressive small-fiber degeneration as the basis for CRPS has gained some ground. This has primarily resulted from the work of Oaklander and Fields.[41] Oaklander and colleagues[42] demonstrated for the first time through a morphometric analysis performed on skin biopsies that CRPS I is associated with small-fiber axonal degeneration.

Since CRPS is a heterogeneous disorder, multiple mechanisms, including inflammatory and neuropathic, are likely involved in complex interactions, resulting in this chronic painful and potentially debilitating disorder.

Electrical Neurostimulation for Complex Regional Pain Syndrome

Management of Complex Regional Pain Syndrome

A number of treatment approaches are available for CRPS. These approaches can be categorized as pharmacological, interventional, physical/occupational therapy, and psychological techniques. Physical therapy is the first-line and the mainstay treatment for CRPS.

However, it is often limited by the pain itself, and pain-control interventions are often essential to enable full patient participation.[43,44] Interventional approaches are very useful and are applied usually in combination with pharmacological measures to enhance patient compliance with physical therapy (PT). Various sympathetic blocks, intravenous regional blocks, and epidural blocks can be provided on an outpatient basis. However, the response to sympathetic blocks varies and appears to be more effective than placebo in duration but not magnitude of pain relief.[45] In general, pharmacological pain treatment is similar to that of managing neuropathic pain and would include antidepressants (particularly tricyclics and serotonin-noradrenalin reuptake inhibitors), antiepileptics (e.g., gabapentin), and occasionally muscle relaxants and topical analgesics.[37] Opioids may have a limited role in refractory CRPS patients. Steroids, given their anti-inflammatory function, may be effective in improving inflammatory signs, especially early on.[46] Antioxidants and free radical scavengers may be effective given that hypoxic phenomena in the affected limb can enhance the production of free radicals. In the Netherlands free radical scavengers such as dimethylsulfoxide (DMSO)[47] and N-acetylcysteine (NAC) are widely applied in the treatment of CRPS. Bisphosphonates have shown promise to significantly improve symptoms of CRPS in randomized clinical trials.[48,49] By reducing local acceleration of bone remodeling, bisphosphonates may alleviate pain by effects on nociceptive primary afferents in bone. Psychological treatment in CRPS involves cognitive behavioral techniques and biofeedback and relaxation training. Even though there are no studies to support its use in CRPS, in the general chronic pain population psychological treatment is an effective treatment modality,[37] and it may be used in CRPS to improve coping skills and facilitate rehabilitation.

Electrical Neurostimulation for Complex Regional Pain Syndrome

The idea of electrical stimulation for pain control was based on the initial description of the gate control theory by Melzak and Wall[50] whereby electrical stimulation of Aβ (A beta) fibers in dorsal columns would result in closing the "gate" and obliterating onward central transmission from peripheral nociceptors (C fibers). Varying methods of neurostimulation have been developed, depending on target tissue. In CRPS there is solid evidence for effectiveness of spinal cord stimulation (SCS) and to a lesser extent for peripheral nerve stimulation (PNS) and motor cortex stimulation (MCS).

Spinal Cord Stimulation for Complex Regional Pain Syndrome

Dorsal column electrical stimulation or SCS has been applied to a variety of pain disorders. The mechanism of action of SCS is described elsewhere in this volume. However, focusing on CRPS, SCS theoretically could act on various pathogenetic mechanisms such as (a) direct inhibitory actions on central sensitization mechanisms, (b) restoration and sustainability of blood flow (microcirculation) to the affected extremity by increasing the release of vasoactive mediators such as CGRP and SP,[51] and (c) decreasing sympathetic output by antidromic effects.[52] Even though there are no firm data to support these hypotheses, some recent animal data and clinical observation are emerging that could indicate how SCS could influence various biological functions in CRPS.[51,53-55]

Evidence of Spinal Cord Stimulation Effectiveness in Complex Regional Pain Syndrome

A plethora of reports supports the use of SCS in treating neuropathic pain conditions in general and CRPS in particular. Of note, the Neuromodulation Therapy Access Coalition found substantial

evidence to recommend the use of SCS for treatment of CRPS.[56] However, as of early 2010, literature search reveals only one SCS randomized controlled trial (RCT), three prospective long-term trials (**Table 9-2**), and 12 retrospective studies and multiple case reports and case series.

The only RCT of SCS for CRPS was performed by Kemler and associates[57] and was initially presented in 2000. Investigators designed a prospective, randomized trial to examine the effects of SCS on a group of 54 patients with refractory CRPS who had persistent pain even after surgical sympathectomy.[57-60] Patients were randomized into two groups in a 2:1 ratio to compare the outcomes of SCS and PT vs. PT alone (36 patients were randomized to receive SCS + PT as active treatment arm, and 18 patients randomized to only receive PT as control). As part of the inclusion criteria most patients recruited for this study had severe disease, with 10 patients requiring wheelchairs, 8 crutches, and 13 upper-extremity splints. CRPS had to be present for at least 6 months and affected unilaterally the entire hand or foot. Inclusion criteria also included pain intensity of at least 5 cm on the visual analog scale (VAS) scale despite pharmacological or psychological therapies. All patients had failed surgical sympathectomy. Outcome measures included quality of life measurements (the Nottingham Health Profile and Sickness Impact Profile), pain measurements (VAS and McGill pain questionnaire), and global perceived effect on a 7-point scale (1 worst ever to 7 best ever). Patients were assessed at 1, 3, and 6 months. Data were analyzed on an intent-to-treat (ITT) basis. Of the 36 patients assigned to SCS and trialed for 7 days, 24 underwent implantation, and 22 of those were available for follow-up at 6 months. At 6 months the ITT analysis results indicated a significant improvement in the 36-patient group assigned to receive SCS and PT ($p < 0.001$; mean reduction of pain intensity on VAS was −2.4 cm) compared with the group that received PT alone (mean change +0.2 cm). The average VAS reduction for the 24 subjects treated with SCS (as-treated analysis) was even greater (−3.6 cm). A significant improvement was also reported in the "much improved" score of the global perceived effect in the subjects assigned to SCS. The authors concluded that there is a beneficial effect of SCS in CRPS at 6 months after implant. These effects were maintained at 2-year follow up (VAS: −2.1 cm vs. 0.0 cm; $p < 0.001$ global perceived effect "much improved" score 43% for the SCS group vs. 6% for the PT group; $p = 0.001$).[61] However, despite a significant improvement in health-related quality of life, no clinically significant improvement in functional status was noted.[61] These findings support the conclusion that SCS results in long-term pain reduction and health-related quality of life improvement in CRPS. The same authors assessed the effectiveness of SCS at 5-year follow up.[60] A statistically significant difference was no longer evident between the SCS + PT group compared to the PT group using an intent-to-treat analysis ($p = 0.25$ at 5 years)[60] with regard to pain relief and other variables. However, an as-treated subgroup analysis looking at patients that were implanted (20 patients) and compared to patients undergoing PT only (13 patients) had a p value near statistical significance ($p = 0.06$) for pain relief, and statistically significant improvement in global perceived effect in the "much improved" subscale ($p = 0.02$). The authors commented that despite the apparently diminishing effectiveness of SCS over time, 95% of implanted patients (19/20) stated they would repeat the treatment for the same result.[60]

In a prospective trial Harke and associates[62] assessed the long-term effects of SCS on pain and improvement of functional status in CRPS patients who had SMP (i.e., their pain responded to blockade of sympathetic efferents). They studied 29 patients with

Table 9-2: Summary of Prospective Studies on Spinal Cord Stimulation for Complex Regional Pain Syndromes

Study Type (Reference Authors)	No. of Patients Enrolled	Indication	Length of Study (Follow-up)	Devices Used	SCS Outcomes/Complication Rate
RCT **SCS + PT vs. PT (2:1 randomization; intent to treat analysis)**					
Kemler et al[57], 2000	54 (24 implants)		6 months		Significant improvement of VAS score (3.6 mm) compared with 0.2 cm increase of control; significant improvement in HQOL Nottingham Health Profile; complication rate 25% at 6 months (most caused by unsatisfactory position of the electrodes)
Kemler et al[61], 2002 (follow-up)	51 (24 implants)	CRPS I (duration ≈40 months)	24 months	Medtronic electrodes; IPG	Significant improvements in SCS+PT group in pain intensity and global perceived effect; no improvement in functional status; HQOL improved only in SCS group; 2-year complication rate 38%
Kemler et al[60], 2008 (follow-up)	44 (20 implants)		60 months		Pain score not significantly different; patient satisfaction significantly higher with SCS; no difference in QOL measures; 5-year complication rate 42% (Two explants)
Prospective studies (nonrandomized)					
Harke et al[62] 2005, SMP	29	SMP CRPS I (RSD) (median duration 3 years)	35.6 months (mean)	Medtronic quadripolar leads; IPG	VAS significantly improved; excellent improvement in allodynia and deep pain; significant improvement in PDI and grip strength (functionality of the limb); excellent improvement in analgesic consumption; psychological screening; generator changes in 16/29 caused by exhaustion
Oakley et al[63], 1999	16	CRPS I (average duration 7.5 months)	7.9 months	Medtronic Pisces-Quad or Quad Plus four contacts; IPG/RG	VAS, QOL measures (sickness impact profile) all significantly improved; BDI trending toward significance; rate of revision 4/19 (lead adjustment or receiver change; one patient accounted for 50% of revisions)
Clavillo et al[65], 1998 SIP	36 (implants; 24 SCS; 7 SCS+PNS; 5 PNS)	CRPS I CRPS II	36 months	Medtronic Pisces II/IPG	Significant improvement in pain intensity; significant decrease in narcotic intake; significant improvement of QOL and 41% return-to-work rate; psychological screening; SIP is an inclusion criterion

BDI, Back Depression Inventory; *CRPS*, Complex regional pain syndrome; *HQOL*, health-related quality of life; *IPG*, implantable pulse generator; *PDI*, Pain Disability Index; *PNS*, peripheral nerve stimulation; *PT*, physical therapy; *QOL*, quality of life; *RG*, radiofrequency generator; *RCT*, randomized controlled trial; *RSD*, reflex sympathetic dystrophy; *SCS*, spinal cord stimulation; *SMP*, sympathetically maintained pain; *SIP*, sympathetic independent pain.

a mean CRPS duration of 5.4 years. All patients received a constant-voltage, fixed-channel system, 16 cervical and 13 thoracic lead placements. The outcomes examined were VAS scores for deep pain and allodynia, changes in Pain Disability Index (PDI) to quantify impairments in activities of daily living, and changes in analgesic medication consumption during SCS therapy. Patients were followed for an average of 35.6 ± 21 months after implant. They reported that all patients had a complete resolution of allodynia at 12 months and a significant improvement in deep pain. Furthermore, nearly three quarters of the patients showed a significant decrease in the PDI with over 50% improvement in scores. However, nearly half of the patients needed battery replacement

secondary to exhaustion (at the time of the study, rechargeable generator systems were not available), and 44.1% underwent surgical revision of the leads. The authors do not describe in detail the reasons for revisions. It is not clear whether the cervical or the thoracic placements were more prone to revision. Of significance, the authors placed the electrodes in the lateral aspects of the canal for cervical lead placement for coverage of shoulders, arms, hands, and midline for thoracic lead placement. Although their rationale was to obtain better coverage and stimulate with low output to conserve energy, this approach could cause stimulation of nerve roots at the entry zones that might lead to uncomfortable stimulation (discomfort threshold or recruitment of motor fibers). Even with the complications encountered, the effectiveness of SCS in CRPS with SMP type is impressive. The complete obliteration of allodynia and the significant increase in grip strength and improvement in functional status and quality of life affirm the effectiveness of SCS in CRPS I patients with SMP. In a prospective study, Oakley and coworkers[63,64] reported on 19 CRPS patients treated with SCS. Sixteen were available at follow-up; 11 were still using their devices; two patients stopped using the system, reporting "no pain"; one died unrelated to the device; and two were unresponsive to therapy. Eight of the 11 patients obtained at least 50% pain relief. Complications identified were minor and were corrected without adverse effect on stimulation parameters or efficacy. In another study by Calvillo and colleagues[65] 36 patients with CRPS affecting the upper extremity were examined following treatment with SCS, SCS and PNS, or PNS alone. The authors report a significant reduction in VAS scores (53%) and 50% reduction in analgesic consumption at 36 months following implant when compared to baseline.[65] They concluded that neurostimulation is an effective and reasonable option when alternative therapies have failed.

Reports of SCS in children and adolescents are limited. CRPS I is not uncommon in children and adolescents, affecting in particular girls with an average age of 11 to 14 years old. It could be associated with minor trauma or sports injury; occasionally a trigger cannot be identified. Although treatment centers around active PT, SCS has been used to facilitate the process by reducing pain intensity. In a case series of seven girls 11 to 14 years of age with significantly incapacitating and therapy-resistant CRPS I, SCS was implemented.[66] Trial stimulation was performed, and optimal coverage was achieved in five of seven cases. Despite a 1- to 2-week delay in onset of pain relief following SCS, pain alleviation was complete in five of seven patients at 2 to 6 weeks after the intervention. SCS therapy was deemed successful in all seven patients (even in two patients in whom the SCS system was removed) since no or minor remaining symptoms were noted at 1- to 8-year follow-up and there were no severe recurrences.

Several retrospective studies have examined the effect of SCS in CRPS. Of note, Bennett and colleagues[67] examined pain reduction in relation to current trends in the use of SCS to treat CRPS. The study specifically examined common factors among patients with successful SCS treatment retrospectively compared to patients implanted with single-lead, four-electrode (quadripolar) systems (with an internal battery) and with those using dual-lead, eight-electrode (octipolar) systems (which at the time required a radiofrequency unit). Data were compiled on 101 CRPS patients who had similar psychological profiles. Patients were divided into two groups: those who had single-lead quadripolar systems and those who had dual-lead octipolar systems. Both groups displayed a significant reduction in VAS pain intensity scores when compared to baseline. The overall satisfaction rate for the group with single quadripolar leads was 70%, whereas for those with dual octipolar leads the rate was 91%. Analysis of variance for improvement in pain scores showed a significantly greater improvement (F-value 56.081, P <0.0001) with dual octipolar leads. There was a mean pain improvement (ΔVAS) in the quadripolar lead group of 3.70 ± 0.79 vs. a mean pain improvement in the dual octipolar lead group of 6.00 ± 1.59. The ability to regain pain control after spontaneous lead movement was significantly different between the two groups. In the quadripolar lead group four patients (3.3%) required surgical revision as a result of spontaneous lead migration, whereas in the dual octipolar group no patients required surgical revision as a result of spontaneous lead migration. The larger number of electrodes available for programming in the dual-octipolar group allowed an increased flexibility when

rostral-caudal changes in positioning occurred; patients who experienced movement of their leads were able to recapture their pain coverage with reprogramming alone. The ability to use higher frequencies (above 250 Hz) in the group with dual octipolar leads (radiofrequency generator unit) allowed some patients to "recapture" pain control. A subset of patients (15.5%) who had lost analgesia in the presence of adequate paresthesia coverage were able to regain pain control when stimulation frequency was increased above 250 Hz (mean 455 ± 104.5 Hz). Although both groups had statistically significant improvements in pain scores and overall satisfaction when compared to baseline, the dual-octipolar group showed greater improvements.[67]

In a case series on 12 patients with upper- and lower-extremity pain, including five CRPS I patients, and using a system delivering multiple independent constant-current output with electrical field-steering capabilities through low cervical epidural SCS leads, Hayek, Veizi, and Stanton-Hicks[68] found a consistent ability to capture and maintain paresthesia coverage in all four extremities that correlated with pain relief.[68] They also reported that the frequency used was relatively low (mean 45 ± 5 Hz). In a recent case report by Williams, Korto, and Cohen[69] complete resolution of CRPS symptoms occurred after 1 month of SCS treatment. Based also on a previous case series reporting resolution without recurrence of CRPS in adolescent girls (11 to 14 years old) following treatment with SCS,[66] the authors argued in favor of central-peripheral neuronal interface ("neuronal switch") that could be modulated by SCS and could lead to complete "cure" of CRPS. Thus a more aggressive treatment strategy, which places neuromodulation therapies early in the treatment algorithm along with the use of more advanced SCS configurations, may prove to be more effective. This hypothesis is promising but requires further research.

Peripheral Nerve Stimulation for Complex Regional Pain Syndrome

Almost in parallel to SCS, PNS was developed in the late 1960s. Whereas SCS targets dorsal columns of the spinal cord, PNS targets fibers of the peripheral nerve along its path. Correct placement of leads close to the nerve trunks requires an incision, nerve exposure, and alignment along or wrapping of the nerve trunk, depending on the leads used. Recent placement of percutaneous leads with ultrasound guidance close to peripheral nerves was touted as potentially safer, possibly reducing risks associated with open dissection.[70,71] The introduction of four electrode contacts coupled with the availability of programmable generators in the early 1980s provided a significant advancement.[72] However, there have been no specific leads developed for PNS, and the procedure is not without complications and not always effective. Although the exact mechanism of action of PNS is not known, it is believed that the principle behind PNS is the same as with SCS but the target is different (peripheral nerves innervating the painful area). Constant peripheral activation of large fibers could provide a consistent block of peripheral nociceptive input allowing the neuronal plasticity to implement changes that could control CRPS-related pain. A recent study demonstrated an increase in brain activity by functional magnetic resonance imaging (fMRI) in the somatosensory cortex on median nerve stimulation, which suggests a central effect as a result of PNS.[72]

Several studies exist on open-dissection PNS placement for chronic pain following peripheral nerve injury. A recent study by Mobbs, Nair, and Blum[73] reviewed the results of a retrospective analysis of 38 patients implanted with PNS systems and followed up for 35 months. The overall results indicated that 61% of the patients reported over 50% pain relief. This recent study compares favorably with previous reports in the literature also reviewed in the same article.[73] In a meta-analysis from previous studies reported, of the 175 implanted patients (studies reviewed from 1975 to 2000), 65.4% reported a successful outcome with good-to-excellent ratings. Efficacy of PNS in CRPS cannot really be assessed with currently available studies. In fact, there is only one study published that specifically examined PNS efficacy over the long term in CRPS. In a prospective study by Hassenbusch and associates,[74] 32 CRPS patients were trialed with PNS systems, and 30 of those had a successful trial with significant pain relief. The study reported a 63% success rate at 3 years after implant in patients with advanced disease that had failed all other modalities except a trial of SCS. Of the 30 patients implanted with permanent PNS systems, 8 (27%) required a revision of the electrode; placement of additional electrodes was carried out in six patients. There were 11 pain relief failures, mostly early on at 1.3 ± 0.1 years. According to this study the best application of PNS appears to be for a small group of patients with localized pain along the distribution of a single major nerve. However, when CRPS spreads and the receptive pain area increases, further surgical revisions might be necessary. Although there might be a place for PNS in the treatment algorithm of CRPS, particularly type II, well-designed randomized trials are necessary to assess its long-term effectiveness.[75] Furthermore, increased effectiveness of this modality may occur with improved design of electrodes.

Motor Cortex Stimulation for Complex Regional Pain Syndrome

Motor cortex stimulation (MCS) may be a promising tool for the treatment of patients with refractory neuropathic pain. The technique consists of implanting epidural electrodes over the motor strip of the parietal lobe. Epidural MCS is safer, less invasive, and easier to perform than deep brain stimulation. The analgesic effects of MCS could be caused either by neuronal activation in the cortical and thalamic areas as demonstrated by positron emission tomography (PET) studies or by activation of descending fibers originating from the motor cortex that control sensory input.[76-78] Although MCS has been shown to be effective in relieving trigeminal neuropathic pain, it has only recently been reported in a few cases with recalcitrant CRPS. MCS resulted in significant relief of pain and allodynia that lasted over 12 months in a patient with CRPS type II of the upper extremity with hemi body allodynia.[79] Velasco and associates[78] reported a case series of five CRPS patients, four of whom benefited from MCS implant. VAS and McGill pain scales diminished significantly throughout the follow-up and worsened when MCS was turned off for 30 days (in a double-blinded fashion). In addition, there was resolution of allodynia and sympathetic signs lasting over 1 year. Nevertheless, randomized, prospective studies are required; technical improvements in areas such as electrode design and stimulation parameters are needed.

Benefits vs. Risks and Complications of Spinal Cord Stimulation in Complex Regional Pain Syndrome

In addition to analgesia, other favorable outcomes of SCS therapy in CRPS range from absence of hyperpathia to normalization of capillary filling, normalization and sustainability of temperature over time, improved quality of life, functional improvement of the diseased limb when SCS is combined with physiotherapy, and a notable decrease in analgesic medication consumption.[59,60,62,80] Currently SCS is the only modality capable of providing sustained pain relief at any treatment stage for CRPS, but it is not effective in all patients. Successful analgesic outcome with SCS has been classically defined as either over 50% pain relief or significant reduction in VAS pain scores. On the basis of these parameters, the success rate of SCS in CRPS I and II derived from of all the studies reported in the literature with a follow-up of at least 6 months is 82% (from 224 cases).[81] Patient satisfaction with SCS is illustrated in the long-term follow-up study of Kemler and associates.[60] Despite no apparent improvement of SCS + PT vs. PT patients at 5 years after implant, 95% of the patients with CRPS I who had undergone SCS implantation stated they would repeat the procedure for similar results.

One of the main criticisms of SCS applications has arisen from the possible role of placebo. Because a patient cannot be blinded to the paresthesias induced by SCS, double-blinded studies evaluating SCS have not been conducted. However, one well-controlled study has shown effectiveness of SCS therapy when compared to placebo in angina.[82]

As an invasive procedure SCS placement carries surgical risks related to the procedure and technical complications related to the implanted device. Risks and complications of SCS are discussed in detail in another chapter of this series. Briefly, risks associated with the procedure that should be discussed with the patients before the trial include mechanical issues such as lead migration or generator problems, infection, spinal fluid leaks, hemorrhage, and neurological injury. Some consequences can be temporary such as cerebrospinal fluid (CSF) leaks; however, others result in explants or even worse in neurological deficits. The typical reported complication rate after SCS varies from 20% to 75% (mean, 42%). On the basis of findings from larger studies, it is known that complications necessitate removal of the system in 5% to 15% of cases.[81] Technical problems (e.g., lead shifting and breaking) seem to be inherent in the treatment with reported incidence of breakage in 9.1% and shifting (migration) in 13.2% (2753 cases).[81] Although complications affect treatment results, cause patient discomfort, and generate costs, these factors rarely cause permanent neurologic deficits (0.03%).[81] CSF leakage occurs after accidental dural puncture with the epidural needle, guidewire, or leads during surgical procedure. A CSF leak can lead to headache, which usually occurs early in the postoperative period. In a large review of the literature (from 1981 to 2004) Cameron[81] found that the incidence of infection was 3.4% (2972 cases) and CSF leak 0.3% (2972 cases).

Specific to CRPS, a varied SCS complication rate is reported. In the RCT study by Kemler and colleagues[60] the complication rate at 2 years that required intervention was 38%, and overall 42% of the patients underwent reoperation 5 years after implant. Most of the complications occurred in the first 2 years after implant (79%), and the annual complication rate after 2 years was fairly low at 5%. Most reoperation in this study was caused by battery replacement, which could be avoided because the technology has advanced and rechargeable batteries are now available. On the other hand, lead migration was clearly high in the first 2 years but was noted in only two cases from the second to the fifth year. Regardless of lead location, cervical or lumbar, the complication rate was comparable.[83] Oakley et al[63] did not report any complication at implant. However, the follow-up complication rate was 21%, with lead repositioning/replacement being the main complication. Overall revision rate was 35% (6 out of 19 patients). In the study of 29 patients by Harke and associates[62] there were 16 battery replacements (55%), 12 lead revision/replacements (41%), and two explants. The relatively high complication rate of SCS should not be an obstacle in treatment consideration but must clearly be communicated to future candidates.

Patient Selection, Trial, and Long-Term Patient Management

Patient Selection

Appropriate patient selection is crucial to the success of SCS therapy for CRPS. Several factors would aid in successful selection of patients that would benefit the most from SCS:

- Applying appropriate diagnostic criteria. The valuable work from IASP special interest groups on CRPS diagnostic criteria is of paramount importance in defining the patient population for treatment clinically and for clinical research studies.
- Psychological factors and behavioral aspects are thought to contribute significantly to CRPS presentation and maintenance.[84-86] But the actual association between psychological factors and CRPS remains controversial because of the lack of methodological high-quality studies. Nonetheless, it is very important that psychological evaluation be performed before patients are considered for SCS therapy.[87]
- Appropriate patient expectations and goal-oriented therapy. An initial clinical interview can also elicit the patient's subjective experience of pain. Discussion with patients should involve clear explanation of the benefits, side effects, and ineffectiveness of the method. It should also be clear that SCS is a part of the complex therapeutic approach together with PT, psychological therapy, and pharmacotherapy working toward the goal of functional rehabilitation of the extremity.
- Since SCS has been used generally at the end spectrum of treatment, it is encouraging that many studies have shown significant pain improvement. Obviously integrating SCS with PT at earlier stages in combination with new implantable systems with enhanced capabilities (multiple electrodes and flexibility in output parameters) might eventually lead to even better outcomes.
- Magnetic resonance imaging (MRI) should be performed in any suspected case of stenosis, disc herniation, or other anatomical abnormality that might explain the patient symptoms or otherwise increase the procedural risk of SCS.[80] Some clinicians rely on MRI to gain information about the depth of epidural space/dorsal CSF and the position of the spinal cord, dimensions that vary among individuals and may affect electrode selection, placement, and adjustment; however, there are no data that show improved technical outcomes following MRI.

Spinal Cord Stimulation Trial

According to the Neuromodulation Therapy Access Coalition, there is excellent evidence that screening trials of SCS provide valid patient selection information.[56] Indeed, one of the advantages of SCS is that trials offer both the physician and patient an opportunity to evaluate SCS before committing to it. The trial should answer two fundamental questions: Is the patient's pain responsive to SCS therapy, and can the patient tolerate the treatment? In CRPS the trial is an opportunity to determine whether the patient can tolerate the interdisciplinary care required for functional rehabilitation (Fig. 9-1). The physician and patient should agree in advance on the goals of the trial and the measures used to assess those goals. In general, candidates should proceed to implantation if their pain can be reduced by at least 50% and they can participate in functional rehabilitation,[44] the area of paresthesia is tolerable and concordant with the area of pain,[88] analgesic medication intake remains stable or can be decreased, and functional improvement has been

assessed (different clinics use different tools for physical evaluation). SCS is effective in nearly two thirds of the CRPS I patients.[88] Generally trials last for 1 week or longer and use externalized lead wires and a temporary external transmitter. Trial period and lead selection varies and is a function of multiple variables detailed elsewhere in this volume. However, a 5- to 7-day home-testing period resulting in at least 50% pain relief is commonly accepted as appropriate. The selection criteria that are currently used do not predict which candidates will continue to respond after implantation of a SCS system. One of the predictors of successful outcomes of SCS in CRPS is the presence of brush allodynia.[89]

Current Treatment Paradigm for Complex Regional Pain Syndrome and the Role of Spinal Cord Stimulation

Functional recovery and rehabilitation of the limb are the essential goals of therapy in CRPS. Physiotherapy is recommended widely in the literature as the mainstay of CRPS treatment. The concurrent implementation of physiotherapy with pain management and psychological therapies is meant to facilitate a sequential progression through the steps of the rehabilitation algorithm (see Fig. 9-1). The point of entry would depend entirely on pragmatic factors such as response to therapy and clinical presentation. It is rational to treat patients who present with CRPS using a multimodal approach. What has not been given competing credence in consensus statements is the place of electrical neuromodulation therapies in CRPS. Although other therapies have been proposed as "more conservative" and therefore "initial" therapies, this rationale is not supported with favorable long-term outcome data (i.e., a change in the course of the condition or significant long-term diminution of pain *and* sequelae of the syndrome). Thus a time-oriented construct that relies on the concept that timely reduction of pain with normalization of blood flow may provide the best environment for functional recovery, may thus favor earlier use of SCS. Mere implantation of a device without rehabilitation is unlikely to produce good functional outcomes. After significant progress has been made, follow-up visits would be scheduled as necessary to ensure a safe and effective use of SCS.

Cost-Effectiveness of Spinal Cord Stimulation in Complex Regional Pain Syndrome

SCS is considered an expensive invasive therapy for chronic pain because of the upfront costs of the screening trial and devices. However, there is a large body of evidence that implanting an SCS system is less costly after 3 years of successful therapy. Kemler and co-workers[57] looked at the economics of conventional treatment vs. SCS for the treatment of CRPS. Even though during the first year the cost of SCS therapy was $4000 higher than non-SCS therapy (PT), in the lifetime analysis SCS was more effective than conventional therapy and less expensive (by $60,000 per patient).[90] These findings are similar to those in a study by Kumar, Malik, and Demeria that compared conventional chronic pain therapies vs. SCS in 104 patients with failed back surgery syndrome.[91] Treatment costs with SCS were higher for the first 2.5 years; thereafter they were approximately one third lower. Furthermore, 15% of the SCS-treated group returned to work. A British trial of patients treated for CRPS I found a lifetime cost savings of approximately U.S. $60,800 for the SCS group when compared to the PT group.[92,93] In a U.S. retrospective study of 222 patients (54% were CRPS I and II patients) Mekhail and colleagues[93] found reduced demand for health care resources by patients receiving neurostimulation, which suggests that, despite the initial costs, PNS and SCS have substantial long-term economic benefits that translate to $17,900 savings per year.

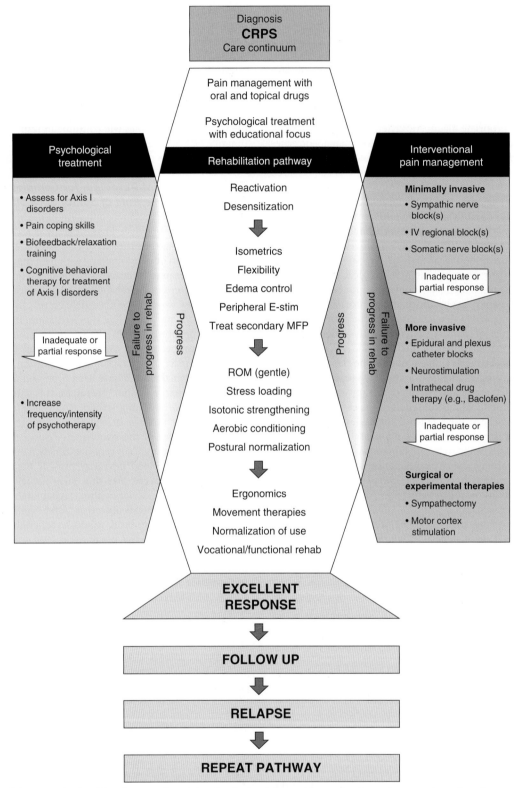

Fig. 9-1 Revised therapeutic algorithm for complex regional pain syndrome with emphasis on therapeutic options in response to patient's clinical progress in the rehabilitation pathway. *CRPS,* Complex regional pain syndrome; *IV,* intravenous; *MFP,* myofascial pain; *ROM,* range of motion.

Conclusions

Appropriate use of implantable technologies for pain management should be based on extensive knowledge of the pathophysiology of pain, clinical presentation of pain syndromes, and evidence of effectiveness of the treatment modality. SCS can provide sufficient analgesia to facilitate early PT and is reversible. Given clinical experience of nearly three decades of SCS, the therapy has no apparent detectable detrimental effect on the nervous system and no significant adverse effects at the usual stimulation levels. SCS has also been shown to be cost-effective or cost neutral over time when compared to ongoing conservative medical management, including physical therapies and medication management. Although SCS appears to be beneficial and cost-effective over the long term in CRPS, multiple questions remain to be answered by well-designed clinical studies. As better tools are developed for early diagnosis, it is of paramount importance to define the role of electrical neuro-modulation early in the disease before significant CNS changes have occurred and significant disease progression has rendered the patient dysfunctional.

References

1. Stanton-Hicks M et al: Reflex sympathetic dystrophy: changing concepts and taxonomy. *Pain* 63:127-133, 1995.
2. Michell SW, Morehouse GR, Keen WW: *Gunshot wounds and other injuries of nerves*, Philadelphia, 1864, Lippincott.
3. Staunton H: Sudeck atrophy. *Ir Med J* 99:313-315, 2006.
4. Evans JA: Reflex sympathetic dystrophy; report on 57 cases. *Ann Intern Med* 126:4174-4226, 1947.
5. Bruehl S et al: External validation of IASP diagnostic criteria for complex regional pain syndrome and proposed research diagnostic criteria: International Association for the Study of Pain. *Pain* 81:147-154, 1999.
6. Harden RN et al: Proposed new diagnostic criteria for complex regional pain syndrome. *Pain Med* 8:326-331, 2007.
7. Harden RN et al: Complex regional pain syndrome: are the IASP diagnostic criteria valid and sufficiently comprehensive? *Pain* 83:211-219, 1999.
8. Stanton-Hicks MD et al: An updated interdisciplinary clinical pathway for CRPS: report of an expert panel. *Pain Pract* 2:1-16, 2002.
9. Sandroni P et al: Complex regional pain syndrome type I: incidence and prevalence in Olmsted county, a population-based study. *Pain* 103:199-207, 2003.
10. de MM et al: The incidence of complex regional pain syndrome: a population-based study. *Pain* 129:12-20, 2007.
11. Schwartzman RJ, Erwin KL, Alexander GM: The natural history of complex regional pain syndrome. *Clin J Pain* 25:273-280, 2009.
12. de MM et al: Referral and treatment patterns for complex regional pain syndrome in the Netherlands. *Acta Anaesthesiol Scand* 53:816-825, 2009.
13. Veldman PH et al: Signs and symptoms of reflex sympathetic dystrophy: prospective study of 829 patients. *Lancet* 342:1012-1026, 1992.
14. Tan EC et al: Complex regional pain syndrome type I in children. *Acta Paediatr* 97:875-879, 2008.
15. Atkins RM, Duckworth T, Kanis JA: Features of algodystrophy after Colles' fracture. *J Bone Joint Surg Brit* 72:105-110, 1990.
16. Schwartzman RJ, McLellan TL: Reflex sympathetic dystrophy: a review. *Arch Neurol* 44:555-561, 1987.
17. Riedl B et al: Autonomic failure after stroke—is it indicative for pathophysiology of complex regional pain syndrome? *Acta Neurol Scand* 103:27-34, 2001.
18. Wasner G, Backonja MM, Baron R: Traumatic neuralgias: complex regional pain syndromes (reflex sympathetic dystrophy and causalgia): clinical characteristics, pathophysiological mechanisms and therapy. *Neurol Clin* 16:851-868, 1998.
19. Herlyn P et al: Frequencies of polymorphisms in cytokines, neurotransmitters and adrenergic receptors in patients with complex regional pain syndrome type I after distal radial fracture. *Clin J Pain* 26:175-181, 2010.
20. van de Beek WJ et al: Susceptibility loci for complex regional pain syndrome. *Pain* 103:93-97, 2003.
21. de MM et al: Estrogens and the risk of complex regional pain syndrome (CRPS). *Pharmacoepidemiol Drug Saf* 18:44-52, 2009.
22. de MM et al: Medical history and the onset of complex regional pain syndrome (CRPS). *Pain* 139:458-466, 2008.
23. Janig W, Baron R: Complex regional pain syndrome: mystery explained? *Lancet Neurol* 2:687-697, 2003.
24. Herrick A et al: Abnormal thermoregulatory responses in patients with reflex sympathetic dystrophy syndrome. *J Rheumatol* 21:1319-1324, 1994.
25. Sherman RA et al: Stability of temperature asymmetries in reflex sympathetic dystrophy over time and changes in pain. *Clin J Pain* 10:71-77, 1994.
26. Eisenberg E et al: Plasma endothelin-1 levels in patients with complex regional pain syndrome. *Eur J Pain* 8:533-538, 2004.
27. Groeneweg G et al: Regulation of peripheral blood flow in complex regional pain syndrome: clinical implication for symptomatic relief and pain management. *BMC Musculoskelet Disord* 10:116, 2009.
28. Drummond PD: Mechanism of complex regional pain syndrome: no longer excessive sympathetic outflow? *Lancet* 358:168-170, 2001.
29. Chemali KR, Gorodeski R, Chelimsky TC: Alpha-adrenergic supersensitivity of the sudomotor nerve in complex regional pain syndrome. *Ann Neurol* 49:453-459, 2001.
30. Gibbs GF et al: Unravelling the pathophysiology of complex regional pain syndrome: focus on sympathetically maintained pain. *Clin Exp Pharmacol Physiol* 35:717-724, 2008.
31. Wasner G et al: Vascular abnormalities in acute reflex sympathetic dystrophy (CRPS I): complete inhibition of sympathetic nerve activity with recovery. *Arch Neurol* 56:613-620, 1999.
32. Weber M et al: Facilitated neurogenic inflammation in complex regional pain syndrome. *Pain* 91:251-257, 2001.
33. Heijmans-Antonissen C et al: Multiplex bead array assay for detection of 25 soluble cytokines in blister fluid of patients with complex regional pain syndrome type 1. *Mediators Inflamm* 2006:283-298, 2006.
34. Kramer HH et al: Inhibition of neutral endopeptidase (NEP) facilitates neurogenic inflammation. *Exp Neurol* 195:179-184, 2005.
35. Wesseldijk F et al: Tumor necrosis factor-alpha and interleukin-6 are not correlated with the characteristics of Complex Regional Pain Syndrome type 1 in 66 patients. *Eur J Pain* 12:716-721, 2008.
36. Vartiainen NV, Kirveskari E, Forss N: Central processing of tactile and nociceptive stimuli in complex regional pain syndrome. *Clin Neurophysiol* 119:2380-2388, 2008.
37. Yung CO, Bruehl SP: Complex regional pain syndrome. *Curr Treat Options Neurol* 5:499-511, 2003.
38. Woolf CJ, Thompson SW: The induction and maintenance of central sensitization is dependent on N-methyl-D-aspartic acid receptor activation; implications for the treatment of post-injury pain hypersensitivity states. *Pain* 44:293-299, 1991.
39. Shiraishi S et al: Cerebral glucose metabolism change in patients with complex regional pain syndrome: a PET study. *Radiat Med* 24:335-344, 2006.
40. Maihofner C et al: Cortical processing of mechanical hyperalgesia: a MEG study. *Eur J Pain* 14:64-70, 2010.
41. Oaklander AL, Fields HL: Is reflex sympathetic dystrophy/complex regional pain syndrome type I a small-fiber neuropathy? *Ann Neurol* 65:629-638, 2009.
42. Oaklander AL et al: Evidence of focal small-fiber axonal degeneration in complex regional pain syndrome-I (reflex sympathetic dystrophy). *Pain* 120:235-243, 2006.
43. Oerlemans HM et al: Adjuvant physical therapy versus occupational therapy in patients with reflex sympathetic dystrophy/complex regional pain syndrome type I. *Arch Phys Med Rehabil* 81:49-56, 2000.
44. Oerlemans HM et al: Do physical therapy and occupational therapy reduce the impairment percentage in reflex sympathetic dystrophy? *Am J Phys Med Rehabil* 78:533-539, 1999.
45. Price DD et al: Analysis of peak magnitude and duration of analgesia produced by local anesthetics injected into sympathetic ganglia of complex regional pain syndrome patients. *Clin J Pain* 14:216-226, 1998.
46. Christensen K, Jensen EM, Noer I: The reflex dystrophy syndrome response to treatment with systemic corticosteroids. *Acta Chir Scand* 148:653-655, 1982.
47. Perez RS et al: The treatment of complex regional pain syndrome type I with free radical scavengers: a randomized controlled study. *Pain* 102:297-307, 2003.

48. Robinson JN, Sandom J, Chapman PT: Efficacy of pamidronate in complex regional pain syndrome type I. *Pain Med* 5:276-280, 2004.

49. Varenna M et al: Intravenous clodronate in the treatment of reflex sympathetic dystrophy syndrome: a randomized, double blind, placebo controlled study. *J Rheumatol* 27:1477-1483, 2000.

50. Melzack R, Wall PD: Pain mechanisms: a new theory. *Science* 150:971-979, 1965.

51. Tanaka S et al: Low intensity spinal cord stimulation may induce cutaneous vasodilation via CGRP release. *Brain Res* 896:183-187, 2001.

52. Wu M, Linderoth B, Foreman RD: Putative mechanisms behind effects of spinal cord stimulation on vascular diseases: a review of experimental studies. *Auton Neurosci* 138:9-23, 2008.

53. Gao J et al: Effects of spinal cord stimulation with "standard clinical" and higher frequencies on peripheral blood flow in rats. *Brain Res* 1313:53-61, 2010.

54. Wu M et al: Extracellular signal-regulated kinase (ERK) and protein kinase B (AKT) pathways involved in spinal cord stimulation (SCS)-induced vasodilation. *Brain Res* 1207:73-83, 2008.

55. Wu M et al: Sensory fibers containing vanilloid receptor-1 (VR-1) mediate spinal cord stimulation-induced vasodilation. *Brain Res* 1107:177-184, 2006.

56. North R et al: American Academy of Pain Medicine: practice parameters for the use of spinal cord stimulation in the treatment of chronic neuropathic pain. *Pain Med* 8(suppl 4):S200-S275, 2007.

57. Kemler MA et al: Spinal cord stimulation in patients with chronic reflex sympathetic dystrophy. *N Engl J Med* 343:618-624, 2000.

58. Kemler MA et al: Pain relief in complex regional pain syndrome due to spinal cord stimulation does not depend on vasodilation. *Anesthesiology* 92:1653-1660, 2000.

59. Kemler MA et al: Impact of spinal cord stimulation on sensory characteristics in complex regional pain syndrome type I: a randomized trial. *Anesthesiology* 95:72-80, 2001.

60. Kemler MA et al: Effect of spinal cord stimulation for chronic complex regional pain syndrome type I: five-year final follow-up of patients in a randomized controlled trial. *J Neurosurg* 108:292-298, 2008.

61. Kemler MA et al: The effect of spinal cord stimulation in patients with chronic reflex sympathetic dystrophy: two years' follow-up of the randomized controlled trial. *Ann Neurol* 55:13-18, 2004.

62. Harke H et al: Spinal cord stimulation in sympathetically maintained complex regional pain syndrome type I with severe disability: a prospective clinical study. *Eur J Pain* 9:363-373, 2005.

63. Oakley J, Weiner RL: Spinal cord stimulation for complex regional pain syndrome: a prospective study of 19 patients at 2 centers. *Neuromodulation* 2:47-50, 1999.

64. Burchiel KJ et al: Prospective, multicenter study of spinal cord stimulation for relief of chronic back and extremity pain. *Spine* 21:2786-2794, 1996.

65. Calvillo O et al: Neuroaugmentation in the treatment of complex regional pain syndrome of the upper extremity. *Acta Orthop Belg* 64:57-63, 1998.

66. Olsson GL, Meyerson BA, Linderoth B: Spinal cord stimulation in adolescents with complex regional pain syndrome type I (CRPS-I). *Eur J Pain* 12:53-59, 2008.

67. Bennett DS et al: Spinal cord stimulation for complex regional pain syndrome I (RSD): a retrospective multicenter experience from 1995 to 1998 of 101 patients. *Neuromodulation* 2:202-210, 1999.

68. Hayek SM, Veizi IE, Stanton-Hicks M: Four-limb neurostimulation with neuroelectrodes placed in the lower cervical epidural spac. *Anesthesiology* 110:681-684, 2009.

69. Williams KA, Korto K, Cohen SP: Spinal cord stimulation: "neural switch" in complex regional pain syndrome type I. *Pain Med* 10:762-786, 2009.

70. Huntoon MA et al: Feasibility of ultrasound-guided percutaneous placement of peripheral nerve stimulation electrodes and anchoring during simulated movement: part two, upper extremity. *Reg Anesth Pain Med* 33:558-565, 2008.

71. Huntoon MA, Burgher AH: Ultrasound-guided permanent implantation of peripheral nerve stimulation (PNS) system for neuropathic pain of the extremities: original cases and outcomes. *Pain Med* 10:1369-1377, 2009.

72. Slavin KV: Peripheral nerve stimulation for neuropathic pain. *Neurotherapeutics* 5:100-106, 2008.

73. Mobbs RJ, Nair S, Blum P: Peripheral nerve stimulation for the treatment of chronic pain. *J Clin Neurosci* 14:216-221, 2007.

74. Hassenbusch SJ et al: Long-term results of peripheral nerve stimulation for reflex sympathetic dystrophy. *J Neurosurg* 84:415-423, 1996.

75. Maleki J et al: Patterns of spread in complex regional pain syndrome, type I (reflex sympathetic dystrophy). *Pain* 88:259-266, 2000.

76. Maihofner C et al: The motor system shows adaptive changes in complex regional pain syndrome. *Brain* 130:2671-2687, 2007.

77. Swart CM, Stins JF, Beek PJ: Cortical changes in complex regional pain syndrome (CRPS). *Eur J Pain* 13:902-907, 2009.

78. Velasco F et al: Motor cortex electrical stimulation applied to patients with complex regional pain syndrome. *Pain* 147:91-98, 2009.

79. Son UC et al: Motor cortex stimulation in a patient with intractable complex regional pain syndrome type II with hemibody involvement: case report. *J Neurosurg* 98:175-179, 2003.

80. North R et al: American Academy of Pain Medicine: Practice parameters for the use of spinal cord stimulation in the treatment of chronic neuropathic pain. *Pain Med* 8(suppl 4):S200-S275, 2007.

81. Cameron T: Safety and efficacy of spinal cord stimulation for the treatment of chronic pain: a 20-year literature review. *J Neurosurg* 100:254-267, 2004.

82. Eddicks S et al: Thoracic spinal cord stimulation improves functional status and relieves symptoms in patients with refractory angina pectoris: the first placebo-controlled randomised study. *Heart* 93:585-590, 2007.

83. Forouzanfar T et al: Spinal cord stimulation in complex regional pain syndrome: cervical and lumbar devices are comparably effective. *Br J Anaesth* 92:348-353, 2004.

84. Szeinberg-Arazi D et al: A functional and psychosocial assessment of patients with post-Sudeck atrophy amputation. *Arch Phys Med Rehabil* 74:416-418, 1993.

85. Galer BS et al: Course of symptoms and quality of life measurement in complex regional pain syndrome: a pilot survey. *J Pain Symptom Manage* 20:286-292, 2000.

86. Eisenberg E et al: Evidence for cortical hyperexcitability of the affected limb representation area in CRPS: a psychophysical and transcranial magnetic stimulation study. *Pain* 113:99-105, 2005.

87. Beltrutti D et al: The psychological assessment of candidates for spinal cord stimulation for chronic pain management. *Pain Pract* 4:204-221, 2004.

88. Oakley JC: Spinal cord stimulation for the treatment of chronic pain. In Follet KA, editor, *Neurosurgical Pain Management*. Philadelphia, 2004, Saunders, pp 131-144.

89. van EF et al: Brush-evoked allodynia predicts outcome of spinal cord stimulation in complex regional pain syndrome type 1. *Eur J Pain* 14:164-169, 2010.

90. Kemler MA, Furnee CA: Economic evaluation of spinal cord stimulation for chronic reflex sympathetic dystrophy. *Neurology* 59:1203-1209, 2002.

91. Kumar K, Malik S, Demeria D: Treatment of chronic pain with spinal cord stimulation versus alternative therapies: cost-effectiveness analysis. *Neurosurgery* 51:106-115, 2002.

92. Taylor RS, Van Buyten JP, Buchser E: Spinal cord stimulation for complex regional pain syndrome: a systematic review of the clinical and cost-effectiveness literature and assessment of prognostic factors. *Eur J Pain* 10:91-101, 2006.

93. Mekhail NA, Aeschbach A, Stanton-Hicks M: Cost benefit analysis of neurostimulation for chronic pain. *Clin J Pain* 20:462-468, 2004.

10 Spinal Cord Stimulation for Peripheral Vascular Disease

Krishna Kumar and Rita Nguyen

CHAPTER OVERVIEW

Chapter Overview: Electrical stimulation of the spinal cord (SCS) can be used for relief of neuropathic pain and for several indications of nociceptive pain. These include the ischemic pain that results from peripheral vascular disease (PVD), particularly in cases that are beyond surgical revascularization. This chapter addresses the ways that SCS works to alleviate the pain—and the underlying condition—of PVD. PVD causes a progressive atherosclerosis of the arteries of the lower extremities and may present initially as claudication (i.e., pain or discomfort with walking that is relieved by rest). Left untreated, PVD progresses to muscle ischemia that leads to ischemic neuropathy and muscle deterioration, denervation, and eventually limb loss. SCS emerged as a treatment for PVD when studies in the 1970s indicated that it could improve vasodilation at the target tissue. Three main mechanisms are thought to underlie the efficacy of SCS for PVD, although they are incompletely understood. First, the usual gate theory mechanism is thought to provide pain relief (i.e., that stimulation of large-diameter afferent neurons "gates" the system to reduce pain signaling). SCS is thought to increase peripheral vasodilation in two ways: by suppression of sympathetic nerve activity (which causes vasoconstriction) and by antidromic stimulation of afferent nerves, leading to peripheral release of potent vasodilators, including calcitonin gene-related peptide (CGRP). Careful consideration of patient selection and technical details of implantation and stimulation can improve the chances of SCS success, which includes reduced pain, increased microcirculation, and ultimately limb survival.

Important Points:
- SCS is an effective alternative treatment for nonreconstructible critical limb ischemia.
- SCS improves pain, microcirculation, limb survival, and clinical stage compared to conservative treatment.

Clinical Pearls:
- When selecting patients, the improvement in the transcutaneous partial pressure of oxygen ($TcpO_2$) and pain relief during trial stimulation is a predictor of outcome.
- Increase of $TcpO_2$ of 10 mm Hg (minimum), preferably >15 mmHg, is a prognostic indicator for both limb salvage and pain relief; however, there is no linear correlation.
- If the regional perfusion index (RPI) improves 0.2 or more from the baseline and is sustained, the limb salvage rate could reach up to 90%.

Clinical Pitfalls:
- If SCS is implanted in cases where trial stimulation produces less than 80% coverage of the area of pain, results will be less than satisfactory.
- If $TcpO_2$ does not rise over 100 mm Hg during trial stimulation, installation of an SCS in such cases will not produce improvement in rest pain, claudication, or limb salvage.
- If the degree of benefit decreases after initial success, prior to blaming the development of tolerance, please exclude other causes of hardware failure.

Establishing Diagnosis

Peripheral vascular disease (PVD) results from progressive atherosclerosis of the arteries of the lower extremities. The presence of PVD signals an increased likelihood of disease in other regions of the body, resulting in cardiovascular and cerebrovascular morbidity and mortality. PVD affects 10% to 15% of the U.S. population; the prevalence increases with advancing age.[1] Risk factors for PVD include smoking, diabetes, hypertension, dyslipidemia, age greater than 40 years, being of African origin, and previous cardiac and cerebrovascular disease.

Most patients with PVD are initially asymptomatic. However, in some patients the early presenting symptom may be intermittent claudication. Classic intermittent claudication is only present in 10% of patients with PVD, and presents as exercise-induced pain; cramping; or discomfort in the hip, buttock, thigh, calf, or foot that is relieved with rest. One of the main differential diagnoses to be considered in vascular claudication is neurogenic claudication, which results from spinal compression caused by conditions such as spinal stenosis, herniated disc, and spondylolisthesis. The pain of neurogenic claudication results from ischemia and swelling of nerve roots at the site of compression. Neurogenic claudication can be differentiated from vascular claudication by the following features:

- Neurogenic claudication is more commonly bilateral.
- The pain associated with neurogenic claudication is relieved by bending over while walking.

■ The individual with neurogenic claudication who walks for a long time is able to walk shorter and shorter distances at the expense of longer and longer periods of rest. This is in contrast to the patient with vascular claudication, who can walk the same distance with equal rest periods in between.

The severity of the symptoms in vascular claudication is governed by the amount of stenosis, presence of collateral circulation, and vigor of exercise. The classification systems used to stage severity of disease are the Fontaine and the Rutherford systems, with the Fontaine system used more widely (**Table 10-1**). Stenoses in the arterial tree secondary to atherothrombosis are responsible for the underlying pathophysiology of this disease. As the disease advances, the resistance in the vascular system increases, and the system is unable to provide oxygenation to the muscles, especially during exercise. This results in claudication, ischemia, ulceration, and eventual loss of limb if left untreated.[2] Skeletal muscle ischemia affects muscle metabolism with the accumulation of lactate and intermediates of oxidative metabolism (acylcarnitines). This in turn causes muscle deterioration, denervation, and atrophy.[3] Chronic ischemia leads to ulceration and gangrene. Pain resulting from ulcers and gangrene is caused by ischemic neuropathy and necrosis of the sensory nerves at the site of the lesion. Severe necrosis of the sensory nerves can paradoxically make gangrenous lesions insensate and anesthetic.

Investigations

In the initial stages of PVD clinical history and physical examination are generally unreliable, with the diagnosis being missed more than 90% of the time based on these two factors alone. To make an early diagnosis of PVD, measurement of the ankle-brachial index (ABI) is helpful. The ABI is a ratio of the systolic blood pressure in the ipsilateral dorsalis pedis and posterior tibial arteries to that in the brachial artery (higher of bilateral brachial pressures), measured with a handheld continuous wave Doppler in the supine position. Normal ABI ranges between 1.0 and 1.3. An ABI <0.9 is 95% sensitive and 100% specific for PVD. Angiograms completed in these patients show more than 50% stenosis in one or more major blood vessels.[4] The lower the ABI score, the more severe the PVD, with ABI <0.4 representing advanced ischemia. Segmental limb pressure, segmental volume plethysmography, duplex ultrasonography, computed tomography (CT) angiography, and magnetic resonance (MR) angiography are additional modalities for evaluation of the level and extent of disease (**Fig. 10-1**).

The goals of treatment for patients with PVD are to relieve claudication, improve walking capacity, and improve quality of life. Initial management of PVD includes modification of risk factors such as smoking cessation, glycemic control, blood pressure normalization, and dyslipidemia management. Exercise rehabilitation has also been shown to be beneficial in reducing the symptoms of intermittent claudication by improving collateral circulation and thus improving functional status. Medical treatment of PVD

Table 10-1: Fontaine Classification of PAD	
Stage	**Clinical**
I	Asymptomatic
IIa	Mild claudication
IIb	Moderate-severe claudication
III	Ischemic rest pain
IV	Ulceration or gangrene

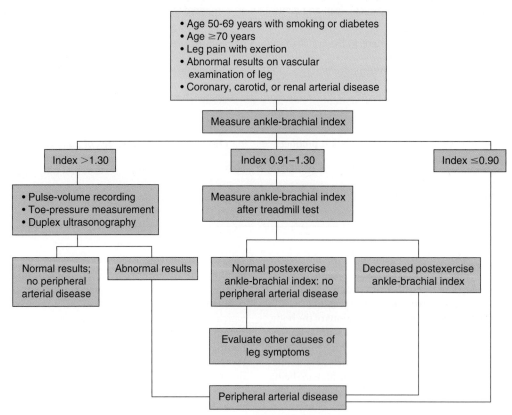

Fig. 10-1 Evaluation of patients with suspected peripheral vascular disease. Adapted from Hiatt WR et al.: Medical treatment of peripheral arterial disease and claudication, *N Engl J Med* 344:1608, 2001. Copyright 2001 Massachusetts Medical Society.

includes antiplatelet and vasodilatory drugs. Revascularization is indicated when ischemic pain is severe, indicated by disabling claudication that prevents the patient from performing daily activities of living, rest pain, ischemic ulcers, or gangrene. Amputation is indicated in approximately 5% of patients with nonreconstructible critical limb ischemia and extensive tissue necrosis or life-threatening infection.[5]

Spinal cord stimulation (SCS) was first shown to be effective in relieving claudication symptoms and increasing blood flow to lower extremities by Cook and associates[6] in 1976, who were using SCS to treat limb pain in patients with multiple sclerosis. During the late 1980s to early 1990s, the use of SCS as an alternative treatment measure for PVD rapidly advanced, especially in Europe. Currently SCS is the most promising neuromodulatory treatment for ischemic pain, and the overall beneficial effects last for at least 1 year in 80% of patients and for up to 5 years in 60% of patients.[7] The beneficial effects of SCS in the treatment of ischemic pain include pain relief, ulcer healing, decreased oxygen requirement, and increased claudication distance.

Basic Science

There are no established animal models with PVD that give rise to ischemic pain. Therefore normal Sprague-Dawley rats are used for research into the mechanisms of action of SCS for PVD. These rats are used to study acute changes in peripheral blood flow during SCS. SCS intensity in the rat is determined by the motor threshold (MT), which is the stimulation required for muscle contraction to be observed. Experimental SCS is performed at 30%, 60%, 90%, and 300% of MT. Stimulation at 30% MT is the minimum stimulus that produces vasodilation, with 60% MT being the level that approximates the stimulation parameters in clinical applications in humans. SCS at the upper lumbar spinal segments such as L2-L3 produces the largest increase in cutaneous blood flow in the lower limbs in the rat.[8] There are several proposed theories as to the mechanism of action of SCS in the treatment of PVD:

- With regard to pain control, the action of SCS falls back on the Wall-Melzack gate control theory of pain, which proposes that stimulation of large diameter afferent fibers such as those in the dorsal columns of the spinal cord would close notional gates in lamina V of the dorsal horn. This would prevent the ascent of impulses that mediate pain and that originate in small-diameter afferents from ascending to higher levels.[9] Relief from pain decreases the vasoconstriction that occurs as a reflex response.
- SCS-induced vasodilation occurs via suppression of sympathetic activity. The sympathetic nervous system causes vasoconstriction via stimulation of α_1- and α_2-adrenoreceptors. Linderoth, Herregodts, and Meyerson[10] observed that cutaneous vasodilation after SCS in the rat hind paw was eliminated by complete surgical sympathectomy. Administration of ganglionic blocker, hexamethonium, or neuronal nicotinic ganglionic blocker, chlorisondamine, had the same effect. High-dose adrenergic receptor blockers phentolamine and prazosin also suppressed SCS-induced vasodilation. Inhibition of vasodilation was not observed after administration of muscarinic receptor antagonists. However, there are conflicting data with the sympathetic mechanism because some patients demonstrate vasodilation with SCS even after chemical or surgical sympathectomy[11] and some incompletely sympathectomized rats in Linderoth, Herregodts, and Meyerson's study still retained the effects of SCS.

- The antidromic mechanism was first proposed by Bayliss in 1901,[12] who noted that dorsal root stimulation at high intensity induced peripheral vasodilation mediated by thin fibers. SCS antidromically activates afferent fibers in dorsal roots, causing the peripheral release of calcitonin gene-related peptide (CGRP), a powerful microvascular vasodilator. Since this time there has been intensive research into the types of fibers that mediate vasodilation and the vasodilators that are released during SCS. CGRP is found in small, myelinated $A\delta$ fibers and unmyelinated C fibers in dorsal root ganglia. By stimulating at various thresholds and blocking C-fiber conduction with the application of capsaicin, Tanaka and colleagues[13] determined that SCS-induced vasodilation at ≤60% MT is mediated by antidromic activation of myelinated fibers, whereas vasodilation at ≥90% is mediated by both myelinated and unmyelinated C-fibers.[13] Wu and associates[14] further characterized that SCS-induced vasodilation is predominantly mediated by those sensory fibers that contain transient receptor potential vanilloid-1 (TRPV1).[14]

Several vasodilators, including CGRP, are contained within the terminals of TRPV1 sensory nerve endings. Antidromic activation and depolarization of these nerve endings cause release of vasodilators into muscle tissue. CGRP is a potent vasodilator that is tenfold more powerful than prostaglandins and 100 to 1000 times more effective than other typical vasodilators such as acetylcholine, adenosine, and substance P.[15] CGRP binds to CGRP-1 receptor of smooth muscle cells and causes direct relaxation or can bind to CGRP-1 receptor of endothelial cells, which causes release of nitric oxide, which leads to vasodilation. Adrenomedullin is a peptide that co-localizes with CGRP in perivascular nerves and dorsal root ganglia and is involved with angiogenesis and endothelial protection.[8]

Despite the intense research into the mechanisms of action of SCS for the treatment of PVD, the theories are incompletely understood, and there is much more to explore. It is very likely that reduction in pain transmission, the sympathetic theory, and the antidromic theory act in concert to provide pain relief and vasodilation in patients suffering from PVD. The relative weight of one mechanism over another may depend on the patient's personal set of risk factors, sympathetic activity, and stimulation parameters. The mechanisms of SCS on the peripheral vascular system are summarized in **Fig. 10-2.**

Indications and Contraindications

General criteria for consideration of a spinal cord stimulator include[16]:

- Nonmalignant cause of pain.
- Failure of medical management.
- Remedial surgical procedure not feasible.
- Absence of a major psychiatric disorder, including somatization of symptoms.
- Elimination of inappropriate drug use before implantation.
- Absence of unresolved issues of secondary gain or litigation that potentially could be central to the propagation of the pain complaint.
- Capacity to give informed consent for the procedure.

SCS is considered specifically for PVD when critical limb ischemia becomes surgically nonreconstructible. Critical limb ischemia is defined as the presence of rest pain or tissue necrosis (ulceration or gangrene) with an ankle systolic pressure of ≤50 mm Hg or a

MECHANISMS OF SCS EFFECTS ON PERIPHERAL VASCULAR SYSTEM IN LIMBS AND FEET OF THE RAT MODEL

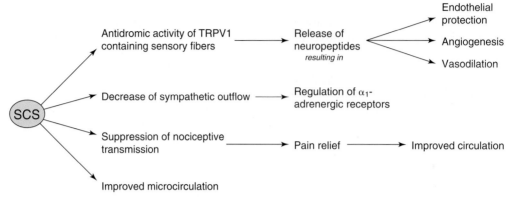

Fig. 10-2 Proposed mechanisms of action of spinal cord stimulation. *SCS,* Spinal cord stimulation; *TRPV1,* transient receptor potential vanilloid-1. From Wu et al: Putative mechanisms behind effects of spinal cord stimulation on vascular diseases: a review of experimental studies, *Autonomic Neurosci* 138:14, 2008.

toe pressure of ≤30 mm Hg. In patients in whom it is not possible to obtain pressure measurements, absence of lower-extremity pulsations on physical examination qualifies as selection criteria. Critical limb ischemia corresponds to Fontaine stages III and IV, in addition to the blood pressure criteria. Surgically nonreconstructible disease is characterized by ischemia in which angioplasty and bypass grafting is not possible, ABI <0.4, or great toe pressures <30 mm Hg. Patients being considered for SCS also must have ischemic rest pain that persists for more than 2 weeks.

SCS is not indicated in PVD for patients who have[17]:

- Ulcerations deeper than the fascia or gangrene with a diameter larger than 3 cm^2.
- Superimposed infections on ulcerations or gangrene.
- Co-morbid disease restricting life expectancy to less than a year.
- Presence of a cardiac pacemaker.
- Poor compliance caused by psychological or social incompetence.

Based on a critical review of available literature on the topic of SCS for PVD, Spincemaille and associates[18] have proposed an algorithm for successful patient selection. This has been adapted and modified (**Fig. 10-3**). The patient selection algorithm has not been tested by a randomized controlled trial.

Technique

SCS hardware consists of an electrode lead, an extension lead, and an implantable pulse generator. There are two main types of electrodes used:

- Cylindrical electrodes with multiple contact points can be introduced in the epidural space percutaneously using a Tuohy type needle. The commonly used percutaneous leads have four or eight contact points.
- Because of their larger size, surgical or paddle electrodes need a small laminotomy for the introduction into the epidural space. These electrodes also can have multiple contact points in various types of configurations. These electrodes can have 4, 8, or 16 contact points (**Fig. 10-4**).

The procedure for insertion of a cylindrical lead is performed in the operating room under sterile conditions with local anesthesia

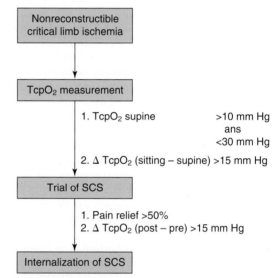

Fig. 10-3 Proposed selection criteria for patients considering treatment with SCS for PVD. Adapted from Spincemaille GH et al: The results of spinal cord stimulation in critical limb ischaemia: a review, *Eur J Vascular Endovascular Surg* 20:103, 2001.

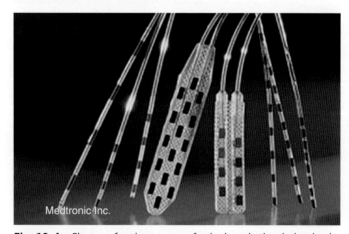

Fig. 10-4 Cluster of various types of spinal cord stimulation leads. Types of leads used may be percutaneous, quadripolar or octipolar, or a surgical paddle lead. These can be used for the treatment of peripheral vascular disease. Image provided courtesy of Medtronic Inc.

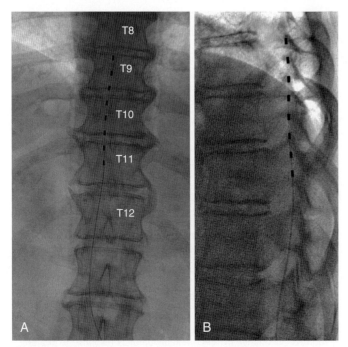

Fig. 10-5   A, Quadripolar percutaneous lead implanted in epidural space, in case of peripheral vascular disease, left leg, anteroposterior view. **B,** Lateral view.

supplemented by conscious sedation. Access to the epidural space is gained with a Tuohy needle, introduced either at L2-L3 or L4-L5 space. A paramedian approach is preferred over a midline approach. Entry into the epidural space is judged by loss of resistance technique and confirmed by taking a lateral x-ray film of the spine.

Positioning of the lead must be performed under fluoroscopic control with lead placement either in the midline if the pain is bilateral, or slightly off of midline to the symptomatic side (**Fig. 10-5**). Intraoperative stimulation is then carried out. The tip of the electrode position should be such that stimulation induces paresthesias. For best results the stimulation-induced paresthesias should cover the entire territory of the pain. Results may be less than satisfactory if stimulation covers <80% of pain territory. The Tuohy needle and the stylet of the electrode are removed, and the lead is then fixed into the deep fascia. For this purpose an anchoring device is used. The lead is then externalized, and a trial of stimulation is initiated. The trial period in North America usually lasts approximately 1 week. In certain European countries (e.g., Belgium) by law the trial must last for 4 weeks.

There is controversy in the literature whether or not a trial of stimulation is beneficial. An analysis of multiple pathologies treated with SCS showed that approximately 18% to 20% of patients fail trial stimulation in spite of the best efforts in selecting candidates for SCS therapy.[16] This emphasizes the importance of screening with trial stimulation before permanent implantation. This approach reduces the rate of failed permanent implants and improves cost-effectiveness. The trial stimulation also allows for a period of patient adjustment to stimulation-induced paresthesia and counseling by the neurosurgical team. The main disadvantages of this process are that it is an added procedure with associated costs and minimal risks such as root irritation, hematoma, or infection, which may add to the hospital stay.

If trial stimulation is successful in relieving at least 50% of pain and in improving microcirculatory status, the lead is internalized by connecting to a pulse generator, which is implanted

subcutaneously in the anterior abdominal wall or in the gluteal region in the area of the hip pocket below the belt line.

Effective stimulation parameters vary with each patient and can range from amplitudes between 1.5 and 6 V, frequencies of 55 to 60 Hz, and pulse widths of 210 to 300 ms. Stimulation can be performed continuously or with cyclical use to preserve the life of the pulse generator battery. Kumar and colleagues[19] found that optimal results were achieved with a cycling mode of 1 minute on, 2 minutes off.[19] With the advent of rechargeable pulse generators, this issue has been resolved. The new pulse generators also allow for multiple programming.

Patient Management and Evaluation

Several parameters are used to evaluate the efficacy of SCS for PVD. Improvements in macrocirculation can be measured by (1) Doppler peak blood flow velocities at the common femoral, popliteal, and dorsalis pedis arteries and the digital arteries in the great toe; (2) pulse volume recording at the midthigh, calf, foot, and big toe; (3) ABIs; and (4) claudication distance evaluated by walking on a treadmill with no incline at 2 miles/hr. Microcirculation is assessed using the transcutaneous partial pressure of oxygen ($TcpO_2$) over the dorsum of the foot with a portable oximeter. Improvement in circulation can also be monitored by documenting healing of ulcers and gangrene.

Pain relief is usually assessed using a visual analog scale and monitoring the patient's narcotic and nonnarcotic analgesic use.

Patients with spinal cord stimulators require lifelong evaluation to review the adequacy of pain relief and address concerns such as fractured or displaced electrodes, hardware malfunction, or exhausted battery life. Stimulation parameters may also require adjustment and refinement at follow-up appointments to better meet the patient's evolving pain experience.

Tolerance is defined as a progressive loss of efficacy in the presence of functional hardware. Gradual loss of pain control after a successful period is a multifactorial problem involving physiological, pathological, and psychological factors. Development of tolerance is most common in the first 2 years of implantation, but it can occur at any point in treatment. Tolerance remains a challenge to the maintenance of high rates of long-term success, regardless of early successful results. Tolerance may be caused by plasticity of pain pathways in the spinal cord, thalamus, or cortex. Fibrosis around the stimulating tip has also been implicated but has not been proven by autopsy or surgical exploration.

A review of the literature fails to provide an adequate explanation or guidance in treatment of tolerance. Stimulation "holidays" of up to 6 weeks have met with minimal success, and addition of adjuvant medications, such as amitriptyline or L-tryptophan, has also been met with equally poor results.[16]

Outcome Evidence

Outcome measures commonly evaluated in clinical studies include pain reduction, macrocirculatory and microcirculatory data, percentage of limb salvage, and clinical improvement in Fontaine classification.

Pain

Several studies show a marked decrease in pain symptoms following SCS (**Table 10-2**). In two separate randomized controlled trials by Spincemaille and associates[20] and Jivegard and colleagues,[21] pain relief is significantly better in the SCS group compared to nontreatment groups at 3 and 12 months. A critical review of the European

Table 10-2: Summary of Selected Articles

Author	Year	Study Type	Number of Patients	Follow-up Period	Conclusions
Augustinsson et al[30]	1985	Prospective study	34	15 months	SCS is very promising in severe limb ischemia when reconstructive surgery is impossible or has failed. The main benefit of SCS is pain relief.
Horsch and Claeys[31]	1994	Prospective study	177	35.6 months	A TcpO$_2$ increase of more than 50% within the first 3 months after implantation is predictive of success. TcpO$_2$ changes are correlated with the presence of adequate paresthesias in the painful area during trial stimulation.
Jivegard et al[21]	1995	Randomized-controlled trial, SCS vs. analgesics	51 26 control vs. 25 treatment	18 months	SCS provided long-term pain relief, but limb salvage at 18 months was not significantly improved by SCS in this rather small study. The results suggest that SCS may reduce amputation levels in patients with severe inoperable leg ischemia and be most effective in patients without arterial hypertension.
Claeys and Horsch[23]	1996	Randomized-controlled trial, SCS + PGE1 vs. PGE1	86	12 months	SCS is beneficial for lesion improvement in patients with nonreconstructible Stage IV PAD. TcpO$_2$ >10 mm Hg responds better to stimulation therapy.
Gersbach et al[25]	1997	Prospective study	20	14 months	Change in TcPO$_2$ reliably predicts response to SCS and may obviate the need for trial stimulation.
Kumar et al[19]	1997	Prospective study	46	21.2 months	Trial stimulation parameters of excellent pain relief combined with an increase in TcpO$_2$ of 10 mm Hg or greater and an increase in peak flow velocity of 10 mm or more give significant predilection for long-term success of SCS. SCS seems to be an efficacious treatment for arteriosclerotic peripheral vascular disease in certain patients who respond favorably to trial stimulation.
Klomp et al[28]	1999	Randomized-controlled trial, SCS + best medical treatment vs. best medical treatment	120	605 days	Adding SCS to best medical care does not prevent amputation in patients with critical limb ischemia. Pain was decreased significantly in both treatment groups at 1 month and 3 months (p <0.001) and did not differ between groups.
Ubbink et al[32]	1999	Randomized-controlled trial, SCS	111 55 control vs. 56 treatment	18 months	SCS possibly is beneficial in a subgroup of patients with chronic critical limb ischemia. The subgroup that might have profited from SCS had an intermediate skin microcirculatory perfusion and an amputation frequency half as high as in the standard group after 12 months. Microcirculatory investigations are worthwhile to screen the suitability of the patients and the effectiveness of the treatment.
Amann et al[26]	2003	Prospective controlled trial	112 41: SCS-Match 71: SCS-Failed stimulation and conservative treatment	18 months	SCS treatment of nonreconstructible critical leg ischemia provides a significantly better limb survival rate compared with conservative treatment when combined with appropriate patient selection using TcpO$_2$ and trial stimulation.

PAD, peripheral artery disease; *PGE1*, prostaglandin E1; *SCS*, spinal cord stimulation; *TcpO$_2$*, transcutaneous partial pressure of oxygen.

literature showed that 70% to 80% of patients achieve >75% of pain relief, which is lost with lead displacement, fracture, or depletion of the pulse generator battery, indicating that pain relief is unlikely a placebo effect.[22]

Macrocirculation

Kumar and associates[19] studied improvement in macrocirculation by measuring blood flow velocities, pulse volume recordings, claudication distance, and ABI. Blood flow velocities at the common femoral artery were most valid in patients with PVD who had undergone previous vascular surgery. In patient in whom SCS was a success, the blood flow velocity increased on average by 40.4 cm/second. The increase in blood flow velocity was directly proportional to increases in TcpO$_2$.

Pulse volume recording measurements showed significant improvements when all patients were considered. Pre-stimulation

Table 10-3: Microcirculation Data

Prospective Studies

Author	Mean Baseline TcpO$_2$ at Rest—Supine (mm Hg)	Mean Change in TcpO$_2$ at Last Follow-up (mm Hg)
Horsch	16	>12
Gersbach	19.5	>16
Kumar	>30	7.2
	<30	45.5
Amann	36	18.4

Randomized-Controlled Trials

Author	Mean Baseline TcPO$_2$ at Rest —Supine (mm Hg)	Percent Change in TcpO$_2$ at Last Follow-up
Claeys		
SCS	10	+213%
Control	11	−2%
Ubbink		
SCS	10	+70%
Control	9	0

Table 10-4: Limb Salvage Data

Author	Limb Survival (%)	Author	Limb Survival (%)
Horsch	66	Klomp	
Gersbach	63	*SCS*	55
Ubbink	60	*Control*	46
Jivegard		Amann	
SCS	62	*SCS*	78
Control	45	*Control*	45

pulse volume recording at the metatarsal and great toe was 5.9 and 2.5, respectively, which improved to 13.4 (p < 0.01) and 7.6 (p < 0.05) after stimulation. The subgroup of successful patients showed similar improvements, with prestimulation metatarsal and great toe pulse volume recordings of 5.6 and 2.8 and post-stimulation results of 13.1 (p < 0.05) and 8.2 (p < 0.05). Successful patients demonstrated an increase in claudication distance, but this difference was not statistically significant. ABI did not show any consistent change with stimulation.

Microcirculation

Since increased circulation is one of the most desirable and beneficial effects of SCS for the disease process, investigators measure improvement in microcirculation using TcpO$_2$. In a randomized controlled trial, Claeys and Horsch[23] compared SCS with optimal medical treatment (OMT) with prostaglandin. There was no significant difference between the initial mean value of TcpO$_2$ between SCS and OMT (10 vs. 11 mm Hg). At 12 months TcpO$_2$ was 21 vs. 11.4 mm Hg (p < 0.0001) between the SCS and OMT, respectively. An increase in TcpO$_2$ greater than 10 mm Hg was a predictor of long-term success. **Table 10-3** summarizes the results of several studies on the measurement of TcpO$_2$.

Limb Salvage

A meta-analysis on SCS for PVD by Ubbink and colleagues[24] revealed significant effects on limb salvage. Pooled results of all trials showed favorable results for SCS after 12 months. The calculated number needed to treat to prevent one major amputation was eight (CI$_{95}$% 5 to 25). Proper selection and screening of patients is helpful in predicting successful outcomes with respect to limb salvage. In the study by Gersbach and associates,[25] patients who had excellent pain relief and a change in TcpO$_2$ >15 mm Hg after 1 week of trial stimulation had an 83% rate of limb salvage vs. 63% for the overall patient population. Amann and associates[26] also found that SCS treatment of nonreconstructible critical leg

ischemia provides a significantly better limb survival rate compared with conservative treatment. Patient selected based on TcpO$_2$ and the results of trial screening further increased the probability of limb survival after SCS therapy. Individual data of several studies with respect to limb salvage is presented in **Table 10-4**.

Clinical Improvement

Using the Fontaine classification, SCS has been shown to improve a patient's clinical status. A number needed to treat analysis performed by Ubbink and colleagues[24] showed that one needs to treat three patients for one patient to improve to Fontaine stage II from Fontaine stage IV (CI$_{95}$% 2 to 5).

The most recent Cochrane review of 2009 analyzed six studies comprising nearly 450 patients.[27] The study concluded that limb salvage after 12 months was significantly higher in the SCS group (CI$_{95}$% 0.56 to 0.90). Pain relief was more impressive in the SCS group, and patients required significantly fewer analgesics. More patients reached Fontaine stage II in the SCS group than in the conservative group (CI$_{95}$% 2.0 to 11.9). Two studies reported on the healing of ischemic ulcers.[23,28] Claeys[23] found that SCS had a significantly better effect on wound healing than conservative treatment (p = 0.013). However, Klomp and Cochrane[28] pooled data showed no significant difference on ulcer healing between the two treatment groups.

Spinal Cord Stimulation for Nonatherosclerotic Peripheral Vascular Disease

SCS also has beneficial effects in the treatment of nonatherosclerotic PVD such as Buerger disease or Raynaud phenomenon. Unfortunately there are only a few published studies on this topic, and the studies do not have large samples of patients. In a prospective study by Donas and colleagues,[29] patients with Buerger disease received SCS treatment. Microcirculation was measured using the regional perfusion index (RPI), which is the ratio between the foot and chest transcutaneous oxygen pressure. Baseline RPI was recorded to be 0.27, which improved to 0.41 at 3 months, and was sustained at 1 and 3 years at 0.49 and 0.52, respectively. Limb survival rate was 93.1%. Claudication symptoms were also improved, and healing of trophic lesions was noted. Thus SCS can also be considered as an alternative treatment for patients with vascular disorders of nonatherosclerotic origin.

Little data are available in the literature with respect to SCS for Raynaud phenomenon, except for several case reports that report successful results.

Risk and Complication Avoidance

Complications with SCS are generally related to the hardware and are similar, regardless of the indication for treatment. In a retrospective analysis of 410 patients over a period of 22 years, Kumar, Hunter, and Demeria[16] found the following types and incidence of complications: displaced electrode (21.5%), fractured electrode (5.9%), other hardware malfunction (8.1%), subcutaneous hematomas (4.4%), infection (3.4%), cerebrospinal fluid leak (0.5%), rotation of the pulse generator (0.7%), and discomfort at the pulse generator site (1.2%). The most common fracture site was distal to the point of anchor where the lead exits from the deep fascia; a bend or kink is created at this point, increasing the stress on the lead. In cases of lead migration, the need for surgical revision is decreasing because of the use of octipolar leads and multichannel pulse generators.

Summary

SCS is currently the most promising neuromodulatory measure for the treatment of PVD. The mechanism of action behind SCS for PVD is still incompletely understood. The theories of reduction in pain transmission, sympathetic suppression, and antidromic activity likely act in concert to provide the beneficial effects of SCS.

Overall SCS has been shown to be an effective alternative for the treatment of nonreconstructible critical limb ischemia. SCS significantly improves pain, microcirculation, limb survival, and Fontaine clinical stage compared to conservative treatment. Selection of patients using improvement in $TcpO_2$ and pain relief during trial stimulation can further improve the success of SCS. However, there is no linear correlation between the degree of pain relief and improvement in $TcpO_2$. It appears that the use of SCS is more effective in patients with rest pain before ulceration takes place.

References

1. Aslam F et al: Peripheral arterial disease: current perspectives and new trends in management. *South Med J* 102:1141-1149, 2009.
2. Ouriel K: Peripheral arterial disease. *Lancet* 358:1257-1264, 2001.
3. Levy PJ: Epidemiology and pathophysiology of peripheral arterial disease. *Clin Cornerstone* 4:1-15, 2002.
4. Belch JJ et al: Critical issues in peripheral arterial disease detection and management: a call to action. *Arch Intern Med* 163:884-892, 2003.
5. Imparato AM et al: Intermittent claudication: its natural course. *Surgery* 78:795-799, 1975.
6. Cook AW et al: Vascular disease of extremities. electric stimulation of spinal cord and posterior roots. *NY State J Med* 76:366-368, 1976.
7. Deer TR, Raso LJ: Spinal cord stimulation for refractory angina pectoris and peripheral vascular disease. *Pain Physician* 9:347-352, 2006.
8. Wu M, Linderoth B, Foreman RD: Putative mechanisms behind effects of spinal cord stimulation on vascular diseases: a review of experimental studies. *Auton Neurosci* 138:9-23, 2008.
9. Melzack R, Wall PD: Pain mechanisms: a new theory. *Science* 150:971-979, 1965.
10. Linderoth B, Herregodts P, Meyerson BA: Sympathetic mediation of peripheral vasodilation induced by spinal cord stimulation: animal studies of the role of cholinergic and adrenergic receptor subtypes. *Neurosurgery* 35:711-719, 1994.
11. Jacobs MJ et al: Epidural spinal cord electrical stimulation improves microvascular blood flow in severe limb ischemia. *Ann Surg* 207:179-183, 1988.
12. Bayliss WM: On the origin from the spinal cord of the vasodilator fibers of the hind-limb and on the nature of these fibers. *J Physiol* 26:173-209, 1901.
13. Tanaka S et al: Role of primary afferents in spinal cord stimulation-induced vasodilation: characterization of fiber types. *Brain Res* 959:191-198, 2003.
14. Wu M et al: Sensory fibers containing vanilloid receptor-1 (VR-1) mediate spinal cord stimulation-induced vasodilation. *Brain Res* 1107:177-184, 2006.
15. Brain SD, Grant AD: Vascular actions of calcitonin gene-related peptide and adrenomedullin. *Physiol Rev* 84:903-934, 2004.
16. Kumar K, Hunter G, Demeria D: Spinal cord stimulation in treatment of chronic benign pain: challenges in treatment planning and present status, a 22-year experience. *Neurosurgery* 58:481-496, 2006.
17. De Vries J et al: Spinal cord stimulation for ischemic heart disease and peripheral vascular disease. *Adv Tech Stand Neurosurg* 32:63-89. 2007.
18. Spincemaille GH et al: The results of spinal cord stimulation in critical limb ischaemia: a review. *Eur J Vasc Endovasc Surg* 21:99-105, 2001.
19. Kumar K et al: Improvement of limb circulation in peripheral vascular disease using epidural spinal cord stimulation: a prospective study. *J Neurosurg* 86:662-669, 1997.
20. Spincemaille G et al: Spinal cord stimulation in patients with critical limb ischemia: A preliminary evaluation of a multicentre trial. *Acta Chir Austriaca* 32:49-51, 2000.
21. Jivegard LE et al: Effects of spinal cord stimulation (SCS) in patients with inoperable severe lower limb ischaemia: a prospective randomised controlled study. *Eur J Vasc Endovasc Surg* 9:421-425, 1995.
22. Claeys L: Spinal cord stimulation for peripheral vascular disease: A critical review—European series. *Pain Digest* 9:337-341, 1999.
23. Claeys LG, Horsch S: Transcutaneous oxygen pressure as predictive parameter for ulcer healing in endstage vascular patients treated with spinal cord stimulation. *Int Angiol* 15:344-349, 1996.
24. Ubbink DT et al: Systematic review and meta-analysis of controlled trials assessing spinal cord stimulation for inoperable critical leg ischaemia. *Br J Surg* 91:948-955, 2004.
25. Gersbach P et al: Discriminative microcirculatory screening of patients with refractory limb ischaemia for dorsal column stimulation. *Eur J Vasc Endovasc Surg* 13:464-471, 1997.
26. Amann W et al: Spinal cord stimulation in the treatment of nonreconstructible stable critical leg ischaemia: Results of the European peripheral vascular disease outcome study (SCS-EPOS). *Eur J Vasc Endovasc Surg* 26:280-286, 2003.
27. Ubbink DT, Vermeulen H: Spinal cord stimulation for non-reconstructable chronic critical leg ischaemia. *Cochrane Database Syst Rev* 004001, 2005.
28. Klomp HM et al: Spinal-cord stimulation in critical limb ischaemia: a randomised trial. ESES study group. *Lancet* 353:1040-1044, 1999.
29. Donas KP et al: The role of epidural spinal cord stimulation in the treatment of Buerger disease. *J Vasc Surg* 41:830-836, 2005.
30. Augustinsson LE et al: Epidural electrical stimulation in severe limb ischemia. pain relief, increased blood flow, and a possible limb-saving effect. *Ann Surg* 202:104-110, 1985.
31. Horsch S, Claeys L: Epidural spinal cord stimulation in the treatment of severe peripheral arterial occlusive disease. *Ann Vasc Surg* 8:468-474, 1994.
32. Ubbink DT et al: Microcirculatory investigations to determine the effect of spinal cord stimulation for critical leg ischemia: the Dutch multicenter randomized controlled trial. *J Vasc Surg* 30:236-244, 1999.

11 Spinal Cord Stimulation for Refractory Angina and Peripheral Vascular Disease

David Barrows and Sean Mackey

CHAPTER OVERVIEW

Chapter Synopsis: Electrical stimulation of the spinal cord (SCS) can provide pain relief and improve the underlying ischemic condition in certain indications, including angina and peripheral vascular disease (PVD). This chapter examines the ways that SCS can improve these conditions, which affect people in staggering numbers that are likely to climb in the coming years. SCS is indicated for angina that is refractory (i.e., it does not respond to pharmacological or mechanical therapies). Although SCS can improve cardiac vascularization and relieve the underlying ischemia, it is not a treatment for advanced cardiovascular disease. Evidence of success of SCS in patients with angina include a decreased need for short-acting oral nitrates, improved cardiac function, and improved quality of life. SCS reduces angina pain as it does in other indications according to the gate theory: by increasing stimulation of Aβ fibers, competing pain signaling from nociceptors is reduced. It also appears that SCS causes release of several biologically active substances in the periphery that can decrease pain and reduce the underlying ischemia, notably including β-endorphin. SCS also seems to improve ischemic conditions by affecting microcirculation within the heart, although these mechanisms have not been entirely elucidated. This may be achieved by redirecting blood flow or oxygen demand via manipulation of intracardiac neurons (ICNs). Patient selection and technical considerations can improve the chances of success of SCS in treatment of refractory angina. The chapter provides further considerations for SCS in the treatment of PVD.

Important Points:

- Stable angina typically arises during physical or emotional stress secondary to severe stenotic lesions affecting more than 70% of the affected coronary artery lumen of one or more arteries that causes myocardial ischemia. Unstable angina involves acute formation of a thrombosis within an already stenotic coronary vessel, which may or may not immediately lead to a myocardial infarction. Refractory angina (RA) is marked by severe chronic chest pain for more than three months secondary to coronary insufficiency; it occurs in patients who have failed to obtain or undergo appropriate control via other modalities including medical therapy, percutaneous revascularization, and CABG, yet who continue to have a reversible ischemia.

- Patients who are unlikely candidates for SCS include patients with RA, who typically have failed either percutaneous coronary interventions (PCIs), CABG, or who have not been candidates for either procedure because of poor coronary anatomy, prior surgical repairs not amenable to further manipulation, impaired left ventricular function, co-morbid noncardiac disease compounding their cardiovascular status, or advanced age.

- Before choosing SCS as a treatment modality, the patient must be properly assessed according to various diagnostic algorithms, ideally ones that have been standardized. The evaluation team must include at a minimum the following specialists: a pain physician and/or a neurosurgeon, an anesthesiologist, a cardiologist, and a psychologist.

- Although pain relief and limb salvage are the primary goals of SCS in PVD, careful patient selection must be undertaken to maximize the likelihood of success, while minimizing inappropriate use of the device and health care resources.

Clinical Pearls:

- Patients who develop unstable angina after SCS implantation will manifest angina that breaks through the SCS-imposed pain relief. Increased mortality with SCS in patients with RA has not been observed in several studies, thus indicating that the use of this device is safe in this patient population.

- SCS use has not demonstrated any arrhythmogenic effects leading to adverse coronary events. Secondarily, the observed perceived decrease in arrhythmogenic events may be related to decreased ischemia with the use of SCS.

- Prior to implanting a SCS it is absolutely imperative that all causes of angina, both intrinsic and extrinsic, be ruled out prior to labeling a patient with RA.

- Be aware that RA may be not only secondary to a lack of medical, procedural, or surgical options, but also secondary to a patient that is in a location where such options are not available or the patient chooses not to partake in them.

- The key to successful employment of a SCS relies on a multidisciplinary approach to these complex patients, whether they have RA or PVD with CLI. For those with RA it is critical that the cardiologist and pain physician maintain excellent communication first to determine feasibility and then to optimize the complex cardiac patient prior to implantation of the SCS.

Introduction

As technologies and research into the treatment of cardiovascular disease and peripheral vascular disease (PVD) advance, applications of treatment regimens not only reduce morbidity and mortality, but they also can lead to undesirable, unintentional consequences—the development of a population of patients who no longer respond to the therapies that initially prolonged their lives, increased their functional capacity, or increased their quality of life. Neuromodulation via spinal cord stimulation (SCS) may be a partial answer to the challenge being faced for patients with refractory angina (RA) or irreparable PVD. It has not been Food and Drug Administration (FDA)–approved for use in either RA or PVD as of yet in the United States. Originally used to treat a patient with cancer pain by Shealy, Mortimer, and Reswick in 1967,[1] SCS therapy has been extended to many other areas with varying amounts of success. Not everyone is a candidate for this technique. But appropriately screened patients who meet appropriate diagnostic and psychological criteria may benefit from SCS, which may alleviate chronic pain while adding an anti-ischemic benefit so patients' quality of life and functional capacity improve.

This chapter discusses RA in its first section and PVD in its second. After the section on epidemiology, each section contains these parts: establishing diagnosis, anatomy, indications, basic science mechanisms, guidelines, equipment and techniques, outcomes, and complications. Ideally this chapter will provoke further thought and research into this novel application of neuromodulation, leading to eventual FDA approval for using SCS in RA and expanded use in PVD.

Epidemiology: Coronary Artery Disease and Peripheral Vascular Disease

Coronary artery disease (CAD) remains the number one cause of morbidity and mortality in the United States, yet the prevalence of RA in the population has not been well-defined in the literature. Several estimates have been proposed. According to the American Heart Association's Heart Disease and Stroke Statistics—2010 Update, approximately 10.2 million people suffer from angina pectoris. Currently the annual incidence is estimated to be approximately 500,000.[2] In 1999 Mukherjee and associates[3] attempted to estimate the incidence of RA. Their approximation of 12% of the total population of those with angina is based on the percentage of people undergoing angiography at tertiary referral centers who ultimately are not eligible for percutaneous or coronary artery bypass graft (CABG) revascularization procedures.[3] This percentage is also endorsed by Mannheimer and associates,[4] who remarked on the paucity of data but noted that one study they reviewed had a prevalence of 5% to 15% of the population as having RA. In 2002 Holmes[5] noted that approximately 2.4 million people in the United States suffer from CAD untreatable by either percutaneous revascularization or CABG. With a large and ever-expanding population, the demand for novel treatments will certainly climb. This demand will undoubtedly be mirrored in the population that suffers from PVD.

PVD likely affects more than 10 million people in the United States according to Vallejo et al estimates in 2006, and it affects 12% to 20% of the population aged 65 and older.[6] Of the people who develop PVD with signs of intermittent claudication, approximately 20% are believed to develop chronic critical limb ischemia (CLI); 25% of CLI sufferers require an amputation.[7] The mortality for this population also is quite high, ranging from 25% to 30% at 2 years and increasing to 50% to 75% at 5 years after the onset of CLI. Although the amputation rate and mortality are significant in this subpopulation, the implementation of SCS shows promise in alleviating some of the suffering and morbidity and mortality of this disease.

Establishing Diagnosis: Angina and Role of Spinal Cord Stimulation

An imbalance between myocardial oxygen delivery and its consumption rapidly results in ischemic conditions within the heart that may progress to infarction if not corrected. This imbalance may or may not be associated with symptoms of angina pectoris because some patients develop silent ischemia. Besides being a harbinger of a potentially serious condition, angina not only presents significant acute or chronic discomfort, but it also typically causes psychological stress that may impact a person's quality of life and functionality.

As defined by the American Heart Association in 1999,[8] angina comprises a clinical syndrome of pain and discomfort in the chest, jaw, shoulder, back, or arm that may be exacerbated by physical exertion or emotional stress. Although angina typically is associated with CAD involving the epicardial vessels and subsequent ischemia, a more robust differential diagnosis of angina must be considered from both a cardiac and noncardiac standpoint. Cardiovascular origins of angina may also include valvular heart disease, severe hypertension, hypertrophic cardiomyopathies, acute aortic dissection, acute pericarditis, severe aortic stenosis, coronary vasospasm, and cardiac syndrome X (CSX).[8-10] CSX patients present similarly to those with CAD-related angina. Although patients with CSX tend to feel pain with exertion and their electrocardiograms (ECGs) may show ST-segment depression during exercise stress tests that induce angina, these patients do not have signs of obvious CAD on angiography; in fact, in some patients, evidence suggests that ischemia may not be a causative factor.[11] Proposed mechanisms for CSX include estrogen deficiency, abnormal function and distribution of adenosine receptors, and coronary microvascular dysfunction.[9,11,12] Noncardiac origins of chest pain include trauma and esophageal conditions, including reflux and motility disorders, biliary colic, costochondritis, and pulmonary embolism or pulmonary hypertension.

In addition, angina may be classified as *stable* or *unstable*. *Stable angina* typically arises during physical or emotional stress secondary to severe stenotic lesions affecting more than 70% of the affected coronary artery lumen of one or more arteries that causes myocardial ischemia.[13] Conversely, *unstable angina* involves acute formation of a thrombosis within an already stenotic coronary vessel, which may or may not immediately lead to a myocardial infarction (MI). Unstable angina is of greatest concern since it predicts an elevated short-term risk of a cardiac event[8] and necessitates immediate coronary revascularization to alleviate. Unstable angina is beyond the scope of this chapter; however, episodes of unstable angina pain manifest even in patients with spinal cord stimulators for RA, as discussed in the following paragraphs.

To improve clinical classification of angina, the Canadian Cardiovascular Society (CCS)[8,14] modified the New York Heart Association's (NYHA) Functional Classification (**Box 11-1**). Campeau and Letter[14] developed four classes—I through IV. In class I angina patients perceive angina only with strenuous activity. Class II patients experience only slight limitation of activity secondary to

angina. Class III patients experience marked limitation of normal activity, and in class IV they experience angina with any activity, including being at rest. MI falls within classes III and IV.

RA is marked by severe chronic chest pain for more than 3 months secondary to coronary insufficiency; it occurs in patients who have failed to obtain or undergo appropriate control via other modalities, including medical therapy, percutaneous revascularization, and CABG, yet who continue to have a reversible ischemia.[9,15,16] RA occurs when all reversible causes for ischemia have been ruled out. SCS has been used successfully to target RA—decreasing the frequency and severity of the episodes and improving patient functionality and quality of life.

Anatomy: Pain Pathway for Angina

Signals for angina pain are initiated at both the chemosensitive and mechanoreceptive nociceptors in the adventitia of the coronary arteries and myocardium.[16] Because the majority of these nerves are slow-conducting C fibers, the predominant pain experienced is of a dull, aching, heavy, and squeezing type.[8] Aδ fibers that carry stabbing and sharp pain are typically not involved in angina. On their activation these nociceptors release a variety of chemical mediators, including adenosine, bradykinin, prostaglandins, and others, which initiate signals in the sympathetic and parasympathetic (vagal) afferent pathways to dorsal spinal cord and parasympathetic ganglia located from C7 to T5.[17,18] The pain experienced by the patient during an episode of angina is related to the convergence of common pathways at the dorsal spinal cord between C7 and T5, where afferent myocardial inputs and cutaneous nociceptors converge on the same interneurons at the same level within the spinal cord.[16] Thus the pain perceived by the patient is distributed within the dermatome from where the cutaneous afferents converge on the same spinal segment as from the heart.

Indications: Spinal Cord Stimulation and the Alternative Therapies Available for Refractory Angina

As previously mentioned, neuromodulation has treated RA successfully; however, before choosing SCS as a treatment modality, the patient must be properly assessed, and all other modalities pursued. SCS provides analgesia and anti-ischemic effects, but it does not cure advanced cardiovascular disease. This section briefly reviews therapies for angina and establishes a framework within which SCS should be considered as an alternative.

As medical, interventional, and operative treatment modalities for angina and occlusive vascular disease have developed along with an aging population, so has the portion of the population with angina that lacks viable options for further improvement, despite optimization from one of the novel or improved therapies. This subgroup contains patients with RA who typically have failed either percutaneous coronary interventions (PCIs) or CABG, or who have not been candidates for either procedure because of poor coronary anatomy, prior surgical repairs not amenable to further manipulation, impaired left ventricular function, co-morbid noncardiac disease compounding their cardiovascular status, or advanced age.[19,20] Jolicoeur and associates[19] also mentioned that a person with RA may fall into the category of "nonrevascularization" secondary to either their geographical location where practitioners may not have the expertise or the patients lack of interest in pursuing a particular therapeutic path.

Multiple pharmacological and nonpharmacological (mechanical intervention) therapies for RA are reviewed in the following

---

Box 11-1: Grading of Angina of Effort by the Canadian Cardiovascular Society

I. "Ordinary physical activity does not cause ... angina," such as walking and climbing stairs. Angina with strenuous, rapid, or prolonged exertion at work or recreation.

II. "Slight limitation of ordinary activity." Walking or climbing stairs rapidly; walking uphill; or walking or stair climbing after meals, in cold or wind, under emotional stress, or only during the few hours after awakening. Walking more than two blocks on the level and climbing more than one flight of ordinary stairs at a normal pace and in normal conditions.

III. "Marked limitation of ordinary physical activity." Walking one to two blocks on the level and climbing one flight of stairs in normal conditions and at normal pace.

IV. "Inability to carry on any physical activity without discomfort—angina syndrome *may be* present at rest."

From Campeau L: Letter: Grading of angina pectoris, *Circulation* 54(3):13, 1976.

paragraphs. The reviews are based primarily on Jolicoeur and colleagues' report of the working group on clinical and research issues regarding chronic advanced CAD.[19] Although their reviews are not comprehensive, they highlight the current management options for RA.

Pharmacological agents mitigate angina symptoms by a variety of mechanisms so the patient has reduced myocardial oxygen demand and increased supply via a reduction in heart rate (HR), decreased afterload, and decreased contractility. Agents with antianginal properties that are helpful in accomplishing these changes include β-blockers, nitrates, calcium channel blockers, and opioids. Each provides angina relief via different mechanisms, but each is not without side effects that lead to dose limitation or intolerance. Antithromboembolic agents such as aspirin and clopidogrel (Plavix) target the platelets; whereas antihyperlipidemics such as statins promote vessel patency, thus decreasing risk for myocardial ischemia and resultant angina. Ranolazine (Ranexa) is a relatively new drug with direct antianginal and anti-ischemic properties. A debate as to its mechanism of action exists; however, it permits an increase in exercise performance without changing HR or blood pressure.[21] In addition, ranolazine improves angina and exercise threshold when used as a monotherapy and in combination with more traditional therapies listed previously.[21,22]

Mechanical interventions are also available for RA: percutaneous stent placement, transmyocardial laser revascularization, and CABG. Despite these interventions, people continue to have angina symptoms, and some people are not candidates for such therapies. Chronic total occlusion (CTO) recanalization via the percutaneous approach has been conducted after the development of chronic occlusions (greater than 3 months) with a substantial improvement in 10-year survival.[19] The reported success of revascularization achieved by CTO recanalization remains a stable 71% despite attempts at canalizing longer lesions, whereas reported complications of the procedure range from 3.8% to 5.1%.[23-25] Technical advances may eventually make this technique more effective and safe.[19]

Another mechanical technique sometimes used is enhanced external counterpulsation (EECP), approved by the FDA in 1995 for angina. In EECP three bilateral lower extremity cuffs are inflated sequentially during diastole to provide increased venous return and diastolic augmentation.[26] Currently this technique requires 35 consecutive days of 1-hour sessions to show some lasting benefit of decreased angina symptoms and a longer time to greater-than–1-mm ST depression on an exercise stress test.[26] EECP has not been studied in a large, randomized controlled setting; and it has side effects, including edema, bruising, and pain in the lower extremities. According to Soran and associates,[27] patients undergoing EECP noted a substantial improvement in the quality of life; 72% improved from severe to mild or moderate angina, 52% stopped nitroglycerin use, and at 2 years 55% of the patients reported a maintained decrease in their angina.

Before choosing SCS as a treatment modality for RA, the patient must be properly assessed according to various diagnostic algorithms, ideally ones that have been standardized. One such algorithm for assessing a person's appropriateness for SCS was proposed by the European Society of Cardiology.[20] First a team of cardiologists and cardiac surgeons should determine if a patient's angina is of ischemic origin and evaluate him or her for revascularization. A recent angiogram should be used to rule out newly treatable coronary pathology. In addition, all other forms of chest pain should be eliminated. For example, the differential diagnosis of chest pain should include noncardiac origins of chest pain, including esophageal pain, gastroesophageal reflux, musculoskeletal pain,

costochondritis, anemia, uncontrolled hypertension, atrial fibrillation, and thyroid disorder.[19,20] Once these criteria have been met, the patient's medical therapy must be optimized. After an appropriate diagnosis has been established and subsequent medical and surgical optimization has occurred, the focus shifts to psychological evaluation to determine if the patient's perception of pain has a significant co-morbidity of depression or anxiety that should be treated before SCS implantation or if the person should be evaluated on the basis of compliance with other treatments. Finally, risk factor management and cardiac rehabilitation must continue.

Basic Science: Mechanism of Action of SCS for Angina

SCS for angina enables both antianginal and anti-ischemic effects to be integrated to achieve pain relief. The severity of the angina decreases; and cardiac function improves, as evidenced by the following: decreased need for short-acting oral nitrates and 24-hour cardiac monitoring and markers of functional status and increased perceived quality of life.[28] Multiple mechanisms have been proposed to explain these effects, a number of which are outlined here. NOTE: What follows is not an exhaustive review of the literature on this topic.

Given the benefits of the antianginal and anti-ischemic effects of SCS, one should also consider its safety for patients with RA. An early concern was that SCS could mask angina pain associated with myocardial ischemia and eliminate a patient's subjective sensation of RA. This concern has not been borne out in several studies.[28] Instead, SCS merely raises the patient's threshold for sensing angina, thus permitting the patient to increase exercise capacity. Investigators have not noted any resultant increase in morbidity and mortality with SCS.

The following mechanisms have been suggested.

Direct Suppression of Pain

The antianginal effect of the SCS may be caused by direct suppression of pain. According to the gate control theory proposed by Melzack and Wall in 1965,[29] fast-conducting myelinated A fibers modulate slow-conducting unmyelinated C fibers via a negative feedback mechanism at the level of the dorsal horn of the spinal cord. Thus applying neuromodulation techniques to the dorsal column of the spinal cord at the level where input from nociceptors occurs inhibits signals ultimately responsible for achieving the decreased sensation of pain. The electricity of the SCS provides a continuous, selective, low-level activation of the sensitive afferent A fibers, which in turn inhibits the Aδ and C fibers of nociception presynaptically.[9] Chandler and associates'[30] support of this mechanism comes in their studies of SCS on anesthetized monkeys. They demonstrated that SCS of the dorsal column decreased the output of spinothalamic tract neurons that were triggered by electrical stimulation of cardiac sympathetic afferent fibers with sensory endings in the ventricles. These spinothalamic tract cells also received somatic input from the chest and upper extremities; this type of input is also blocked with SCS. Chandler and associates[30] also demonstrated that intracardiac injection of bradykinin, which duplicates the effects of either cardiac sympathetic or somatic nociception, is blocked by the use of an SCS.[30] What was not resolved was whether suppression of the spinothalamic tract is a direct effect or a decrease in information from nociceptive afferent.[31]

Molecular Mechanism

More recently a molecular mechanism leading to reduced angina has been investigated. Excitatory amino acids involved in transmitting signals within the dorsal horn include glutamate and aspartate. The release of these neurotransmitters has been shown to decrease in the presence of elevated gamma aminobutyric acid (GABA) that occurs during neuromodulation of the dorsal horn.[32] Cui and associates[32] further pointed out that this observed effect was transiently reversed with the addition of a GABA β-receptor antagonist placed at the dorsal horn. In addition, Oldroyd and colleagues[33] found that β-endorphins are released from the pituitary in response to myocardial ischemia.[33] The significance of these findings is that β-endorphins may participate in pain reduction through their action as endogenous opioids. In addition, β-endorphins may affect the regulation locally at the level of the myocardium by directly aiding in decreased oxygen consumption.[34] According to Eliasson and associates,[34] β-endorphin release at the myocardium increased with the use of SCS during conditions of rest and during pacing to angina in humans. They suggest that the data be interpreted cautiously since they conducted their study by applying an accepted method of evaluation of myocardial ischemia involving the myocardial lactate extraction ratio and using it to look at myocardial turnover of peptides. While conducting the study, they derived a wide range of individual values.[34] Thus one current hypothesis suggests that SCS promotes release of biologically active molecules that may have both direct and indirect effects on angina pain and myocardial ischemia.

Central Nervous System Mechanism

A central mechanism of pain control may be triggered by the use of neuromodulation. According to Eckert and Horstkotte,[16] functional neuroimaging has been used to examine areas of cerebral blood flow in patients with known CAD. In such patients angina and ECG changes are elicited by dobutamine infusion. According to Hautvast and colleagues,[35] dynamic positron emission tomography (PET) scans during such periods of chemically induced ischemia demonstrated areas of varying regional cerebral blood flow. When using SCS, Zonenshayn and associates[36] noticed corresponding changes of increase and decrease in cerebral blood flow during periods with and without stimulation, respectively. Eckert and Horstkotte[16] pointed out that, when they examined the two groups, they saw similarities in increased cerebral blood flow to the hypothalamus bilaterally and the periaqueductal grey area, and decreased cerebral blood flow in the posterior insular cortex that modulates sympathetic nervous system (SNS) activity. Thus SCS may be influencing pain perception and processing in the central nervous system. These findings suggest that the thalamus may be acting as a filter for afferent pain signals.

Anti-Ischemic Mechanisms

It is important to recognize that the antianginal benefits of SCS are enhanced by its anti-ischemic effect as demonstrated by improvements in patients' ECGs during stress testing and 24-hour Holter monitoring. In addition, by decreasing their subjective experience of angina, patients can exercise more, thus improving cardiac conditioning. This suggestively leads to the benefits of improved functionality and quality of life. As with antianginal mechanisms, several mechanisms have been proposed for anti-ischemic effects as well.

One hypothesis to explain this decreased ischemia suggests that coronary blood flow (CBF) is redistributed to areas of poor perfusion, likely secondary to collateral flow.[28] It has been suggested that SCS improves myocardial perfusion via vasodilation of microvessels within the myocardium, alleviating angina pain in patients who continue to have a small amount of coronary reserve, despite the ischemia. SCS may eliminate this reserve. Many techniques (i.e., intracoronary pressure and flow measurements, stress echo, myocardial scintigraphy, and PET scanning) have been attempted to evaluate possible mechanisms to explain why the SCS has an anti-ischemic effect, but they have not been entirely successful in elucidating such mechanisms. These techniques may not be able to fully identify the changes in microcirculation that result in decreased angina symptoms.[16]

The ability of neuromodulation to promote blood flow change remains controversial since evidence is lacking and somewhat contradictory. Mobilia and associates[37] used PET to evaluate CBF and suggested that the SCS promoted increased CBF and allowed for redistribution from areas of high and low flow.[37] SCS promotion of increased CBF was contradicted by Norrsell and colleagues[38] who demonstrated an anti-ischemic effect independent of CBF velocity. Studies on dogs with normal hearts did not show an increase in local flow or a redistribution.[39] Wu, Linderoth, and Foreman[31] also point out that long-term use of SCS has been shown to decrease myocardial ischemia, perhaps because of better coronary collateralization secondary to increased physical activity of the patients.[31]

Remodeled Neural Pathways

The myocardium contains intracardiac neurons (ICNs) that are the primary integrators of the nervous system within the heart.[40] Neuromodulation with an SCS has been suggested to "remodel the neural pathways" by altering the firing rate of the intracardiac neurons and stabilizing their activity during ischemia.[41] Hypothetically decreases in angina secondary to SCS allow patients to increase and prolong their exercise. Initially SCS was believed to modulate the sympathetic branch of the SNS with respect to the perception of pain; however, this is likely not the case because there is no change in HR variability or in epinephrine and norepinephrine metabolism.[28] Instead it is hypothesized that SCS acts on the myocardium via the ICNs to permit a redistribution of blood flow from the areas of normal perfusion to areas of ischemia.[42] Speculation exists as to how this blood flow redistribution occurs. Possibilities include angiogenesis, collaterals, and preconditioning.

Intrinsic Cardiac Nervous System

Another working hypothesis suggests that the SCS neuromodulates the intrinsic cardiac nervous system. Wu, Linderoth, and Foreman[31] witnessed decreased magnitude of ST-changes in the ECG and decreased risk for development of arrhythmias secondary to ischemia in patients with functioning SCSs.[31] The intrinsic cardiac nervous system is comprised of parasympathetic and sympathetic efferent nerves, sensory afferents, and interconnecting local neurons. It resides in the cardiac ganglion plexi of the pericardial fat pads near and within the myocardium.[43] According to Armour,[40] these neurons interact both locally and regionally, which allows "reflex coordination" of autonomic neuronal outflow to the heart. It is important to note that SCS effects are blocked by stellectomy.[44] Wu, Linderoth, and Foreman[31] point out that SCS is believed to stabilize the activity of the intrinsic cardiac nervous system typically activated by ischemia.

In addition, it has been shown that SCS has decreased pain and O_2 consumption in similar HRs in atrial-paced studies.[45] Those who develop myocardial ischemia will still experience angina with a quality and distribution similar to that of their original symptoms.[9] There has been no demonstrated arrhythmogenic effect associated with SCS.[46] Furthermore, the perceived decrease in arrhythmic events may be secondary to the decreased myocardial ischemia from the use of the SCS. This observation may also be associated with the hypothesis that the SCS stabilizes the intracardiac neurons so the chance for an arrhythmic event is lessened as noted previously.

Early work by Mannheimer and colleagues[47] suggested that SCS does not manifest changes at rest; instead, under conditions of stress, its effects occur. It has been proposed that SCS does not decrease cardiac sympathetic activity, leading to its anti-ischemic effect. Instead, it has been suggested that SCS globally decreases SNS activity, which leads to a decreased oxygen demand.[45] According to Mannheimer and colleagues[47], the total body norepinephrine spillover, but not that of the myocardium, was reduced, suggesting that SCS affects global sympathetic activity. During stress the SCS can lower HR, which counters the increase in activity in the intrinsic nervous system that would otherwise lead to dysrhythmias.[48] This activation of the intrinsic neurons leads to changes in the system that persist after cessation of the SCS, which suggests that a remodeling exists that may limit the excitatory input induced by ischemia.

Murray and colleagues[49] point out that 53% of those with RA responding to SCS have a history of sustaining a non-Q wave MI, whereas only 20% to 30% of all MIs are characterized by this.[49] These patients are unique because they survive despite severe CAD; consequently they have further problems such as RA. To account for the difference in non-Q wave MIs between the two groups, Ganz and Braunwald[50] note that these patients typically have severe CAD yet extensive collateral flow. This difference may reflect an advantage to this population, because subendocardial ischemia is believed to be aggravated by adenosine-mediated myocardial steal. Neuromodulation may promote the redistribution of myocardial blood flow from nonischemic to ischemic areas by reducing the adenosine-mediated steal phenomena.[49] Thus patients who respond well to SCS may be doing so via adenosine antagonism, whereby blood is drawn from the extensive collateral reservoir and shifted to areas of ischemia.

In summary, although much research has been conducted, the exact mechanism has yet to be fully elucidated. However, this fact does not preclude this modality from being a viable option for well-selected patients.

Guidelines: Patient Selection for Spinal Cord Stimulation in Refractory Angina

Careful consideration of a patient's candidacy for implantation involves a multidisciplinary approach to assess the patient's cardiovascular status and other issues typically faced with SCS implantation. The evaluation team must include at a minimum the following specialists: a pain physician and/or a neurosurgeon, an anesthesiologist, a cardiologist, and a psychologist.[28,51] De Vries and associates[28] suggest a series of inclusion and exclusion criteria to determine patients' suitability for SCS in RA (**Box 11-2**).

The cardiologist's evaluation is the most critical one, because the pain physician should operate under the assumption that the angina is not refractory until proven otherwise. The cardiologist evaluates the patient's cardiac status to determine whether the patient suffers from RA or a nonoptimized cardiac condition. If the cardiologist finds the patient to be an SCS candidate, he or she can also comment on the patient's cardiac stability in terms of blood pressure, ejection fraction, and other parameters that aid the anesthesiologist in determining the risk and tolerability for the patient to undergo anesthesia. The cardiologist's other significant contribution is to optimize the patient's drugs that impact bleeding, including aspirin, warfarin (Coumadin), and medications that alter platelet function[51] (**Table 11-1**). Use of blood thinners must be stopped secondary to the risk of surgical bleeding and, more important, the risk of epidural hematoma that may lead to paralysis. The cardiologist must determine the feasibility of stopping

---

Box 11-2: Inclusion and Exclusion Criteria: Spinal Cord Stimulation for Ischemic Heart Disease

Inclusion Criteria
1. Severe chest pain (New York Heart Association classes III-IV or visual analog scale score >7)
2. Optimal tolerated pharmacological therapy
3. Significant coronary artery disease (i.e., >1 stenosis of 75%)
4. Not eligible for percutaneous transluminal intervention or coronary artery bypass surgery
5. No prognostic benefit from surgical revascularization (according to guidelines)
6. Patient considered intellectually capable to manage the spinal cord stimulation device
7. No acute coronary syndrome during last 3 months

Exclusion Criteria
1. Myocardial infarction within the last 3 months
2. Uncontrolled disease such as hypertension or diabetes mellitus
3. Personality disorders or psychological instability
4. Pregnancy
5. Implantable cardioverter-defibrillator and pacemaker dependency
6. Local infections
7. Insurmountable spinal anatomy
8. Contraindication to withheld antiplatelet agents or warfarin
9. Addictive behavior

From De Vries J et al: Spinal cord stimulation for ischemic heart disease and peripheral vascular disease, *Adv Tech Stand Neurosurg* 32:71, 2007.

Table 11-1: Drug Recommendations

Drug	Recommendation
Warfarin	Off 3 days before implant with normal INR
Clopidogrel and similar drugs	10 days and until the trial lead is removed
Baby aspirin	Most physicians do not recommend stopping baby aspirin
Conventional aspirin and NSAIDs	Physician discretion

From Deer, T.R (ed): Spinal cord stimulation for the treatment of angina and peripheral vascular disease. *Curr Pain Headache Rep* 2009, pp. 20. *INR*, International normalized ratio; *NSAID*, nonsteroidal antiinflammatory drug.

---

these medications for the period of device implantation. The patient may remain on baby aspirin but should be off warfarin for a minimum of 3 days with an international normalized ratio (INR) check before the time of trial or implantation. Clopidogrel and associated drugs should be stopped for 10 days. If there is a question about continued alteration of platelet function caused by clopidogrel, a platelet function assay should be considered. Because placement of an SCS device is an elective procedure, the injunction, "Do no harm to the patient," takes precedence. If taking a patient off these medications causes excessive risk, the procedure should not be attempted. If it is a concern that the patient is off medications, he or she may be a candidate for hospital admission for initiation of heparin therapy, which may be stopped 6 hours before surgery and restarted 6 hours afterward. Low–molecular weight heparin should be avoided secondary to the increased risk of epidural bleeding after SCS lead placement for patients on this therapy.

Even if a patient is cleared from a cardiac standpoint, the implanting physician must evaluate him or her to determine tolerance for such a device, comprehension of its function, and understanding of how to use the available programs to self-treat. If the patient fails to understand the purpose and functionality of SCS, even after appropriate training, he or she should be excluded from implantation. Also important are the patient's expectations about pain relief. To avoid unrealistic expectations and eventual failure of SCS therapy, the physician should point out that the SCS technique may reduce but probably not eliminate the pain. In addition, a psychological evaluation is imperative to elucidate personality disorders or psychological barriers to having or using such a device.

Equipment and Technique for Spinal Cord Stimulation in Refractory Angina

With implantation of SCS in any patient, the most critical step is placement of the SCS leads at the proper level and location to achieve paresthesias over the area the patient experiences the angina. Typically the tip of the stimulator lead should be placed, under fluoroscopic guidance, at the C7 level in the dorsal epidural space since the afferent fibers are located from approximately T1 to T4. Most successful placement involves stimulation between T1 and T2.[46,48,52] For percutaneous placement the 14-gauge Tuohy needle usually used for insertion should be introduced at approximately the T4-T5 to T6-T7 levels, depending on the patient's anatomy. The further down the vertebral column a needle is introduced, the more difficult it may become to advance the percutaneous stimulator lead. Because the most common cause of failure is improper position of the stimulator electrode,[9,51] care should be taken to direct one stimulator lead slightly to the left of midline and one at midline to capture most of the angina pain.

Other considerations exist. One is whether the patient has a pacemaker; an automatic implantable cardioverter-defibrillator (AICD) is a contraindication to SCS. SCS compatibility with the pacemaker should be confirmed before implantation, and the pacemaker should be interrogated before and after implantation of the final device. Because of the acuity of this patient population, another consideration is how to trial the patient. If the patient requires titration on and off of blood thinners and/or has difficult lead placement, he or she may be a candidate for implanting trial leads so the leads don't have to be reintroduced if the trial is successful; instead the patient may go directly to generator placement. Deer[51] points out that no outcome studies have been published to elucidate a better trial technique.

Another consideration is careful review with the patient of pocket placement before implantation. Available sites include the low back above the beltline, buttock, lateral abdominal wall, and anterior chest wall on the right side, opposite to where a pacemaker would be placed. Patient involvement in the selection of the location is critical, not only to promote a sense of autonomy, but also because the patient's level of function and occupation may suggest the optimal location. From a practical standpoint an object of similar size and shape may be used to demonstrate the future presence of the device at a location and aid the patient in the decision process.

Outcomes for Spinal Cord Stimulation and Refractory Angina

Since SCS was introduced in 1987 as a treatment modality for RA, no large or long-term randomized controlled clinical trials have been conducted to examine its efficacy, likely because of the cost. Instead, several observational, retrospective, and small randomized

controlled trials (RCTs) have been done, each measuring different primary and secondary endpoints, excluding any common standardized outcome measures. In addition, as Mannheimer and associates[53] pointed out in their study, patients enrolled for SCS caused by RA must be considered in relation to the medical knowledge and technology at that time. Studies conducted over too long a period potentially lead to differences between early and late enrollees secondary to advancing surgical, interventional, and anesthetic techniques.[53]

Most of the outcomes literature comes from European studies, which focused on the following measures: exercise capacity, ischemic burden, nitrate drug consumption, functional class of angina, health-related quality of life, adverse events and SCS-related complications, cost, reduced frequency and severity of angina, change in pain scores, sleep, and morbidity and mortality. To put many of these outcome measures into perspective, Taylor and associates[54] prepared a systematic literature review and meta-analysis of SCS use for RA as of February 2008. Following the methods outlined in the *Cochrane Handbook for Systematic Reviews of Interventions*, the team ultimately examined 11 papers involving seven RCTs with similar inclusion criteria: all patients developed RA despite medical optimization, they were not candidates for revascularization, and they were included in NYHA angina classes III and IV. All seven trials were short term, except for the electrical stimulation versus coronary artery bypass surgery study (ESBY) in severe angina pectoris conducted by Mannheimer and associates[53] and the open label, single-centre, randomized trial of spinal cord stimulation versus percutaneous myocardial laser revascularization in patients with refractory angina pectoris (SPiRiT trial) conducted by McNab and associates[55] that followed up beyond 1 year.[55]

Taylor and colleagues[54] examined seven specific outcome categories across the seven RCTs: exercise capacity, ischemic burden, nitrate drug consumption, functional class of angina, health-related quality of life, adverse events and SCS-related complications, and cost. The RCTs reviewed included one that examined SCS implantation vs. no implantation conducted by de Jongste et al in 1994.[56] Four of the RCTs involved an SCS on state vs. an SCS off state with all patients in the study being implanted.[52,57-59] The ESBY study compared CABG to SCS.[53] The SPiRiT trial examined percutaneous myocardial laser revascularization vs. SCS.[55] Much of the following discussion is based on Taylor and associates' findings with respect to these investigations. Adverse events and SCS-related complications are addressed in a different section, and cost is examined last within this section from the perspective of investigators other than Taylor and colleagues.

According to Taylor and associates, investigators in six RCTs studied exercise capacity. However, investigators in only three RCTs found statistical significance between baselines and follow-up with the SCS out of four studies that looked at change in exercise capacity within the SCS group. The authors pointed out that in the fourth, the ESBY study, the investigators turned off the stimulator while the patients were undergoing evaluation for exercise capacity; thus the patients did not demonstrate any significant change in work capacity. They stated that a pooled analysis demonstrated an improvement in exercise capacity in the SCS-on vs. SCS-off state (p = 0.03) but noted no difference when compared to CABG or percutaneous myocardial laser revascularization (PMR) to SCS and exercise capacity.[54]

Next the authors evaluated ischemic burden in four of the studies they examined. This burden was measured in these studies by evaluating the patient's 24- or 48-hour ECG monitoring for the frequency and magnitude of ST depression.[54] No statistical difference with regard to ischemic burden was noted between SCS and

CABG (p = 0.44), and only a trend favored SCS when compared to no SCS or nonoperating SCS (p = 0.12).

When the authors examined the third category, nitrate consumption, they reported that three RCTs individually noted a statistically significant reduction in short-acting nitrate use when comparing SCS patients to controls. However, when pooling the data, this decrease in nitrate consumption within the SCS group was not borne out. Furthermore, when they examined 6-month and 2-year follow-up data, Taylor and associates reported no difference in short-acting nitrate consumption between the SCS and the CABG groups.

Only two RCTs evaluated a change functional class of angina by using the CCS angina classification (similar to NYHA). At 3 and 12 months, McNab and associates[55] reported an improvement in CCS class (lower) of p = 0.049 and p = 0.093, respectively, when compared to patients receiving PMR. But a decrease in CCS class was only statistically significant at 3 months.[55] The other study by Eddicks and associates[58] was statistically significant with p = 0.002, with a mean decrease in CCS functional class of 1.6.

Quality of life was ascertained by five of the studies analyzed by Taylor and associates. Four of the studies demonstrated improved quality of life when comparing the SCS to either the no implant state or the SCS off, but no difference when compared to either CABG or PMR.

Taylor and colleagues concluded that SCS is a viable option for patients with RA citing the significant improvement in both exercise capacity and health related quality of life in most of the RCTs they evaluated.[54] Although they noted that none of the parameters differed tremendously from CABG or PMR, it must be pointed out that these techniques have not been very beneficial for patients with RA. Not one of the randomized controlled trials in the literature use change in pain (any scale) as a primary outcome measure. Instead, all primary outcomes are linked to either exercise capacity in five studies, and ischemic burden in one study. The focus on these outcome measures points to the importance of SCS use for RA to improve primarily function and quality of life as opposed only to pain.

Before the review by Taylor and associates,[54] the American College of Cardiology and American Heart Association 2002 Guideline Update on Chronic Stable Angina classified SCS as class IIb (usefulness/efficacy is less well established by evidence/opinion).[60] Up to the time the guidelines were written, only two small RCTs had been conducted. Since that time, no multiple large-scale RCTs have been conducted demonstrating intermediate and long-term benefit that would elevate the use of SCS to level IA data.

A recent review by Simpson and associates[61] out of the United Kingdom evaluated clinical and cost-effectiveness of SCS for both neuropathic and ischemic pain. Their review uses four of the same studies analyzed by Taylor and associates. From a clinical standpoint Simpson and associates come to a similar conclusion. In addition, they went on to assess the cost-effectiveness of SCS as a treatment. Because the paucity of data available to determine comparative efficacy to other treatments, including medical management, CABG, or PCI, Simpson and associates[61] conducted a threshold analysis to determine what the cost benefit would be with the choice of SCS instead of one of the other treatments. Each analysis suggested that each comparison examined would require the patient receiving SCS to live longer to achieve benefit for a life year group. Besides a lack of evidence for comparison, the comparison does not take into account the fact that the suggested use of SCS is for patients who would not be candidates for one of the other interventions on account of the fact that their RA is not amenable to other such treatments.

In addition, several studies by investigators other than Taylor and colleagues have demonstrated cost-effectiveness with the use of SCS. In a study by Rasmussen and associates,[62] use of the device was shown to save approximately 30% on medical costs because of decreased invasive testing alone. In addition, in a retrospective study by Yu and associates[63] the cost of the total SCS procedure was recuperated within 16 months, which they point out was less than 40% of the life span of the device as of 2004. Murray and associates[49] noted that rehospitalization and length of stay after SCS when compared to revascularization was significantly lower (p = 0.002). All of these studies have been observational or retrospective; none have been prospective RCTs.

After approximately a decade of use, a study by TenVaarwerk and colleagues[64] demonstrated in a retrospective clinical outcome study that the use of SCS in RA did not lead to any increase in the rate of adverse events when compared to populations that did not undergo SCS implantation. This retrospective study evaluated 517 patients by questionnaire at 14 centers in Europe. They concluded that the patients died from either events unrelated to heart disease or coronary events linked to lower ejection fraction and the severity of CAD, not the presence of the SCS. In addition, when compared to patients receiving medical management, there was no change in mortality.

Complications for Spinal Cord Stimulation and Refractory Angina

Whenever SCS is implanted, several complications are possible—from the most common, lead migration, to a variety of others, including loss of paresthesia, electrode failure, premature battery exhaustion, and infection. Buchser and Durrer[65] stated that the combined rate of complication is 6.8%. Simpson and associates[61] reported that four studies totaling 403 patients showed a 1% incidence for device removal secondary to infection and a 5%- to 38%-range for device complications in studies with follow-ups greater than 2 months. They suggested such a range for device complications because of the variable sizes of studies, different follow-up periods, or clinical circumstances.

Establishing Diagnosis: Peripheral Vascular Disease and Role of Spinal Cord Stimulation

PVD most commonly develops secondary to advancing atherosclerosis; however, a variety of other conditions lead to the final common pathway, but for brevity's sake they are not discussed here.[66] If left unchecked, PVD progresses to CLI and eventual infarction secondary to a decrease in blood flow rate necessary to maintain tissue metabolic function. Patients suffering from PVD typically first notice symptoms of vascular claudication or intermittent pain with ambulation that resolves at rest. If left untreated, the disease progresses to infarction and gangrene, ultimately requiring amputation if other measures fail.

Establishing a CLI diagnosis is critical for selecting patients for various therapies. The second European consensus conference on chronic CLI recommended two ways to identify and define CLI. First, in patients with and without diabetes CLI may be defined by either of two criteria: (1) persistently recurring ischemic rest pain requiring regular adequate analgesia for more than 2 weeks, with an ankle systolic pressure ≤50 mm Hg and/or a toe systolic pressure of ≤30 mm Hg; or (2) ulceration or gangrene of the foot or toes, with an ankle systolic pressure ≤50 mm Hg and/or a toe systolic pressure of ≤30 mm Hg.[7] Second, the conference recommended a more precise way to identify and define CLI (i.e., use

Table 11-2: Classification of Peripheral Arterial Disease: Fontaine Stages and Rutherford Categories

Fontaine		Rutherford		
Stage	Clinical	Grade	Category	Clinical
I	Asymptomatic	0	0	Asymptomatic
IIa	Mild claudication	I	1	Mild claudication
IIb	Moderate-severe claudication	I	2	Moderate claudication
		I	3	Severe claudication
III	Ischemic rest pain	II	4	Ischemic rest pain
IV	Ulceration or gangrene	III	5	Minor tissue loss
		IV	6	Ulceration or gangrene

Reprinted from Dormandy JA, Rutherford RB: Management of peripheral arterial disease (PAD), *J Vasc Surg* 31(S1-S296), for the TransAtlantic Inter-Society Consensus (TASC) Working Group. Copyright 2000 with permission from Elsevier.

angiography to identify large-vessel disease, take toe arterial pressure, and use methods such as transcutaneous partial pressure of oxygen ($TcpO_2$) to delineate local microcirculation.[7] It is important to note that not every patient with CLI falls within these definitions, despite having severe disease. Best clinical judgment must be used to evaluate all patients for extent of disease.

For those patients with concomitant diabetes, a few important factors must be considered during patient evaluation. First, because patients with diabetes may also suffer from painful diabetic neuropathy, their neuropathic pain should be distinguished from their CLI pain at rest. In addition, as the consensus conference points out, because patients with diabetes may have falsely high ankle systolic pressures, pressure readings with a toe cuff should be taken.[7] Patients with diabetes may also lack palpable pulses or be so weak that observer variability may affect diagnosis. Thus the consensus conference suggested evaluating absolute pressure at the ankle or toe as a more appropriate method of determining extent of disease than the standard ankle/arm pressure index.

Two classification systems, Fontaine stages and Rutherford categories, have been developed to help determine the extent of CLI in PVD (**Table 11-2**). The Fontaine classification helps assess limb ischemia and the severity of PVD. In stage I the patient is asymptomatic; in stage II the patient demonstrates intermittent claudication; in stage III the patient develops pain at rest; and in stage IV the patient has evidence of tissue loss, including ulcers and gangrene, and pain at rest.[10,67] Fontaine stages III and IV (Rutherford categories 4, 5, and 6), along with the associated blood pressure criteria noted later in the paragraph, define CLI.[28,66] Although these definitions help categorize the extent of CLI, they do not aid in prognosis for the affected limb. According to De Vries and associates,[28] no consensus currently exists as to how to most accurately determine prognosis. Patients with Fontaine stages III or IV disease have affected macrocirculation and microcirculation, each of which is evaluated differently. According to Jacobs and Jorning, [68] macrocirculation is best evaluated by systolic ankle/arm pressure measurements at rest and after treadmill exercise. Microcirculatory (cutaneous) blood flow may be evaluated by tissue oxygen pressure measurement, laser Doppler flowmetry, and radioisotope clearance.[28,68] Ubbink and associates[69] evaluated prognostic capabilities of these methods. They determined that microcirculatory classification predicted the need for eventual amputation; but Fontaine stage, ankle blood pressure, or diabetes did not. The combination of toe blood pressure of 38 mm Hg and $TcpO_2$ of 35 mm Hg supine was of good prognostic value.[28,70]

Anatomy: Pain Pathway for Peripheral Vascular Disease

Pain within the lower-extremity distribution is believed to be transmitted by a combination of Aδ and C fibers of the somatic nervous system. The pain is also likely to be partially mediated by the SNS. In addition, the pain experienced may have both ischemic and neuropathic origins.

Indications: Spinal Cord Stimulation and the Alternative Therapies Available for Peripheral Vascular Disease

A variety of modalities have been used to treat and alleviate the symptoms of CLI in PVD. As in the case of angina, medical, interventional, and surgical techniques are used to curtail the progression of the disease. SCS is an alternative for patients with inoperable lesions who are facing the prospect of amputation.

Conservative therapies include a variety of pharmacological agents, but options are sparser than for the treatment of angina. As of 2005 several drugs were under investigation to treat CLI. Pentoxifylline (Trental), a xanthine derivative with vasodilator and hemorrheologic properties, did not demonstrate any significant benefit for patients with CLI. Cilostazol, approved for intermittent claudication patients, as of 2005 had not been demonstrated as effective in patients with CLI.[66] According to Hirsch and associates,[66] three prostaglandins (PGs)—PGE-1, iloprost, and ciprostene—with vasodilatory properties have undergone multiple trials in patients with inoperable CLI without success. More traditional conservative therapies, including analgesics, vasodilators, or anticoagulants, either slightly limit the progression or aid in alleviating the symptoms of the disease.[71]

Many patients with CLI are candidates for revascularization procedures before being considered for SCS. Approximately 5% of the patients with intermittent claudication develop CLI, and approximately half of those require revascularization.[66] Revascularization may be conducted by either endovascular stenting or surgical arterial vascular reconstruction. According to Hirsh and associates,[66] the mortality associated with surgical revascularization ranges from 0% to 6%, whereas the mortality for amputation is 4% to 30% during the first 30 days. Furthermore, if patients do undergo amputation, they are at greater risk for other complications, especially with decreased mobility in the elderly population. Thus, if at all possible, revascularization by one technique or another should be considered as the primary mode of treatment for patients with CLI. Not all of them are candidates for revascularization for one reason or another, but they may benefit from SCS implantation.

Basic Science: Mechanism of Action for Peripheral Vascular Disease

PVD develops through a process of slowly narrowing blood vessels, especially in the lower extremities. Eventually decreased vascular patency progresses to distal tissue ischemia and resultant limb pain. This limb pain is likely a combination of nociceptive pain from the ischemic process and neuropathic pain. Neuromodulation has been used successfully to relieve pain from tissue ischemia; but, more important, it promotes enhanced blood flow via vasodilation to the extremities.[72,73] Promotion of blood flow was first demonstrated by Cook and associates[72] in 1976, who observed ulcer healing in patients with lower extremity PVD and attributed the improvement to increased vascular flow.

Those who suffer from PVD typically present with a history of claudication after having walked a fixed distance. As the disease progresses, claudication occurs even at rest; a condition known as *CLI*. CLI can be followed by infarction and the need for amputation. The ischemia that develops in the limbs occurs during a switch from aerobic to anaerobic metabolism.

As is the case of using neuromodulation to treat patients with RA, the mechanism of action for treating ischemic limb pain has not been fully elucidated. Despite this, two significant plausible mechanisms have been proposed.[31] First, stimulation activates sensory fibers via an antidromic mechanism, resulting in a release of vasodilators. Second, neuromodulation decreases sympathetic outflow, resulting in vasodilation of distal arterial vessels.

The Antidromic Mechanism

Bayliss[74] initially proposed the antidromic mechanism in 1901 when he observed that high-intensity, dorsal root stimulation caused peripheral vasodilation mediated by thin fibers. His proposal was confirmed by others who have significantly clarified the antidromic mechanism over the past decade.[31] Tanaka and colleagues[75] investigated antidromic activation of $A\delta$ fibers or C fibers of primary afferent nerves by SCS.[75] They used capsaicin to determine if C fibers were responsible for peripheral blood flow changes by SCS. Their results demonstrated that after capsaicin application, before SCS, vasodilation was decreased at higher levels of stimulation (percent of motor threshold [MT]), whereas vasodilation at lower levels (30% and 60% MT) was not affected. This result suggested that capsaicin blocked the unmyelinated fibers and thus prompted a decrease in the amount of calcitonin gene-related peptide (CGRP) to be released. CGRP may be antidromically released by small myelinated and unmyelinated fibers, and it is a potent vasodilator.[76,77] The fact that vasodilation still occurred at 30 and 60% MT suggested that small myelinated fibers are also involved in vasodilation.[31]

Wu and colleagues[78] further investigated the antidromic mechanism and demonstrated that transient receptor potential vanilloid-1 (TRPV-1)–containing sensory fibers mediate vasodilation when stimulated via SCS.[78] In another study they determined that the SCS antidromically activated TRPV-1–containing sensory fibers, which in turn promoted the release of CGRP, the peptide involved in vasodilation.[79] A review by Wu and colleagues[31] discusses a possible mechanism for the vasodilation that is initiated by the SCS. CGRP is one of the most potent vasodilators; it targets the CGRP-1 receptor on vascular smooth muscle. In addition, it is proposed that the CGRP also activates nitric oxide (NO) release from endothelial cells, prompting further vasodilation.

The Sympathetic Mechanism

The second proposed mechanism is that SCS induces peripheral vasodilation via stimulation, which inhibits the efferent SNS. The evidence for this mechanism stems from the fact that sympathectomies or sympathetic blocks help with pain relief and vasodilation.[28,31,80] On the basis of their understanding that vascular tone is maintained by the SNS via autonomic ganglia, Linderoth, Herregodts, and Meyerson[81] evaluated this mechanism by applying various pharmacological agents that affect the SNS in the setting of SCS. Acetylcholine targets postsynaptic nicotinic receptors, which eventually trigger the peripheral adrenergic receptors that lead to vasoconstriction. They demonstrated that hexamethonium, a nonspecific ganglionic-blocking agent, and chlorisondamine, a neuronal nicotinic ganglionic blocker, both eliminated the vasodilation created by SCS. In addition, they pointed out that complete sympathectomy prevents the actions of SCS. However, most sympathectomies performed in humans are subtotal; thus SCS may still be efficacious.[31,81]

To reconcile these two seemingly independent mechanisms, Tanaka and associates[82] examined whether temperature differentials affected the two mechanisms because they noted that Linderoth, Herregodts, and Meyerson[81] rats were in a cooler climate, suggesting elevated peripheral sympathetic tone compared to their rats. When Linderoth, Herregodts, and Meyerson[81] and Tanaka and colleagues[82] conducted a collaborative study in which they examined SCS-caused vasodilation on cooled extremities in the presence of hexamethonium and CGRP (8-37), a CGRP-1 receptor antagonist, the results demonstrated that both the antidromic and sympathetic mechanisms likely are involved and that the antidromic mechanism likely occurs at moderate temperatures (25° to 28° Celsius).[82] They further pointed out that the threshold for the sympathetically mediated mechanism is likely higher. According to Wu and associates,[31] the mechanism that predominates likely relates to level of sympathetic activity, level of SCS, and the individual's genetic variability.

In their review Wu and colleagues[31] pointed out that other mechanisms have also been proposed (i.e., vasodilator improvement of endothelial function, stimulation of angiogenesis from released substances that would lead to long-term improvement in ischemic tissue, improved blood flow through collaterals to further tissue healing, and potential release of endogenous opioids with SCS).

Guidelines: Patient Selection for Spinal Cord Stimulation in Peripheral Vascular Disease

Although pain relief and limb salvage are the primary goals of SCS in PVD, patients must be selected carefully to maximize the likelihood of success and minimize inappropriate use of the device and health care resources. Patients deemed candidates for this modality should meet several criteria: have a CLI diagnosis (Fontaine stage III or IV) that is currently not evolving rapidly over a period of days or weeks,[28] have failed conservative measures, have been considered unsuitable for endovascular or surgical revascularization, or have already failed such interventions. Furthermore, De Vries and associates[28] suggest that ulcers or other skin lesions should not exceed 3 cm^2 since lesions beyond this size suggest a more advanced stage of disease that typically cannot be reversed with SCS. Patients should also meet macrovascular and microvascular criteria, especially the latter. If patients have a Doppler ankle systolic pressure ≤50 mm Hg or an ankle/brachial index ≤35 mm Hg and TcpO$_2$ between 10 and 35 mm Hg,[9] they can be included. NOTE: Patients with TcpO$_2$ ≤10 mm Hg are at greater risk for impending

Table 11-3: Lead Placement

Site of Ischemia	Lead Placement
Chest, arm, jaw, shoulder	C7, T1, T2
Upper extremity	C3 to C6
Lower extremity, including foot	T10 to L3
Failure to get foot stimulation with conventional placement	L5 or S1 foramen

From Deer TR, editor: Spinal cord stimulation for the treatment of angina and peripheral vascular disease, *Curr Pain Headache Rep* 13(1):19, 2009.

amputation because of significantly decreased microvascular reserve, whereas patients with TcpO$_2$ $\geq$30 mm Hg are likely to improve without the SCS.[83]

Exclusion criteria should be considered in the decision as well. Patients not suitable for implantation include those without at-rest pain, gangrene, or ulceration; and those with infection, cancer, a vascular disease other than atherosclerosis, and a psychological or social incompetence, as outlined in **Box 11-3**.

Equipment and Technique for Spinal Cord Stimulation in Peripheral Vascular Disease

SCS for PVD requires epidural placement of the device leads at a level that will enable the patient to feel paresthesias over the same area as their pathology. Usually leads are introduced epidurally at a level two to three below the final resting place of the tip of the lead.[28] For example, to cover lower-extremity PVD, placement typically is targeted at the T10 level initially and adjusted from there (see **Table 11-3** for the complete listing suggested by Deer). Again, placement should be attempted at a 45-degree angle to minimize the risk of dural puncture with the Tuohy needle and to allow a smooth insertion of the stimulator lead, both for the trial and for the placement of the permanent lead. The patient should be sedated lightly enough to be aware of paresthesias as the lead is advanced.

By confirming paresthesias of the affected areas, the patient can aid the physician in determining proper placement of the lead. Once paresthesias are confirmed, the lead may be tunneled laterally to minimize movement and decrease infection risk during the trial period.

To determine if the technique will be successful, Petrakis and Sciacca[70] suggested that a trial time of up 2 weeks be conducted. Their suggestion is based on the finding that limb salvage was achieved in their patients who demonstrated a significant increase in their TcpO$_2$ measured at the foot within 2 weeks of the trial and a 50% increase in TcpO$_2$ after 2 months of implantation.

Drug regimens that impact blood clotting before trial and implantation should be optimized, as is also the case for SCS in RA.

Outcomes for Spinal Cord Stimulation and Peripheral Vascular Disease

Recently Ubbink and Vermeulen[65] reviewed the available literature on SCS for nonreconstructible chronic CLI for the Cochrane Collaboration. They conducted a meta-analysis based on 10 papers encompassing six randomized or controlled trials that met their selection criteria. The investigators picked studies that involved patients of advanced age and CLI secondary to arthrosclerosis that was considered nonreconstructible. The randomized trials picked by Ubbink and Vermeulen[65] included those by Suy and associates, Jivegard and associates, Claeys and Horsch, Klomp and associates, and Spincemaille and associates; the controlled trial was by Amann and associates.[84-93] Combined, these studies pooled 444 patients between 1994 and 2006. The primary outcome noted in all studies was limb salvage (defined as no major amputation of foot or higher after 12 months).[94] Limb amputation leads to significant further morbidity caused by decreased mobility in the elderly population, which translates to an overall increased mortality. Secondary end points reviewed included pain relief, clinical improvement, change in macrocirculation and microcirculation, quality of life, SCS complications (see next section), and costs.

Ubbink and Vermeulen[83] focused on limb salvage, the primary end point of the reviewed studies first. They noted that the overall amputation prevalence was 50% no matter what treatment was provided. However, they did note that all the studies that reviewed the SCS groups demonstrated a tendency toward improved limb salvage, especially if the patients were selected based on initial TcpO$_2$. In addition, normotensive patients with SCS implanted had a lower amputation rate.[86] They also proposed that, on the basis of their meta-analysis of pooling the results after 12 months, the number needed to treat to prevent one major amputation was nine.[83]

In terms of the secondary outcome of pain relief, Ubbink and Vermeulen[83] noted that data from the selected studies could not be pooled secondary to lack of standard deviations.[83] They did point out that with two studies pain was significantly better at 3 and 12 months with the SCS groups than with the medically treated groups by Jivegard and associates[86] and Spincemaille and colleagues,[91] respectively. In addition, a study by Spincemaille and colleagues[90] noted that patients with SCS implantation for CLI used significantly less opioid and nonopioid analgesics, suggesting lower pain levels.

The next outcome examined was clinical improvement. The studies by Suy and associates[93] and Claeys and Horsch[85] showed clinical stage (measured by use of the Fontaine stages) improvement from CLI to intermittent claudication (p = 0.0014) when compared to those receiving medical treatment alone.[65] When

Ubbink and Vermeulen[65] pooled the data, they showed that the number of patients who needed treatment to convert from rest pain to intermittent claudication was three. Two of the reviewed studies evaluated wound healing; but, when the data were pooled, no significant differences between the groups were determined. In addition, no significant differences were noted between patients with and without diabetes.[85]

To determine the effects of SCS on circulation, investigators have looked for improved macrocirculation (measured by the ankle/brachial pressure index [ABPI]) and microcirculation. In the Cochrane review SCS-treated patients in Claeys' study demonstrated improved ABPI of 10% with SCS and a decrease of 17% in the medically treated group ($p < 0.02$), whereas Jivegard and associates did not demonstrate a difference.[85,86] Ubbink and Vermeulen[94] reported that they were not able to pool the data for these studies. When evaluating the studies for an improvement in microcirculation (change in $TcpO_2$), no determination of significant improvement in $TcpO_2$ values over medical management could be made. However, when looking at individual studies, significant increases in microcirculation were observed (Claeys: $p < 0.001$; Ubbink and associates: $p < 0.05$).[85,95]

Investigators in each of the studies evaluated quality of life in only a few of the studies. Unfortunately their different methods of evaluation of outcomes prevented overall compilation and analysis of data. When looking at the reviewed studies individually, the study by Amann and colleagues[84] demonstrated no overall decrease in quality of life. Spincemaille and colleagues[90] demonstrated quality of life significantly improved in patients treated with SCS ($p < 0.01$). In addition, some of the study groups evaluated only the SCS arm and not the conservatively treated one. Spincemaille and colleagues[92] used the Nottingham Health Profile, which demonstrated improved quality of life in both the conservative and SCS groups, but the mobility score was significantly improved in the SCS group ($p < 0.01$).

Only one study reviewed,[90] done in Europe, compared costs between the two groups at 2 years. The SCS group cost substantially more than the conservative group ($p < 0.009$), even when adjusted for mortality ($p < 0.002$).

Complications for Spinal Cord Stimulation and Peripheral Vascular Disease

In Ubbink and Vermeulen's review,[94] they noted no differences between the mortality of medically managed and SCS groups. SCS implantation complications in patients with PVD included implantation difficulties (inability to place lead) approximately 8% of the time, increasing to 12% in multicenter trials. This level of difficulty suggests the need for better-trained specialists in this technique. Other complications included battery failure, infection of lead or generator pocket, and lead fracture—all of which may potentially occur with any patient undergoing an SCS implantation.

Conclusions

If patients are selected carefully, SCS appears to be an excellent modality with multifaceted results for treating RA and/or PVD. Patients with RA not only gain pain relief, but they also improve cardiac outcome as their capacity for exercise increases. This may lead to an improved functional capacity and increased quality of life. Furthermore, SCS is advantageous because it does not mask the symptoms of acute angina from a new event or chronic angina pain. As the population of angina patients who fail a multitude of other medical and interventional approaches grows, the role of SCS

will likely become more prominent. Similarly, for equally debilitating PVD, SCS promises improved pain relief, clinical improvement of disease, improved limb salvage, and better quality of life. These outcomes occur with relatively low complication rates and reasonable cost benefit.

For both disease states more research must be pursued to develop standardized patient-inclusion criteria so the possible outcomes of this expensive, highly specialized modality can be optimized and long-term efficacy may be confirmed.

References

1. Shealy CN, Mortimer JT, Reswick JB: Electrical inhibition of pain by stimulation of the dorsal columns: preliminary clinical report. *Anesth Analg* 46(4):489-491, 1967.
2. Lloyd-Jones D et al: Heart disease and stroke statistics—2010 update: a report from the American Heart Association. *Circulation* 121(7):e46-e215, 2010.
3. Mukherjee D et al: Direct myocardial revascularization and angiogenesis—how many patients might be eligible? *Am J Cardiol* 84(5):598-600, 1999.
4. Mannheimer C, Camici P, Chester MR et al: The problem of chronic refractory angina: report from the ESC joint study group on the treatment of refractory angina. *European Heart Journal* 23:355-370, 2002.
5. Holmes DR, Jr: Treatment options for angina pectoris and the future role of enhanced external counterpulsation. *Clin Cardiol* 25(12sSuppl 2):II22-25, 2002.
6. Vallejo R et al: Spinal neuromodulation: a novel approach in the management of peripheral vascular disease. *Tech Regional Anesthes Pain Management* 10:3-6, 2006.
7. Second European Consensus Document on chronic critical leg ischemia. *Eur J Vasc Surg* 6(suppl A):1-32, 1992.
8. Gibbons RJ et al: ACC/AHA/ACP-ASIM guidelines for the management of patients with chronic stable angina: a report of the American College of Cardiology/American Heart Association Task Force on Practice Guidelines (Committee on Management of Patients With Chronic Stable Angina). *J Am Coll Cardiol* 33(7):2092-2197, 1999.
9. Buchser E, Durrer A, Albrecht E: Spinal cord stimulation for the management of refractory angina pectoris. *J Pain Symptom Manage* 31(4 Suppl):S36-S42, 2006.
10. Erdek MA, Staats PS: Spinal cord stimulation for angina pectoris and peripheral vascular disease. *Anesthesiol Clin North Am* 21(4):797-804, 2003.
11. Sestito A et al: Spinal cord stimulation normalizes abnormal cortical pain processing in patients with cardiac syndrome X. *Pain* 139(1):82-89, 2008.
12. Panting JR et al: Abnormal subendocardial perfusion in cardiac syndrome X detected by cardiovascular magnetic resonance imaging. *N Engl J Med* 346(25):1948-1953, 2002.
13. Latif OA, Raj PP: Spinal cord stimulation: a comparison of efficacy versus other novel treatments for refractory angina pectoris. *Pain Pract* 1(1):36-45, 2001.
14. Campeau L: Letter: Grading of angina pectoris. *Circulation* 54(3):522-523, 1976.
15. Management of stable angina pectoris: recommendations of the Task Force of the European Society of Cardiology. *Eur Heart J* 18(3):394-413, 1997.
16. Eckert S, Horstkotte D: Management of angina pectoris: the role of spinal cord stimulation. *Am J Cardiovasc Drugs* 9(1):17-28, 2009.
17. Bolser DC et al: Effects of intracardiac bradykinin and capsaicin on spinal and spinoreticular neurons. *Am J Physiol* 257(5 Pt 2):H1543-H1550, 1989.
18. Selzer M, Spencer WA: Interactions between visceral and cutaneous afferents in the spinal cord: reciprocal primary afferent fiber depolarization. *Brain Res* 14(2):349-366, 1969.
19. Jolicoeur EM et al: Clinical and research issues regarding chronic advanced coronary artery disease: part I: Contemporary and emerging therapies. *Am Heart J* 155(3):418-434, 2008.

20. Mannheimer C et al: The problem of chronic refractory angina; report from the ESC Joint Study Group on the Treatment of Refractory Angina. *Eur Heart J* 23(5):355-370, 2002.

21. Chaitman BR et al: Anti-ischemic effects and long-term survival during ranolazine monotherapy in patients with chronic severe angina. *J Am Coll Cardiol* 43(8):1375-1382, 1004.

22. Chaitman BR et al: Effects of ranolazine with atenolol, amlodipine, or diltiazem on exercise tolerance and angina frequency in patients with severe chronic angina: a randomized controlled trial. *JAMA* 291(3):309-316, 2004.

23. Abbott JD et al: Recent trends in the percutaneous treatment of chronic total coronary occlusions. *Am J Cardiol* 97(12):1691-1696, 2006.

24. Olivari Z et al: Immediate results and one-year clinical outcome after percutaneous coronary interventions in chronic total occlusions: data from a multicenter, prospective, observational study (TOAST-GISE). *J Am Coll Cardiol* 41(10):1672-1678, 2003.

25. Suero JA et al: Procedural outcomes and long-term survival among patients undergoing percutaneous coronary intervention of a chronic total occlusion in native coronary arteries: a 20-year experience. *J Am Coll Cardiol* 38(2):409-414, 2001.

26. Sinvhal RM, Gowda RM, Khan IA: Enhanced external counterpulsation for refractory angina pectoris. *Heart* 89(8):830-833, 2003.

27. Soran O et al: Two-year clinical outcomes after enhanced external counterpulsation (EECP) therapy in patients with refractory angina pectoris and left ventricular dysfunction (report from The International EECP Patient Registry). *Am J Cardiol* 97(1):17-20, 2006.

28. De Vries J et al: Spinal cord stimulation for ischemic heart disease and peripheral vascular disease. *Adv Tech Stand Neurosurg* 32:63-89, 2007.

29. Melzack R, Wall PD: Pain mechanisms: a new theory. *Science* 150(699):971-979, 1965.

30. Chandler MJ et al: A mechanism of cardiac pain suppression by spinal cord stimulation: implications for patients with angina pectoris. *Eur Heart J* 14(1):96-105, 1993.

31. Wu M, Linderoth B, Foreman RD: Putative mechanisms behind effects of spinal cord stimulation on vascular diseases: a review of experimental studies. *Auton Neurosci* 138(1-2):9-23, 2008.

32. Cui JG et al: Spinal cord stimulation attenuates augmented dorsal horn release of excitatory amino acids in mononeuropathy via a GABAergic mechanism. *Pain* 73(1):87-95, 1997.

33. Oldroyd KG et al: Beta endorphin release in patients after spontaneous and provoked acute myocardial ischaemia. *Br Heart J* 67(3):230-235, 1992.

34. Eliasson T et al: Myocardial turnover of endogenous opioids and calcitonin-gene-related peptide in the human heart and the effects of spinal cord stimulation on pacing-induced angina pectoris. *Cardiology* 89(3):170-177, 1998.

35. Hautvast RW et al: Relative changes in regional cerebral blood flow during spinal cord stimulation in patients with refractory angina pectoris. *Eur J Neurosci* 9(6):1178-1183, 1997.

36. Zonenshayn M, Mogilner AY, Rezai AR: Neurostimulation and functional brain imaging. *Neurol Res* 22(3):318-325, 2000.

37. Mobilia G et al: Effects of spinal cord stimulation on regional myocardial blood flow in patients with refractory angina: a positron emission tomography study. *G Ital Cardiol* 28(10):1113-1119, 1998.

38. Norrsell H et al: Effects of spinal cord stimulation on coronary blood flow velocity. *Coron Artery Dis* 9(5):273-278, 1998.

39. Kingma JG, Jr et al: Neuromodulation therapy does not influence blood flow distribution or left-ventricular dynamics during acute myocardial ischemia. *Auton Neurosci* 91(1-2):47-54, 2001.

40. Armour JA: Myocardial ischaemia and the cardiac nervous system. *Cardiovasc Res* 41(1):41-54, 1999.

41. Lathrop DA, Spooner PM: On the neural connection. *J Cardiovasc Electrophysiol* 12(7):841-844, 2001.

42. Hautvast RW et al: Effect of spinal cord stimulation on myocardial blood flow assessed by positron emission tomography in patients with refractory angina pectoris. *Am J Cardiol* 77(7):462-467, 1996.

43. Ardell JL: Intrathoracic neuronal regulation of cardiac function. In Armour JA, Ardell JL, editors: *Basic and clinical neurocardiology*, 2004, Oxford University Press, pp 118-152.

44. Cardinal R et al: Spinal cord stimulation suppresses bradycardias and atrial tachyarrhythmias induced by mediastinal nerve stimulation in dogs. *Am J Physiol Regul Integr Comp Physiol* 291(5):R1369-1375, 2006.

45. Mannheimer C et al: Effects of spinal cord stimulation in angina pectoris induced by pacing and possible mechanisms of action. *Br Med J* 307(6902):477-480, 1993.

46. Eliasson T, Augustinsson LE, Mannheimer C: Spinal cord stimulation in severe angina pectoris–presentation of current studies, indications and clinical e experience. *Pain* 65(2-3):169-179, 1996.

47. Mannheimer C et al: The effects of transcutaneous electrical nerve stimulation in patients with severe angina pectoris. *Circulation* 71(2):308-316, 1985.

48. Foreman RD et al: Modulation of intrinsic cardiac neurons by spinal cord stimulation: implications for its therapeutic use in angina pectoris. *Cardiovasc Res* 47(2):367-375, 2000.

49. Murray S et al: Spinal cord stimulation significantly decreases the need for acute hospital admission for chest pain in patients with refractory angina pectoris. *Heart* 82(1):89-92, 1999.

50. Ganz P, Braunwald E: Coronary blood flow and myocardial ischemia. In Braunwald E, editor: *Heart Disease*, Philadelphia, 1997, Saunders, pp 1168-1174.

51. Deer TR: Spinal cord stimulation for the treatment of angina and peripheral vascular disease. *Curr Pain Headache Rep* 13(1):18-23, 2009.

52. Hautvast RW et al: Spinal cord stimulation in chronic intractable angina pectoris: a randomized, controlled efficacy study. *Am Heart J* 136(6):1114-1120, 1998.

53. Mannheimer C et al: Electrical stimulation versus coronary artery bypass surgery in severe angina pectoris: the ESBY study. *Circulation* 97(12):1157-63, 1998.

54. Taylor RS et al: Spinal cord stimulation in the treatment of refractory angina: systematic review and meta-analysis of randomised controlled trials. *BMC Cardiovasc Disord* 9:13, 2009.

55. McNab D et al: An open label, single-centre, randomized trial of spinal cord stimulation vs. percutaneous myocardial laser revascularization in patients with refractory angina pectoris: the SPiRiT trial. *Eur Heart J* 27(9):1048-1053, 2006.

56. de Jongste MJ et al: Stimulation characteristics, complications, and efficacy of spinal cord stimulation systems in patients with refractory angina: a prospective feasibility study. *Pacing Clin Electrophysiol* 17(11 Pt 1):1751-1760, 1994.

57. Di Pede F et al: Long-term effects of spinal cord stimulation on myocardial ischemia and heart rate variability: results of a 48-hour ambulatory electrocardiographic monitoring. *Ital Heart J* 2(9):690-695, 2001.

58. Eddicks S et al: Thoracic spinal cord stimulation improves functional status and relieves symptoms in patients with refractory angina pectoris: the first placebo-controlled randomised study. *Heart* 93(5):585-590, 2007.

59. Jessurun GA et al: Clinical follow-up after cessation of chronic electrical neuromodulation in patients with severe coronary artery disease: a prospective randomized controlled study on putative involvement of sympathetic activity. *Pacing Clin Electrophysiol* 22(10):1432-1439, 1999.

60. Gibbons RJ et al: ACC/AHA 2002 guideline update for the management of patients with chronic stable angina–summary article: a report of the American College of Cardiology/American Heart Association Task Force on practice guidelines (Committee on the Management of Patients With Chronic Stable Angina). *J Am Coll Cardiol* 41(1):159-168, 2003.

61. Simpson EL et al: Spinal cord stimulation for chronic pain of neuropathic or ischaemic origin: systematic review and economic evaluation. *Health Technol Assess* 13(17):iii, ix-x, 1-154, 2009.

62. Rasmussen MB et al: Cost-benefit of electric stimulation of the spinal cord in the treatment of angina pectoris. *Ugeskr Laeger* 154(17):1180-1184, 1992.

63. Yu W et al: Spinal cord stimulation for refractory angina pectoris: a retrospective analysis of efficacy and cost-benefit. *Coron Artery Dis* 15(1):31-37, 2004.

64. TenVaarwerk IA et al: Clinical outcome of patients treated with spinal cord stimulation for therapeutically refractory angina pectoris: the working group on neurocardiology. *Heart* 82(1):82-88, 1999.

65. Ubbink DT, Vermeulen H: Spinal cord stimulation for non-reconstructable chronic critical leg ischaemia. *Cochrane Database Syst Rev* 1:1-35, 2009.

66. Hirsch AT et al: ACC/AHA 2005 Practice Guidelines for the management of patients with peripheral arterial disease (lower extremity, renal, mesenteric, and abdominal aortic): a collaborative report from the American Association for Vascular Surgery/Society for Vascular Surgery, Society for Cardiovascular Angiography and Interventions, Society for Vascular Medicine and Biology, Society of Interventional Radiology, and the ACC/AHA Task Force on Practice Guidelines (Writing Committee to Develop Guidelines for the Management of Patients With Peripheral Arterial Disease): endorsed by the American Association of Cardiovascular and Pulmonary Rehabilitation; National Heart, Lung, and Blood Institute; Society for Vascular Nursing; Trans-Atlantic Inter-Society Consensus; and Vascular Disease Foundation. *Circulation* 113(11):e463-e654, 2006.

67. Augustinsson LE, Linderoth B, Mannheimer C, Eliasson T: Spinal cord stimulation in cardiovascular disease. *Functional Neurosurgery* 6(1):157-165, 1995.

68. Jacobs MJ, Jorning PJ: Is epidural spinal cord electrical stimulation indicated in patients with severe lower limb ischaemia? *Eur J Vasc Surg* 2(4):207-208, 1988.

69. Ubbink DT et al: Prediction of imminent amputation in patients with non-reconstructible leg ischemia by means of microcirculatory investigations. *J Vasc Surg* 30(1):114-121, 1999.

70. Petrakis IE, Sciacca V: Epidural spinal cord electrical stimulation in diabetic critical lower limb ischemia. *J Diabetes Complications* 13(5-6):293-299, 1999.

71. Ubbink DT et al: Systematic review and meta-analysis of controlled trials assessing spinal cord stimulation for inoperable critical leg ischaemia. *Br J Surg* 91(8):948-955, 2004.

72. Cook AW et al: Vascular disease of extremities. Electric stimulation of spinal cord and posterior roots. *NY State J Med* 76(3):366-368, 1976.

73. Dooley DM, Kasprak M: Modification of blood flow to the extremities by electrical stimulation of the nervous system. *South Med J* 69(10):1309-1311, 1976.

74. Bayliss WM: On the origin from the spinal cord of the vasodilator fibres of the hind-limb, and on the nature of these fibres. *J Physiol* 26(3-4):173-209, 1901.

75. Tanaka S et al: Role of primary afferents in spinal cord stimulation-induced vasodilation: characterization of fiber types. *Brain Res* 959(2):191-198, 2003.

76. Croom JE et al: Cutaneous vasodilation during dorsal column stimulation is mediated by dorsal roots and CGRP. *Am J Physiol* 272(2 Pt 2):H950-957, 1997.

77. Tanaka S et al: Low intensity spinal cord stimulation may induce cutaneous vasodilation via CGRP release. *Brain Res* 896(1-2):183-187, 2001.

78. Wu M et al: Sensory fibers containing vanilloid receptor-1 (VR-1) mediate spinal cord stimulation-induced vasodilation. *Brain Res* 1107(1):177-184, 2006.

79. Wu M et al: Roles of peripheral terminals of transient receptor potential vanilloid-1 containing sensory fibers in spinal cord stimulation-induced peripheral vasodilation. *Brain Res* 1156:80-92, 2007.

80. Linderoth B, Gunasekera L, Meyerson BA: Effects of sympathectomy on skin and muscle microcirculation during dorsal column stimulation: animal studies. *Neurosurgery* 29(6):874-879, 1991.

81. Linderoth B, Herregodts P, Meyerson BA: Sympathetic mediation of peripheral vasodilation induced by spinal cord stimulation: animal studies of the role of cholinergic and adrenergic receptor subtypes. *Neurosurgery* 35(4):711-719, 1994.

82. Tanaka S et al: Local cooling alters neural mechanisms producing changes in peripheral blood flow by spinal cord stimulation. *Auton Neurosci* 104(2):117-127, 2003.

83. Ubbink DT, Vermeulen H: Spinal cord stimulation for critical leg ischemia: a review of effectiveness and optimal patient selection. *J Pain Symptom Manage* 31(4 Suppl):S30-S35, 2006.

84. Amann W et al: Spinal cord stimulation in the treatment of non-reconstructable stable critical leg ischaemia: results of the European Peripheral Vascular Disease Outcome Study (SCS-EPOS). *Eur J Vasc Endovasc Surg* 26(3):280-286, 2003.

85. Claeys LG, Horsch S: Transcutaneous oxygen pressure as predictive parameter for ulcer healing in endstage vascular patients treated with spinal cord stimulation. *Int Angiol* 15(4):344-349, 1996.

86. Jivegard LE et al: Effects of spinal cord stimulation (SCS) in patients with inoperable severe lower limb ischaemia: a prospective randomised controlled study. *Eur J Vasc Endovasc Surg* 9(4):421-425, 1995.

87. Klomp HM et al: Design issues of a randomised controlled clinical trial on spinal cord stimulation in critical limb ischaemia: ESES Study Group. *Eur J Vasc Endovasc Surg* 10(4):478-485, 1995.

88. Klomp HM et al: Spinal-cord stimulation in critical limb ischaemia: a randomised trial: ESES Study Group. *Lancet* 353(9158):1040-1044, 1999.

89. Klomp HM et al: Spinal cord stimulation is not cost-effective for non-surgical management of critical limb ischaemia. *Eur J Vasc Endovasc Surg* 31(5):500-508, 2006.

90. Spincemaille GH et al: Pain and quality of life in patients with critical limb ischaemia: results of a randomized controlled multicentre study on the effect of spinal cord stimulation: ESES Study Group. *Eur J Pain* 4(2):173-184, 2000.

91. Spincemaille GH et al: Spinal cord stimulation in patients with critical leg ischemia: a preliminary evaluation of a multicenter trial. *Acta Chirurgica Austriaca* 32:49-51, 2000.

92. Spincemaille GH et al: Technical data and complications of spinal cord stimulation: data from a randomized trial on critical limb ischemia. *Stereotact Funct Neurosurg* 74(2):63-72, 2000.

93. Suy R et al: *Spinal cord stimulation for ischemic rest pain. The Belgian randomized study*, Steinhof, 1994, Darmstadt, pp 197-202.

94. Ubbink DT, Vermeulen H: Spinal cord stimulation for non-reconstructable chronic critical leg ischaemia. *Cochrane Database Syst Rev* (3):CD004001, 2005.

95. Ubbink DT et al: Microcirculatory investigations to determine the effect of spinal cord stimulation for critical leg ischemia: the Dutch multicenter randomized controlled trial. *J Vasc Surg* 30(2):236-244, 1999.

12 Spinal Cord Stimulation for Visceral Abdominal Pain

Leonardo Kapural

CHAPTER OVERVIEW

Chapter Synopsis: Visceral abdominal pain is among the many pain states that can be improved by electrical stimulation of the spinal cord (SCS). This chapter examines how SCS works to alleviate visceral pain, including considerations of the unique features of visceral pain transmission, which differ from somatic pain sensations. Spinal afferents from the viscera convey predominantly nociceptive (noxious) information, whereas vagal afferents carry information about the physiological state. Visceral pain is generally poorly localized and referred to somatic areas, although painful responses arising from different visceral organs vary. As in other indications, SCS is thought to relieve chronic visceral pain in several ways. Spinal gating of pain signals from small-fiber afferents may be decreased by continued stimulation of large-fiber, nonnociceptive afferents. Suppression of sympathetic efferents may also reduce the conditions leading to painful states, particularly ischemia. Because the underlying pathophysiology of visceral pain can vary dramatically among patients, it is crucial to determine proper electrode lead placement for implantation specific to the condition. Patient selection is of particular importance in treating visceral abdominal pain with SCS, and the treatment should be incorporated into a multidisciplinary plan.

Important Points:
- Proper patient selection seems to provide better outcome of SCS for visceral abdominal pain.
- Appropriately long trial of SCS is required to objectively assess patient's improvements in pain and function.
- Psychological evaluation and interdisciplinary committee for implantable devices assessment are now frequently required before conducting an SCS trial and are an essential part of the patient selection process.
- Collaboration and consultation with the referring physician (frequently gastroenterologist) and continued exchange of information on implantation techniques should advance our understanding of mechanisms and refine this novel technique of SCS for abdominal visceral pain.

Clinical Pearls:
- In most patients SCS leads are positioned with their tips at the level of the T5 vertebral body.
- Midline position of the leads is most frequently used, and the number of leads used for trialing is not related to the success of the trial.
- Retrograde differential epidural block can assist in proper selection of patients by identifying those who have predominantly visceral abdominal chronic pain.

Clinical Pitfalls:
- On the basis of the currently available data, SCS for abdominal pain may be an exciting therapeutic option for patients with severe visceral pain. Food and Drug Administration (FDA) approval of the new indication for SCS is still required; that process should be initiated as soon as possible in the form of a randomized, prospective clinical trial.
- Patients who require repeated magnetic resonance imaging (MRI) for ongoing monitoring of the disease process should not have SCS leads implanted.
- Although there is no evidence that recurrent inflammatory acute pancreatitis episodes could be concealed with use of SCS, those painful episodes seem to respond poorly to such treatment.

Introduction

Abdominal pain is one of the most frequent complaints to a primary care physician, accounting for nearly 2.5 million office visits a year.[1] In many patients who present with abdominal pain, a definitive diagnosis can be made, but in 35% to 51% of patients, no identifiable cause is found.[2] There are approximately 2 million patients in the United States who currently experience severe abdominal pain. Most of them undergo a multitude of imaging studies and consultations with gastroenterology and surgery before being referred to a chronic pain specialist.[3,4] Despite adequate evaluations by multiple physicians, the etiology of some abdominal pain remains unknown.

Characteristics of visceral pain have been described extensively in literature as poorly localized, referred to somatic structures, and not evoked by all viscera.[5] Visceral nociceptors are capable of responding to a variety of noxious stimuli such as mechanical and chemical stimuli. However, pain is not necessarily evoked from all of the viscera or from visceral injury. Some internal organs lack nociceptors and can be damaged without the individual perceiving pain. Spinal and vagal afferent fibers convey sensory information from the upper gastrointestinal tract to the central nervous system. Vagal afferents transmit predominantly physiological information, whereas spinal afferents transmit noxious information.[6] The dorsal root ganglia of the spinal nerves contain cell bodies of both vagal and spinal afferents. Vagal afferents enter the brainstem, whereas spinal afferents enter the spinal cord, making synaptic connections with second-order neurons, thereby conveying visceral information to the central nervous system. The ascending spinal pathways project to the thalamic nuclei. Afferent fibers with visceral and somatic information converge onto spinothalamic and spinoreticular pathways.

The role of the dorsal column pathway in transmission/amplification of visceral pain has been described more recently by Palacek and Willis[7] and Palacek,[8] and its role as participating in the neuromodulation of visceral painful information by spinal cord stimulation (SCS) has been hypothesized.[9] Still the spinothalamic tracts are considered to be the major pathways for visceral nociception.[10]

Spinal sensitization process following tissue injury is characterized as a leftward shift in pain sensation/behavior (hyperalgesia) and enlargement of receptive fields within cutaneous areas able to activate the dorsal horn neuron (allodynia). This pattern is analogous to the change in functional bowel disorders, where a leftward shift in the stimulation-pain curve and enlargement of the somatic referral area occur.[11] The expansion of convergent cutaneous fields after repetitive distension of a viscus indicates the presence of a central mechanism contributing to the alteration of excitability of central neurons.[12] Brain-gut axis abnormalities can manifest as gastrointestinal motility and functional disorders. Because the neural activity plays a major role in these disorders, interventions aiming to modulate these processes can possibly improve the symptoms.

Spinal Cord Stimulation in Visceral Pain: Possible Mechanisms of Pain Relief

Several possible mechanisms may be involved in the phenomena of chronic abdominal pain relief produced by SCS. Published studies used the model of visceral hyperalgesia by colorectal distention in rats. Suppression of lumbosacral spinal neuron responses to the noxious colorectal stimuli by SCS could be produced by placing the electrical lead either near the lumbar or cervical dorsal column.[13,14] It was suggested that such suppression of the visceromotor reflex (VMR) by SCS may be the result of antidromic activation of primary efferent fibers within the dorsal column.[13,14] Spinal gating mechanisms[15] might also be operant as an explanation for the reduction in pain transmission of small-diameter visceral fibers by stimulating large afferents using relatively low-intensity electrical stimulation.[15]

Although interruption of the recently described midline dorsal column pathway relieves visceral pelvic pain in cancer patients,[7,8,10,11] at this time it is not clear if this visceral pathway can be modulated, excited, or suppressed by SCS.

Suppression of the sympathetic nervous system could play a significant role in control of the abdominal visceral pain;[16] chemical or surgical neurectomy/sympathectomy involving the superior hypogastric or celiac plexus can suppress chronic abdominal pain.[16,17] Suppression of the sympathetic nervous system has been proposed as an important mechanism of pain control in intractable angina.[18] It may be that such sympathectomy by SCS plays a role in suppression of chronic visceral abdominal pain.[19]

Clinical Experience in Using Spinal Cord Stimulation for Chronic Visceral Pain

Compelling data suggest that SCS may decrease pain and improve functional capacity in patients with various visceral chronic pain syndromes (**Table 12-1**). However, it may require years to accumulate sufficient clinical evidence.

The first case report on SCS for the treatment of abdominal pain described the case of a 78-year-old male with chronic, unrelieved severe postprandial pain caused by mesenteric ischemia. The patient experienced full pain relief after a SCS lead was placed epidurally at the T6 vertebral level.[20] The only case report dealing with *irritable bowel syndrome (IBS)* described a female patient who suffered from 11 to 14 diarrheal episodes per day and extreme pain from IBS and who, after placement of a thoracic SCS system, became immediately diarrhea free. However, her initial reduction in pain relief was not sustained.[21]

Khan, Raza, and Khan[22] described five successful cases of patients with nonalcoholic pancreatitis who received both single and dual leads placed at the T5-T7 vertebral height in the posterior epidural space. This report was followed by several others describing improvements in pain and function in patients with severe chronic pancreatitis[23-25] (see **Table 12-1**).

Tiede and associates[26] described improvements in pain scores of patients with gastroparesis, whereas Jackson and Simpson[27] reported improved pain control and swallowing in a patient with a rather complicated history of esophageal problems. A most recently published report describes two cases of familial

Table 12-1: Reported Causes of Severe Chronic Abdominal Pain Treated with Spinal Cord Stimulation

Causes of Abdominal Pain Treated With SCS	Study/Case Series/ Case Report	Number of Patients Studied
Mesenteric ischemia	Ceballos et al, 2000[20]	1
Esophageal dysmotility	Jackson and Simpson, 2004[27]	1
Irritable bowel syndrome	Krames and Mousad, 2005[21]	1
Chronic pancreatitis	Khan et al, 2005[22]	5
Familial Mediterranean fever	Kapur, Mutagi, and Raphael, 2006[28]	2
Pelvic visceral pain	Kapural et al, 2006[19]	6
Gastroparesis	Tiede et al, 2006[26]	2
Chronic pancreatitis	Kapural and Rakic, 2008[23]	1
Chronic pancreatitis	Kim et al, 2009[24]	1
Chronic pancreatitis, abdominal adhesions, gastroparesis, mesenteric ischemia, postgastric bypass pain	Kapural et al, 2010[29]	35
Chronic pancreatitis, postsurgical intraabdominal adhesion, gastroparesis	Kapural et al, 2010[30]	76
Chronic pancreatitis	Kapural and Bensitel, 2010[25]	30

SCS, Spinal cord stimulation.

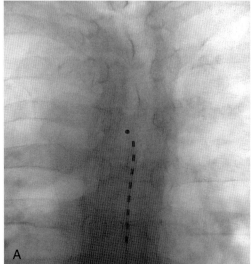

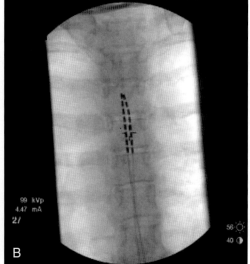

Fig. 12-1 Fluoroscopic anterior-posterior (AP) radiographs of thoracic spine with appropriately positioned leads in midline and with the lead tips positioned anywhere from T4 *(A)* to T6 *(C)*. Used were either 1, 2, or 3 leads *(A,B,C,* respectively) without significant difference in pain score improvements if one, two, or three leads were trialed.[29] (From Kapural L, et al: Spinal cord stimulation for visceral abdominal pain. *Pain Med* 11(3):347–355, 2010.)

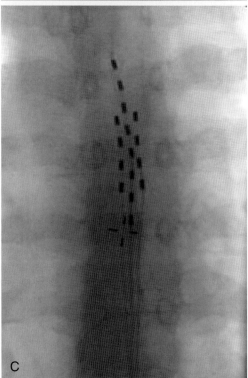

Mediterranean fever (FMF) in which painful abdominal intermittent attacks responded positively to SCS at T8-T9 and T7-T8, respectively.[28]

Despite initial enthusiasm for a novel modality for treatment of severe abdominal pain, interpreting such limited published experience was further complicated by the fact that there was considerable variability in patient selection, lead positioning, and type of hardware used in these reports. Consequently, it remained unclear whether a reasonable fraction of the patients may have long-term benefit from stimulation.

Recently much larger clinical experience using SCS for treatment of chronic abdominal pain has been published.[29] In this study 35 patients were trialed with SCS over 4 to 14 days. Consistent with most previous reports (**Figs. 12-1** and **12-2**), SCS lead tips were positioned at T5 (n = 11) or T6 (n = 10) height within the epidural space. Thirty patients (86%) reported at least 50% pain relief on completion of the trial. Among 28 patients who received permanent implant, 19 were followed at least a year. Their visual analog scale (VAS) pain scores remained low (3.8 ± 1.9 cm; p < 0.001) at 1 year, as was opioid use (138.3 ± 134 to 38 ± 48 mg morphine equivalents [**Fig. 12-3**]). This report for the first time suggested that SCS may provide consistent long-term improvements as a very useful therapeutic option for patients with severe visceral pain.

To initiate the formation of consensus between pain physicians on patient selection and technical aspects of SCS for abdominal visceral pain, a national survey directed to physicians who implant SCS for such pain was conducted recently and collected 76 case reports.[30] Considering so few cases reported by the physicians responding to this survey, SCS for abdominal visceral pain is still rarely used, despite possibly high therapeutic success rate. Causes

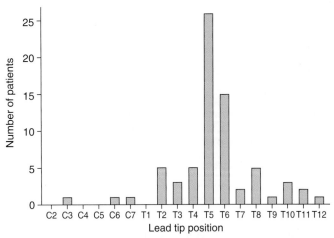

DISTRIBUTION OF LEADS, TIP POSITION IN 70 CASES

Fig. 12-2 The graph illustrates the distribution of the leads' tip position in 70 cases reported in a national survey. The most frequent positions of the tip of the spinal cord stimulation leads where the optimal paresthesias to cover the area of the patients' pain was achieved were at T5 (26 patients) and T6 (15 patients) vertebral level. (From Kapural L, et al: Spinal cord stimulation for visceral abdominal pain: results of the national survey. *Pain Med* 11(5):685-691, 2010.)

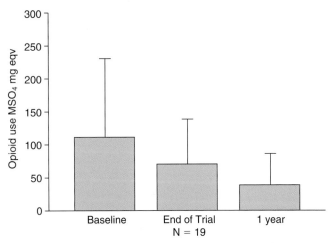

DECREASE IN OPIOID USE IN PATIENTS WITH SCS FOR CHRONIC ABDOMINAL PAIN

Fig. 12-3 The graph illustrates decrease in opioid use in 19 patients with spinal cord stimulation for chronic abdominal pain at 6 months and 1 year follow-up. Significant decrease of opioid use was achieved at 6 months and 1 year in these patients when compared to baseline (p = 0.089). (From Kapural L, et al: Spinal Cord Stimulation for visceral abdominal pain. *Pain Med* 11(3):347-355, 2010.)

for this include very few studies describing basic mechanisms of neuromodulation for long-standing visceral pain, comfort levels by the physicians, and issues with coverage of such treatment by the payers.

The technical aspects of SCS for the treatment of abdominal visceral pain seem to be uniform among physicians who use such technology across the United States and are also consistent with our larger retrospective study described previously.[29,30] In most patients, the SCS leads were positioned with their tips at the level of the T5 (26 patients) or T6 vertebral body (15 patients) (see **Fig. 12-2**). Pain relief exceeded 50% in 66 of 70 patients reported. VAS pain scores before an implant were 8 ± 1.9 cm, whereas after the implant they were 2.49 ± 1.9 cm. The opioid use before an implant was 158 ± 160 mg; at the last office visit after the implant, it was 36 ± 49 mg. The weakness of this survey was that the subgroup of responding physicians may not adequately represent the population of all of the physicians who trialed SCS for chronic visceral abdominal pain but rather those who had largely positive results; therefore results may be biased. However, the aim was to examine technical aspects of SCS for chronic abdominal pain, and this was not an efficacy study.[30]

Spinal Cord Stimulation in the Algorithm for the Treatment of Chronic Abdominal Pain

The definite place for SCS within a pain treatment continuum for chronic visceral abdominal pain is still unclear. Following a multidisciplinary evaluation, possibly within a comprehensive abdominal pain center, an interdisciplinary treatment plan should be established. Such treatments include cognitive and behavioral therapies; pharmacological pain management; adjuvant therapies for co-morbidities, including the management of sleep disturbances; and interventional diagnostic and therapeutic nerve blocks—including retrograde epidural differential block; splanchnic, celiac plexus and hypogastric blocks; and radiofrequency ablation. Based on the limited human experience reported in the literature, SCS might be indicated when conservative therapies fail to improve analgesia and function. Psychological evaluation for implantable devices and case discussion within the interdisciplinary medical team should precede SCS trialing. Only after trial is completed can a decision be made if SCS is an appropriate next step in the therapeutic continuum. Following such a rigorous algorithm would likely produce a smaller group of candidates for an implant. In our published study, only 28 patients received SCS implant from 237 initial candidates.[29] The data in support of SCS for visceral pain presently are encouraging. However, randomized controlled trials need to be initiated to support the role of SCS for long-term treatment of visceral pain.

References

1. Everhart J: Overview. In Everhart J, editor: *Digestive diseases in the United States: epidemiology and impact*, vol. NIH publication no. 94-1447, Washington, DC, 1994, US Department of Health and Human Services, Public Health Service, National Institutes of Health, National Institute of Diabetes and Digestive and Kidney Diseases, pp 3-53.
2. Klinkman MS: Episodes of care for abdominal pain in a primary care practice. *Arch Fam Med* 5:279-285, 1996.
3. Russo MW et al: Digestive and liver diseases statistics. *Gastroenterology* 126:1448-1453, 2004.
4. Derbyshire SW: Imaging visceral pain. *Curr Pain Headache Rep* 11(3):178-182, 2007.
5. Giamberardino MA, Vecchiet L: Pathophysiology of visceral pain. *Curr Pain Headache Rep* 1:23-33, 1997.
6. Grundy D: Neuroanatomy of visceral nociception: vagal and splanchnic afferent. *Gut* 51(suppl I):2-5, 2002.
7. Palecek J, Willis D: The dorsal column pathway facilitates visceromotor responses to colorectal distention after colon inflammation in rat. *Pain* 104(3):501-507, 2003.
8. Palecek J: The role of dorsal columns pathway in visceral pain. *Physiol Res* 53 (suppl. 1):S125-S130, 2004.
9. Krames ES, Foreman R: Spinal cord stimulation modulates visceral nociception and hyperalgesia via the spinothalamic tracts and the

postsynaptic dorsal column pathways: a literature review and hypothesis. *Neuromodulation* 10 (3), 224-237, 2007.

10. Palecek J, Paleckova V, Willis WD: Fos expression in spinothalamic and postsynaptic dorsal column neurons following noxious visceral and cutaneous stimuli. *Pain* 104(1-2):249-257, 2003.

11. Ness TJ, Metcalf AM, Gebhart GF: A psychophysiological study in humans using phasic colonic distension as a noxious visceral stimulus. *Pain* 43:377-386, 1990.

12. Cervero F, Laird JMA, Pozo MA: Selective changes of receptive field properties of spinal nociceptive neurons induced by noxious visceral stimulation in the cat, *Pain* 51:335-342, 1992.

13. Qin C et al: Spinal cord stimulation modulates intraspinal colorectal visceroreceptive transmission in rats. *Neurosci Res* 58:58-66, 2007.

14. Greenwood-Van Meerveld B et al: Attenuation by spinal cord stimulation of a nociceptive reflex generated by colorectal distention in a rat model. *Auton Neurosc-Basic Clin* 104:17-24, 2003.

15. Melzack R, Wall PD: Pain mechanisms: a new theory. *Science* 150:971-979, 1965.

16. Steege JF: Superior hypogastric block during microlaparoscopic pain mapping. *J Am Assoc Gynecol Laparosc* 5:265-267, 1998.

17. Rauck RL: Sympathetic nerve blocks. In Raj PP, editor: *Practical management of pain*, ed 2, St Louis, 1992, Mosby, pp 778-812.

18. Linderoth B, Foreman RD: Mechanisms of spinal cord stimulation in painful syndromes: role of animal models. *Pain Med* 7(S1):S14-S26, 2006.

19. Kapural L et al: Spinal cord stimulation is an effective treatment for the chronic intractable visceral pelvic pain. *Pain Med* 7(5):440-444, 2006.

20. Ceballos A et al: Spinal cord stimulation: a possible therapeutic alternative for chronic mesenteric ischaemia pain. *Pain* 87(1):99-101, 2000.

21. Krames E, Mousad DG: Spinal cord stimulation reverses pain and diarrheal episodes of irritable bowel syndrome: a case report. *Neuromodulation* 8:82-88, 2005.

22. Khan Y, Raza S, Khan E: Application of spinal cord stimulation for the treatment of abdominal visceral pain syndromes: case reports. *Neuromodulation* 8:14-27, 2005.

23. Kapural L, Rakic M: Spinal cord stimulation for chronic visceral pain secondary to chronic non-alcoholic pancreatitis: a case report. *Clin Gastroenterol Hepatol* 42(6):750-751, 2008.

24. Kim JK et al: Spinal cord stimulation for intractable visceral pain due to chronic pancreatitis. *J Korean Neurosurg Soc* 46(2):165-167, 2009.

25. Kapural L, Bensitel T: Spinal cord stimulation for pain management in chronic pancreatitis patients, 2010 American Academy of Pain Medicine Annual Meeting Abstracts, A256.

26. Tiede JM et al: The use of spinal cord stimulation in refractory abdominal visceral pain: case reports and literature review. *Pain Pract* 6(3):197-202, 2006.

27. Jackson M, Simpson KH. Spinal cord stimulation in a patient with persistent oesophageal pain. *Pain* 112:406-408, 2004.

28. Kapur S, Mutagi H, Raphael J: Spinal cord stimulation for relief of abdominal pain in two patients with familial Mediterranean fever. *Br J Anaesth* 97: 866-868, 2006.

29. Kapural L et al: Spinal cord stimulation for visceral abdominal pain. *Pain Med* 11(3):347-355, 2010.

30. Kapural L et al: Spinal cord stimulation for visceral abdominal pain: results of the national survey. *Pain Med* 11(5):685-691, 2010.

13 Nerve Root, Sacral, and Pelvic Stimulation

Erich O. Richter, Marina V. Abramova, Durga Sure, and Kenneth M. Alò

CHAPTER OVERVIEW

Chapter Synopsis: Electrical stimulation of the spinal cord (SCS) can be used to relieve pain that arises from many sources. Conditions that are classified as pelvic pain affect a diverse array of organs and structures and feature primarily neuropathic pain. This chapter covers the anatomical and physiological considerations for implantation of SCS hardware for the treatment of these pelvic conditions. For the most part these pelvic pain conditions are best addressed by stimulation of the sacral nerve roots. SCS may be used as treatment for interstitial cystitis, a painful inflammatory bladder condition, and other conditions of urinary dysfunction. The genitals and reproductive organs are affected in both sexes. Women may suffer from vulvodynia, a chronic neuroinflammatory stinging or burning pain of the external genitalia; whereas men are subject to chronic testicular pain and prostadynia. Coccygodynia is a painful syndrome arising from the coccyx. In addition to alleviating the pain associated with these indications for SCS, treatment can improve the underlying pathophysiology in the periphery, particularly improving bladder function. As in all indications for SCS, proper patient selection can increase the chances of a successful treatment.

Important Points:
- Stimulation of sacral nerve roots from within the spinal canal is an important technique to consider for the treatment of many forms of chronic pelvic pain, including epididymoorchialgia, vulvodynia, and interstitial cystitis; urinary control problems; and other forms of pelvic floor dysfunction and bilateral foot pain.
- A transforaminal placement from a cranial to caudal orientation is often the best way to obtain the stimulation pattern desired with a low migration rate.
- A "laterograde" approach to gain cephalad access is easier to perform and improves the learning curve.

Clinical Pearls:
- The entry site is best at L2-L3. The angle of the thecal sac to the skin is most favorable there.
- The more lateral the entry site, the more shallow is the angle of the needle to the dura, and the easier the access.
- The needle is perpendicular to the skin in craniocaudal orientation—the entire angle is mediolateral.
- When placing bilateral electrodes, allow the needle tips to nearly "kiss" in the midline, then turn the bevels caudally to pass the electrodes.
- For transforaminal placement keep the electrode in the midline until the last minute; then roll laterally into the foramen only about a vertebral level from target.

Clinical Pitfalls:
- In patients with prior lumbar surgery, the epidural space may be obliterated. Get appropriate imaging.
- Many practitioners are less familiar with sacral radiographs. Make use of lateral films to verify level.
- Avoid the tendency to aim the needle caudally at the entry site. The shingling of the laminae makes it difficult to gain entrance this way.
- When placing electrodes transforaminally, do not "wedge" the electrode distally in the foramen. Leave it loosely in the proximal foramen to avoid painful low threshold stimulation.

Introduction

Brindley[1] performed the first implantation of a sacral anterior root stimulator in a patient with multiple sclerosis who suffered from impaired bladder emptying and incontinence in 1976. Since then, sacral neuromodulation has evolved rapidly, with the development of several different anatomic approaches and Food and Drug Administration (FDA) approval of a specific device in 1997 for the treatment of urge incontinence and frequency-urgency syndrome and nonobstructive urinary retention in 1999.[2-6] Sacral neuromodulation has also been shown to be efficacious in the treatment of chronic pelvic pain syndromes such as interstitial cystitis (IC), vulvodynia, prostadynia/epididymoorchialgia, sacroiliac pain, and coccygodynia.

Establishing the Diagnosis

Interstitial Cystitis

Interstitial cystitis (IC) is a chronic, often debilitating condition with symptoms of urinary urgency and frequency associated with suprapubic or pelvic pain with bladder filling in the absence of urinary tract infection (UTI) or other obvious pathology.[7-12] The diagnosis of IC can be made in patients with characteristic cystoscopic findings of glomerulation or Hunner ulcers (10%) along with clinical findings.[12,13] The histological findings are consistent with neurogenic inflammation.[13] The prevalence varies across studies least in part because of differing diagnostic criteria, but it is in the range of 45 to 197 per 100,000 women and 8 to 41 per

100,000 men[14,15] The pathogenesis and natural history are not completely understood but appear to be multifactorial,[12,15] including infection, allergic, immunological, and genetic processes.[12,15] The most popular theory is that a sequence of toxic reactions follows damage to the bladder epithelium, resulting in a severe inflammatory reaction that induces neurogenic pain and bladder irritation.[9,12,16,17] Other chronic pelvic conditions may mimic this process with minimal differences. The European Society for the Study of Interstitial Cystitis (ESSIC) has proposed a new nomenclature and classification system with the name of painful bladder syndrome.[18] Patients without classic cystoscopic or histological findings were included in these criteria.

IC is typically associated with other chronic debilitating conditions such as irritable bowel syndrome (IBS), systemic lupus erythematosus (SLE), migraine, fibromyalgia, asthma, incontinence, or vulvodynia, and is commonly associated with a history of abuse.[12,14,19,20] The differential diagnosis includes a variety of similar conditions such as overactive bladder (OAB), chronic pelvic pain (CPP), vulvodynia, UTI, or even endometriosis.[15]

Vulvodynia

Vulvodynia is a chronic stinging, burning, itching, or irritating pain in the vaginal region without evidence of infectious, inflammatory, or neoplastic causes or any underlying neurologic disorder.[21-23] The estimated prevalence is more than 2 million women in the United States.[24] This chronic condition has debilitating effects on both physical and psychological aspects of the patient's life.[22] The pathology is not well understood. Hormonal and immunologic factors that stimulate nociceptive nerve endings directly or lead to local inflammatory signals can cause neuropathic pain of this kind.[22] Clinical symptoms occur in episodes with irregular intervals. The diagnosis is one of exclusion. Both a gynecologist and urologist should evaluate the patient to make this diagnosis. The mainstays of therapy are dietary changes, physical therapy, psychological and sexual counseling, and oral or local medications under the guidance of pain specialists.[22,23,25]

Chronic Testicular Pain

Chronic testicular pain is pain in the scrotal or testicular area lasting for more than 3 months and interfering with daily activities and quality of life. It is also called *chronic orchialgia, orchiodynia* or *chronic scrotal pain syndrome*.[26,27] It typically occurs in patients with infectious, inflammatory, vascular, postsurgical, or neoplastic conditions. Detailed examination by a urologist with proper investigations to rule out treatable causes is the primary initial focus in patient evaluation.

Prostadynia

Prostadynia is defined as chronic genital or perineal pain associated with urinary urgency and dysuria. It is seen in 5 of every 10,000 outpatient visits. National Institutes of Health (NIH) criteria differentiate this from CPP syndrome based on the presence or absence of leukocytes in expressed prostatic secretions, postprostatic massage urine, or seminal fluid analysis.[13] Some authors suggest that this pathological process in males is similar to IC in females.[28]

Coccygodynia

Coccygodynia is a painful syndrome limited to the coccyx; it may be aggravated by sitting or standing up. The process is commonly attributed to fractures or soft tissue injuries, but many cases are idiopathic.[29] Coccygodynia is extremely challenging to treat. Options include rubber ring cushions, sacrococcygeal rhizotomy, physiotherapy, local injections, coccygectomy, and neuromodulation.[13]

Anatomy

Fibers from the thoracic, lumbar, and sacral segments of the spinal cord all contribute to the formation of the pelvic and sacral plexuses. These fibers include sympathetic (T12-L2 via the superior hypogastric plexus), parasympathetic (S2-S4 via the preganglionic pelvic splanchnic nerves), and somatic components (S2-S4). Afferent fibers in the parasympathetic system (S2-S4) primarily carry sensation from the pelvic viscera. The anterior pelvic floor musculature is primarily controlled by the S3 segment roots. Therefore the S2-S4 nerve roots are the primary targets in nerve root stimulation (NRS).

Basic Science

Spinal cord or nerve root neuromodulation for pain was initially explored based on the gate control theory introduced by Melzack and Wall,[30] which suggested that activation of large-diameter afferent fibers (Aβ) suppressed pain signals travelling to the brain (**Fig. 13-1**). Since its adoption for widespread clinical use, it has become clear that for electrical neuromodulation to be successful, the following criteria must be met:

- The stimulation-induced paresthesia should cover the entire painful area.
- The anatomical distribution of the paresthesia is primarily determined by the location of the cathode, or negative contact, often referred to as the *active contact*.
- Alternative positions of the anode, or positive contact, can "pull" the perceived stimulation in a desired direction or "shield" other areas by hyperpolarizing them.

Shaker and colleagues[31] suggested that neuromodulation acts by inhibiting signal transmission to the central nervous system (CNS) via C fibers, but chronic neuropathic pain conditions can also induce new neural activity in second-order neurons in the CNS, shifting the focus of activity.[13] Matharu and associates[32] showed that successful stimulation may change thalamic metabolism and remodel the intrinsic pain circuits. Thus neuromodulation can be applied to many neuropathic pain conditions.

Pelvic pain syndromes appear to be neuropathic in nature, with characteristics of hyperpathia and allodynia.[13] Histological findings

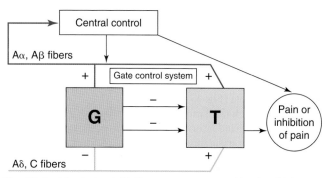

Fig. 13-1 The Aα and Aβ fibers are represented by the thick blue lines running from the dorsal root and traveling to substantia gelatinosa. The Aδ and C fibers are represented by fine pink lines running from the dorsal root to substantia gelatinosa. The fibers synapse with the cells of the substantia gelatinosa (*G*). G cells modulate the activity of transmission cells (*T*) located in the spinothalamic tract. Aα, Aβ, Aδ, and C fibers are excitatory to T cells. Large myelinated fibers (Aα and Aβ) are excitatory to G cells, whereas small myelinated and unmyelinated fibers (Aδ and C fibers) inhibit G cell activity. The G cell in turn inhibits T cell activity.

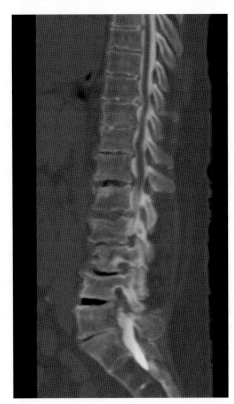

Fig. 13-2   This myelogram demonstrates vacuum changes in multiple discs, indicating that mechanical pain is likely a major issue in this patient. The large disc herniations at multiple levels also raise concerns regarding the safety of passing electrodes over the cord in the epidural space.

in both IC and vulvodynia suggest neurogenic inflammation.[33-35] In addition, 40% of women with IC have a history of hysterectomy, suggesting that injury may lead to transient inflammation, which resembles reflex sympathetic dystrophy.[13]

Imaging

No specific imaging techniques are available that demonstrate the pathological changes that cause neuropathic pain disorders such as CPP and coccygodynia. Imaging is directed at ruling out other causes of the symptoms such as infection or spinal pathology and for delineating anatomical difficulties in applying neuromodulation techniques such as spina bifida, previous surgical sites where the epidural space is obliterated, severe spondylolisthesis, or severe stenosis, which would make placing epidural electrodes more difficult or impossible (**Fig. 13-2**).

Voiding cystourethrogram and cystometrogram are usually performed to assess bladder function in patients with voiding dysfunction. Urodynamic evaluation may also include uroflowmetry and detrusor pressure-flow studies aimed to determine the presence of detrusor overactivity.

Indications/Contraindications

General Indications
Sacral intraspinal NRS is commonly used for[36]:

- CPP
- Epididymoorchialgia
- Vulvodynia

- IC
- Urinary urge incontinence
- Detrusor dysfunction
- Bilateral foot pain
- Postlaminectomy syndrome

The transforaminal approach is commonly used for[36]:

- Ilioinguinal neuralgia
- IC
- Failed back surgery syndrome
- Discogenic back pain

The extraforaminal approach is commonly used for[36]:

- Urinary urge incontinence
- Urgency-frequency syndromes
- Fowler syndrome
- Pelvic floor muscle overactivity
- Fecal incontinence

Careful patient selection and accurate diagnosis are essential for effective treatment. A multidisciplinary approach, including urology, gynecology, and psychiatry is needed to develop an optimal treatment plan. Careful and thorough investigation based on symptomatology is needed to rule out treatable causes of pain. Psychiatric evaluation is particularly useful in the management of these disorders since there is frequently some psychogenic component of the pain. Neuromodulation is an important consideration when conservative methods are ineffective in controlling the pain or improving quality of life. The optimal treatment modality and surgical approach is tailored to each patient based on pain distribution, patient anatomy, and the surgeon's experience with particular techniques.

Absolute Contraindications
- Significant systemic infection
- Any process that obliterates the epidural space is a contraindication to epidural placement over that location (e.g., previous laminectomy at that level). Computed tomography (CT) scan best shows bony removal from previous operation; magnetic resonance imaging (MRI) with gadolinium is the best test to show scar formation.
- Ongoing intravenous drug abuse
- Severe psychiatric disease such as personality disorders, severe depression and other mood disorders, somatoform disorders, or somatization

Relative Contraindications
- Spinal bifida occulta
- Spondylosis
- Spondylolisthesis
- Chronic debilitating conditions with poor prognosis
- Bleeding disorders
- Severe coronary artery disease or other systemic disease
- Minor infection (e.g., minor UTI)
- Morbid obesity
- A demand pacemaker or implanted defibrillator

Equipment

In principle nearly any stimulator could be used to deliver sacral NRS. In practice many centers prefer a cephalocaudal intraspinal approach using standard spinal cord stimulators with percutaneous leads.[37-39] Two devices have received FDA approval for sacral NRS.

- In 1997 the Medtronic InterStim (Medtronic, Inc., Minneapolis, Minn) (**Fig. 13-3**) received the Food and Drug Administration (FDA) approval for the treatment of urge incontinence.
- In 1999 the FDA approved Medtronic InterStim (Medtronic, Inc., Minneapolis, Minn) for the treatment of urinary retention and urgency-frequency.
- In 2002 the FDA approved the revised Medtronic InterStim (Medtronic, Inc., Minneapolis, Minn) to include the term *overactive bladder.*
- The FDA approved Renew radiofrequency (RF)-powered generator (St. Jude Medical, Inc., Plano, Tex) (**Fig. 13-4**) in 1999 for the treatment of chronic pain of the trunk and limbs.

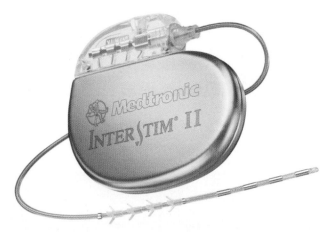

Fig. 13-3 Neurostimulation system for sacral nerve root stimulation. With permission of Medtronic, Inc. 2010.

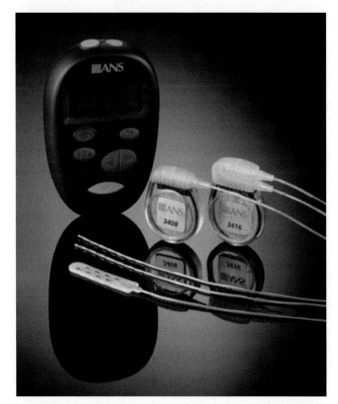

Fig. 13-4 Radio frequency–powered generator with an external power source. With permission of St. Jude Medical, Inc., Plano, Tex.

Brief summary of equipment:

- Tuohy needle—used to access epidural space
- The C-arm portable fluoroscopy machine—used to guide needle placement and electrode steering to the desired final location
- Electrodes, most commonly dual percutaneous quadripolar electrodes (St. Jude Medical, Inc., Plano, Tex)
- Subcutaneous tunneller—used to externalize percutaneous trial lead extensions or to connect the lead to the permanent pulse generator
- Trial stimulator—external generator used during trial stimulation period
- Anchors—to anchor the leads as they exit the fascia or the skin; also prevent migration
- Lead extension—used to connect the epidural leads to the internal pulse generator (IPG) or to extend out to the trial stimulator when the leads are intended to be permanent if the trial is successful
- IPG—implanted programmable power source

Technique

Several techniques for stimulation of lower lumbar and sacral nerve roots have been described in the literature. These include intraspinal, typically transforaminal, NRS; extraforaminal NRS; and trans-spinal NRS. Each may have advantages or disadvantages in various situations.

Intraspinal Nerve Root Stimulation

In these techniques the desired roots are stimulated from the intraspinal epidural space. This can be accomplished via an anterograde or retrograde placement. Anterograde placement is usually used for thoracic and cervical roots, with a traditional entry point in the upper lumbar spine, keeping the electrode in the midline as for a traditional dorsal column stimulator; and then rolling laterally to cover the nerve root in the lateral gutter as it approaches the foramen. This approach is not feasible for the lower lumbar or sacral roots, but entry at the sacral hiatus can be used for anterograde access to these lower roots.[39] Widespread adoption of this technique has been limited by the extremely caudal area of the incision and the personal hygiene issues that are associated with it. The concern for infection with any contamination of the wound in permanent implant situations is considerable, and it is often difficult to place the connections and anchors in this region in such a way that they are not uncomfortable in a seated position when the permanent system is fully implanted. Selective NRS via the retrograde (aka cephalocaudad) percutaneous placement of electrode is also a well-established technique. It has been described by two techniques. Under fluoroscopic guidance the epidural Tuohy needle can be placed in a paramedian fashion and advanced caudally until it reaches the desired interspace. The shingling of the laminae (**Fig. 13-5**) can make access to the epidural space quite difficult from this approach; but, if the electrode can be introduced to the epidural space in this fashion, it can be directed retrograde from this point without difficulty. Because of the technical difficulty of this approach and the steep learning curve, several centers have moved to what is often termed the *laterograde approach.*[40,41] In this technique the Tuohy needle begins initial approach to eventual S2-3 placement more laterally at the L2-L3 interspace, with an entry angle nearly perpendicular to the skin (**Fig. 13-6**). The bevel is then rotated caudally, and the electrode introduced and passed caudally in the midline (**Fig. 13-7**).[42]

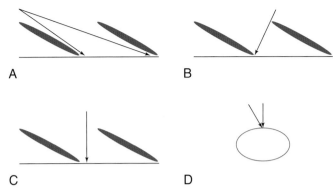

Fig. 13-5   Schematic showing anatomic relationships important in understanding the laterograde approach for craniocaudal electrode placement. Note the "shingled" laminae (blue ovals) and spinous processes. The black line represents the dura, and the black arrows depict trajectories a physician can use to access the epidural space for electrode placement. A, In a traditional anterograde electrode placement, the orientation of the laminae allows a wide variety of trajectories and a very shallow angle of approach, which minimizes the risk of dural penetration. B, In the sagittal plane the orientation of the laminae limits the ability to obtain a shallow angle of approach to the dura in a craniocaudal approach. C, Approaching "straight on" in the sagittal plane provides a wide corridor of entry, but the angle of approach to the dura must be controlled in the axial plane. D, In the axial plane with a midline site of entry, the dura (blue line) is beginning to slope away; and as the needle approach is brought more steeply from lateral to medial, the angle of approach to the dura becomes more shallow. Reprinted with permission from Neuromodulation—Technology at the Neural Interface, 2010.

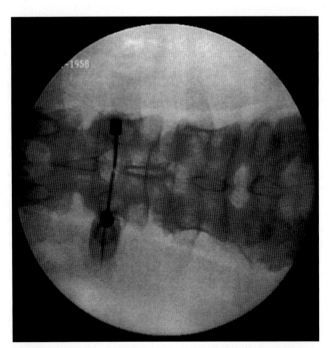

Fig. 13-6   Placement of dual S2-S3 "retrograde" electrodes: the needle placement is bilateral with the needle tips nearly "kissing" in the midline. Reprinted with permission from Deer T: Atlas of implantable therapies for pain management, New York: Springer, 2011.

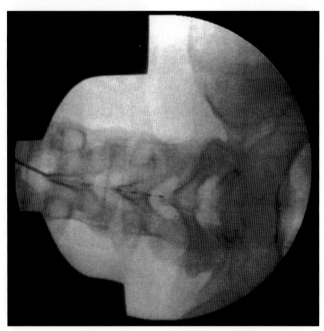

Fig. 13-7   Placement of S2-S3 "retrograde" electrodes: the electrode is directed caudally in the midline. Reprinted with permission from Deer T: Atlas of implantable therapies for pain management, New York: Springer, 2011.

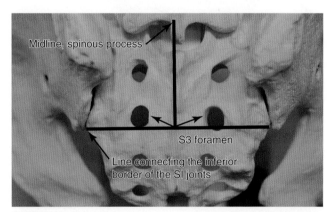

Fig. 13-8   Anatomic landmarks for needle placement at the S3 foramen. The vertical line denotes the midline; the horizontal line connects the inferior limit of the sacroiliac joints. The S3 foramen is generally slightly lateral to the intersection of these two lines. SI, Sacroiliac.

Retrograde Transforaminal Nerve Root Stimulation

To address limited spinal segment pathology, the transforaminal approach for spinal NRS may be used. This can be done through an open laminectomy or through a minimally invasive technique. The electrode is introduced by a retrograde technique; and, when the foramen of interest is approached, the electrode is rotated laterally and passed to just inside the foramen.[42,43]

Extraforaminal Nerve Root Stimulation

This technique is used primarily for isolated S3 stimulation, but it can be applied with modifications at higher levels when dictated by the presence of significant spinal stenosis. Two landmarks are visualized: the spinous processes and the inferior point of the sacroiliac joints. The S3 foramen is located lateral to the intersection of these two lines (Fig. 13-8). The needle is inserted under the fluoroscopic guidance 1 to 4 cm above the foramen. A small paramedian incision is made over the S3 foramen, and a finder needle is

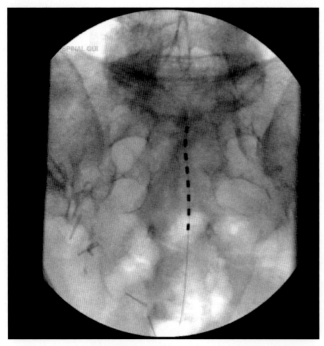

Fig. 13-9 Midline S4-S5 electrode placed by caudal technique for coccygodynia. The entry point is at the sacral hiatus.

inserted. Next, an Angiocath or introducer sheath is advanced over the finder needle. The beveled end of it should not go beyond the S3 foramen. The finder needle is removed, and the permanent electrode (typically the tined Medtronic InterStim (Medtronic, Inc., Minneapolis, Minn) is inserted through the sheath, which is removed.[44] This technique becomes more invasive when surgical exposure is necessary to identify the foramen.[36] Retrograde lead placements have a lower rate of lead migration.[13]

Sacral Nerve Root Stimulation for the Treatment of Coccygodynia or Sacroiliac Joint Pain

To implant the leads over the S4 and S5 roots, a retrograde technique or the approach through the sacral hiatus is required. With a retrograde technique the needle is advanced caudally in the midline until it crosses S3. However, a transforaminal technique is not used, leaving the electrode in the midline caudally. Care must be taken to avoid placing the tip close to the sacral hiatus since undesired stimulation may result in pain (**Fig. 13-9**).

An alternative technique is to place an electrode in a retrograde fashion over the posterior surface of the sacrum to provide peripheral nerve stimulation as depicted in **Fig. 13-10**. Generally this technique is used after mapping the pain generators with RF stimulation via a needle probe, confirmed with a stimulation-guided local anesthetic block. For coccygodynia this is treated with placement of quadripolar electrodes where stimulation leads to coccygeal paresthesia. This activates the S4-S5 roots and lateral transverse branches but avoids the potential discomfort of stimulation at the sacral hiatus. An identical technique with treatment of the lateral transverse branches of L5 to S3 is often effective in the treatment of sacroiliac joint pain. This represents a fairly simple and stable approach to sacroiliac joint pain, which is extraordinarily difficult to cover from the epidural space.

Patient Management/Evaluation

Evaluation begins with a complete history and examination, followed by appropriate preoperative laboratory evaluation and

imaging as discussed previously. All patients should undergo psychological screening before trial stimulation and receive appropriate psychiatric care as indicated. The trial period varies from center to center, but most commonly lasts for the better part of a week. The programming of stimulation electrodes has evolved from the "simple C-stim" program (continuous stimulation) that gave the patient only a single program, to modern devices, which can often offer multiple independent programs across 16 independently programmed electrodes. This programming flexibility, although often critical in dorsal column stimulation, is often not as critical in selective nerve root applications, where the precise position of the electrode over the foramen is of greatest importance. Criteria for a successful trial generally include a greater than 50% relief of pain, reduced use of narcotic pain medications, and improvement in functional daily activity.

Success of the trial must be gauged sequentially by the answers to two questions. Was the trial technically successful? In other words, when the stimulator is activated, does it produce paresthesias that "map" to the areas of pain? If the paresthesias do not cover the painful areas, the trial is a technical failure, and the second question cannot be asked appropriately. If the paresthesia covers the area of pain, the second question is, "Does it help the pain?" The first question is answered immediately after the trial implantation with the first few programming sessions. The remainder of the trial period is devoted to answering the second question, determining the effect of stimulation on the visual analog scale pain score, the quality of life indices, the use of narcotics, and function in activities of daily living.

Outcome Evidence

Treatment of Interstitial Cystitis

Treatment is tailored to each individual patient. First-line treatment includes diet modifications, oral pentosan polysulfate sodium (PPS), hydroxyzine, amitriptyline, gabapentin, prednisone, and cyclosporine A. Intravesical dimethylsulfoxide (DMSO), cystoscopic bladder hydrodistention, and resection of Hunner ulcers are more aggressive options. Intramural botulinum toxin injections and hyperbaric oxygen have been shown beneficial in some patients.[10,15,45] Major reconstructive surgery has been performed as well.[12,45]

In 1997 the FDA approved the Medtronic InterStim (Medtronic, Inc., Minneapolis, Minn) device for urinary urge incontinence, urinary urgency-frequency, and unobstructive urinary retention.[46] Many reports in the literature document the efficacy of neuromodulation in IC.[13,38,42,47-52] These studies have shown significant decreases in urinary urgency-frequency and pelvic pain and decreased antiproliferative factor activity. These findings were established in a multicenter trial.[53] Improvements in muscular activity are clearly seen in these patients.[47] These patients can experience an initial worsening of their typical symptoms with subsequent improvement,[47,49] which can be treated effectively with caudal epidural block or prevented by giving the block before stimulator placement.[47] It is postulated that, if administered early before the muscularis fibrosis phase, caudal block might prevent or reverse the neurogenic inflammation.[47]

Other centers have found that S2-S4 stimulation from an intraspinal approach, either unilateral or bilateral,[47,54,55] may be more effective than isolated S3 stimulation. Alternatively Peters, Feber, and Bennett[46] in a randomized, cross-over trial demonstrated that pudendal nerve stimulation leads to better improvement than S3 root stimulation.

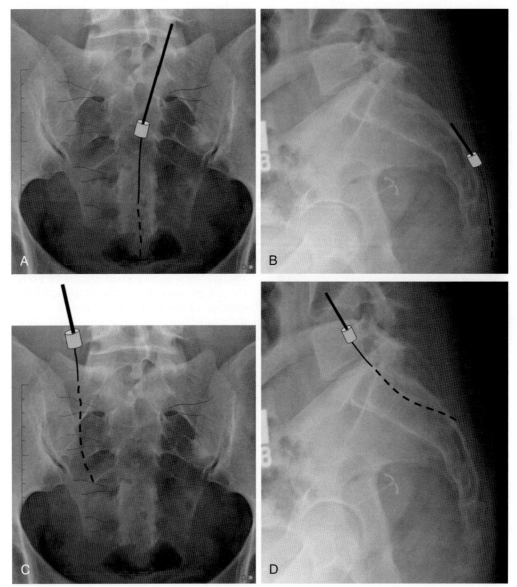

Fig. 13-10 Electrode placement for peripheral nerve stimulation for the treatment of sacroiliac joint pain and coccygodynia. Placement is guided by needle radiofrequency stimulation, followed by confirmation of the pain generator by local anesthetic injection. **A,** AP diagram of placement of a peripheral stimulator for the transverse branches of S4 and S5 to treat coccygodynia. **B,** Lateral diagram of electrode from **A**. **C,** AP diagram of placement to treat the lateral transverse branches from L5 to S3 for sacroiliac pain. **D,** Lateral view of electrode in **C.** *AP,* Anteroposterior. Courtesy of Krista Runge.

Treatment of Vulvodynia

Because of the excellent results in patients with IC, the treatment of vulvodynia has also been explored. Nair and associates[22] reported a patient with vulvodynia treated with bilateral S4 NRS with 90% improvement in symptomatology and overall quality of life.[22] Ramsey, Wright, and Fischer[23] demonstrated an excellent clinical outcome after S3 NRS in a patient with vulvar vestibulitis. The literature for this indication suffers from variable selection of patients, target nerve roots, stimulation systems, and surgical approaches.[13,22,23] Because the disorder is uncommon and difficult to distinguish clearly from other pelvic pain conditions, prospective trials with good outcome scales are very difficult to conduct.

Treatment of Chronic Testicular Pain

Treatment with antibiotics, nonsteroidal antiinflammatory drugs, tricyclic antidepressants, and pudendal nerve blocks is considered

first line for pain management.[26] More invasive methods such as microsurgical denervation of the spermatic cord, epididymectomy, and vasovasostomy have been advocated as the next level of care.[26] When these treatments have failed, the inguinal orchiectomy can be considered. However, sacral nerve stimulation is considered by many to be a less morbid alternative. In a single case McJunkin, Wuollet, and Lynch[27] reported 80% improvement after unilateral S2, S3, and S4 NRS. Feler, Whitworth, and Fernandez[13] demonstrated 75% improvement with sacral NRS at S2-S4 performed via an anterograde approach.

Results Summary

There is a paucity of level I evidence literature on pelvic and sacral NRS for the treatment of CPP and coccygodynia. A review of the literature is summarized in **Table 13-1**.[37,47-49,56-60]

Table 13-1: Literature Review of Outcomes after Sacral Nerve Root Stimulation

Study	Technique	Indication	No. of Patients	Mean Follow-Up (mo)	Outcome, % of Patients With Improvement
Aboseif et al, 2002[37]	Extraforaminal	Idiopathic urinary retention	20	24	90 (Decreased postvoid residual volume and improved quality of life)
Aboseif et al, 2002[56]	Extraforaminal	Voiding dysfunction	64	24	80 (Improvement of presenting symptoms)
Alò, Gohel, and Corey, 2001[57]	Cephalocaudal	Urge incontinence and detrusor dysfunction	1	5	Symptoms resolved
Alò and McKay, 2001[47]	Cephalocaudal	Interstitial cystitis	1	12	Symptoms resolved
Alò et al, 1999[58]	Cephalocaudal	Chronic pelvic pain due to interstitial cystitis, ilioinguinal neuralgia, discogenic low back pain, FBSS, or vulvodynia	5	NS	100 (Achieved paresthesia coverage >75%)
Comiter, 2003[48]	Extraforaminal	Interstitial cystitis	17	14	94 (Improvement in frequency, nocturia, voided volume, and average pain)
Powell and Kreder, 2010[59]	Extraforaminal	Interstitial cystitis	22	60	77 (Improvement in dysuria or pelvic pain)
Sutherland et al, 2007[60]	Extraforaminal	Voiding dysfunction	104	22	69 (>50% Subjective improvement)
Feler, Brookoff, and Powell, 1999[49]	Cephalocaudal	Interstitial cystitis	10	4	70 Responded to treatment (Average reduction in VAS score is 6.6)

FBSS, Failed back surgery syndrome; *mo*, Months; *NS*, not specified; *VAS*, visual analog scale.

Risk and Complication Avoidance

Establishing and practicing strict patient selection criteria are perhaps the most important factors for obtaining positive long-term results. Significant contraindications should be actively searched for, and poor risk patients should not be offered the therapy.

The primary complications are neurological injury, infection, lead migration, and cerebrospinal fluid (CSF) leakage with spinal headache.

The nature of neurological injury is determined by the spinal level of the procedure and the nature of access to the perineural space. As discussed in the section on contraindications, some patients have anatomical abnormalities that increase the risk of complication. For example, spina bifida involves abnormalities of the lamina, and usually of the dura, which makes accurate access of the epidural space and safe steering of the electrodes more difficult. Significant spondylolisthesis changes the alignment of the spinal canal. Large disc herniations or other masses in the spinal canal may be completely asymptomatic but may reduce the volume of the canal to the point that it is no longer possible to place an electrode in the epidural space without neural compromise. The introduction of the Tuohy needle may be traumatic to the neural elements in the setting of severe spinal stenosis or if the needle is passed too deeply by using poor technique in accessing the epidural space.

Meticulous attention to sterile technique and wound closure are the best defenses against infection. It is critical that preoperative antibiotics are administered in such a way that tissue levels are therapeutic at the time of skin incision. The risk of infection is higher at the site of the IPG implantation and is often related to

seroma formation. Avoid making the pocket any larger than necessary since this encourages seroma formation. Wearing an elastic abdominal binder for up to 2 weeks after surgery has been found helpful by many. Women may prefer to find a comfortable girdle with very similar results. If patients find the binder too uncomfortable, any form of gentle pressure after surgery may help to prevent this problem. If a seroma forms and develops significant pressure, it is important to aggressively manage the wound complication quickly, before leakage begins that can lead to infection. Drainage of a seroma and resumption of pressure is one method of addressing this. If the system becomes infected, it must be removed until all evidence of infection is completely resolved, evaluated by imaging and inflammatory markers such as C-reactive protein and erythrocyte sedimentation rate. Some centers routinely keep patients on oral antibiotics for the duration of their externalized trial, but there is no evidence base to support this.

Lead migration, which is a common problem with percutaneous electrodes in general, seems to be somewhat less problematic with intraspinal cephalocaudal placement than with direct extraforaminal techniques, which rely on "tines" on the electrode to prevent backing out (see **Fig. 13-3**) since they pass directly through a significant amount of muscle tissue just before reaching the target. A loss of coverage that is not associated with extremely high impedance (which would indicate a broken lead) is usually caused by migration of the lead. Careful attention to anchoring and formation of a relaxing loop at the midline incision are the technique points to help prevent this complication.[61,62] Particularly with bending and twisting motions of the lower lumbar area, a tension is exerted on the lead or lead extension as it traverses the distance between the entry point to the epidural space and the pulse generator. If this tension is applied repetitively, it can cause lead migration. The mechanics of this process are best avoided by careful attention to the relaxing loop and meticulous attention to anchoring technique. A tension relief loop of at least several centimeters should always be left at the spinal incision. The anchor should attach the lead to the fascia just as it exits the fascia and directly in line with this exit site. When the spine moves in flexion and extension, the distance between the target space and the exit from the fascia changes. When there is a substantial gap between the exit site and the anchor, the electrode may be slightly withdrawn during such movements, but it is quite unlikely to be pushed back through the fascia into position when the movement reverses. This ratcheting phenomenon can lead to electrode migration; but, if the anchor is placed perfectly in line with the exit site and just at the point of fascial exit, these factors are minimized. Some newer anchors have flexible extensions that can be passed through the fascial defect to further minimize this risk.

It is advisable to undermine a small pocket for the relaxing loop above the lumbar fascia to allow the loop to lie flat across the wound. This avoids the tendency for the loop to push up through the wound and risk erosion through the skin.

Most "wet taps," or attempted epidural placement with return of CSF, do not go on to become symptomatic. It is generally not recommended to continue attempting to place the lead in that particular location. Placing two trocars on the same side at a given level or using an adjacent level (typically the level above, to avoid traversing the area) usually allows placement of the electrode and does not aggravate the problem. If the leak becomes symptomatic, a blood patch typically resolves the condition but may slightly increase the risk of infection.

These devices can generally be used safely but cautiously in conjunction with cardiac pacemakers. When used with a cardiac device, they should generally be programmed in bipolar mode, with a frequency of at least 20 Hz. Using caution, with electrocardiogram monitoring during stimulator programming, is advised.[63]

Conclusion

Sacral NRS can be accomplished by a number of techniques, most notably the retrograde intraspinal technique and the direct extraforaminal approach. It is effective for urge incontinence, frequency-urgency syndrome, nonobstructive urinary retention, IC, prostadynia/epididymoorchialgia, vulvodynia, sacroiliac pain, and coccygodynia. Careful attention to precise diagnosis and patient selection, the presence of anatomic abnormalities or significant infection, and meticulous technique maximize patient outcomes and avoid complications.

References

1. Brindley GS: History of the sacral anterior root stimulator, 1969-1982. *Neurourol Urodyn* 12:481-483, 1993.
2. Brindley GS, Polkey CE, Rushton DN: Sacral anterior root stimulators for bladder control in paraplegia. *Paraplegia* 20:365-381, 1982.
3. Brindley GS et al: Sacral anterior root stimulators for bladder control in paraplegia: the first 50 cases. *J Neurol Neurosurg Psychiatry* 49:1104-1114, 1986.
4. Cardozo L et al: Urodynamic observations on patients with sacral anterior root stimulators. *Paraplegia* 22:201-209, 1984.
5. Kohli N, Rosenblatt PL: Neuromodulation techniques for the treatment of the overactive bladder. *Clin Obstet Gynecol* 45:218-232, 2002.
6. Sauerwein D et al: Extradural implantation of sacral anterior root stimulators. *J Neurol Neurosurg Psychiatry* 53:681-684, 1990.
7. Abrams P, Hanno P, Wein A: Overactive bladder and painful bladder syndrome: there need not be confusion. *Neurourol Urodyn* 24:149-150, 2005.
8. Bogart LM, Berry SH, Clemens JQ: Symptoms of interstitial cystitis, painful bladder syndrome and similar diseases in women: a systematic review. *J Urol* 177:450-456, 2007.
9. Butrick CW: Interstitial cystitis and chronic pelvic pain: new insights in neuropathology, diagnosis, and treatment. *Clin Obstet Gynecol* 46:811-823, 2003.
10. Hanno P, Nordling J, van Ophoven A: What is new in bladder pain syndrome/interstitial cystitis? *Curr Opin Urol* 18:353-358, 2008.
11. Marinkovic SP, Gillen LM: Sacral neuromodulation for multiple sclerosis patients with urinary retention and clean intermittent catheterization. *Int Urogynecol J Pelvic Floor Dysfunct* 21:223-228, 2010.
12. Marinkovic SP et al: The management of interstitial cystitis or painful bladder syndrome in women. *Br Med J* 339:b2707, 2009.
13. Feler CA, Whitworth LA, Fernandez J: Sacral neuromodulation for chronic pain conditions. *Anesthesiol Clin North Am* 21:785-795, 2003.
14. Clemens JQ et al: Prevalence and incidence of interstitial cystitis in a managed care population. *J Urol* 173:98-102; discussion 102, 2005.
15. Dell JR, Mokrzycki ML, Jayne CJ: Differentiating interstitial cystitis from similar conditions commonly seen in gynecologic practice. *Eur J Obstet Gynecol Reprod Biol* 144:105-109, 2009.
16. Metts JF: Interstitial cystitis: urgency and frequency syndrome. *Am Fam Physician* 64:1199-1206, 2001.
17. Sant GR, Theoharides TC: Interstitial cystitis. *Curr Opin Urol* 9:297-302, 1999.
18. van de Merwe J et al: Diagnostic criteria, classification, and nomenclature for painful bladder syndrome/interstitial cystitis: an ESSIC proposal. *Eur Urol* 53:60-67, 2008.
19. Peters KM et al: Fact or fiction—is abuse prevalent in patients with interstitial cystitis? Results from a community survey and clinic population. *J Urol* 178:891-895; discussion 895, 2007.
20. Rodriguez MA, Afari N, Buchwald DS: Evidence for overlap between urological and nonurological unexplained clinical conditions. *J Urol* 182:2123-2131, 2009.
21. Moyal-Barracco M, Lynch PJ: 2003 ISSVD terminology and classification of vulvodynia: a historical perspective. *J Reprod Med* 49:772-777, 2004.
22. Nair AR et al: Spinal cord stimulator for the treatment of a woman with vulvovaginal burning and deep pelvic pain. *Obstet Gynecol* 111:545-547, 2008.
23. Ramsay LB, Wright J, Jr, Fischer JR: Sacral neuromodulation in the treatment of vulvar vestibulitis syndrome. *Obstet Gynecol* 114:487-489, 2009.
24. Reed BD: Vulvodynia: diagnosis and management. *Am Fam Physician* 73:1231-1238, 2006.
25. Farage MA, Galask RP: Vulvar vestibulitis syndrome: a review. *Eur J Obstet Gynecol Reprod Biol* 123:9-16, 2005.
26. Granitsiotis P, Kirk D: Chronic testicular pain: an overview. *Eur Urol* 45:430-436, 2004.
27. McJunkin TL, Wuollet AL, Lynch PJ: Sacral nerve stimulation as a treatment modality for intractable neuropathic testicular pain. *Pain Physician* 12:991-995, 2009.
28. Miller JL et al: Prostatodynia and interstitial cystitis: one and the same? *Urology* 45:587-590, 1995.
29. Maigne JY, Guedj S, Straus C: Idiopathic coccygodynia. Lateral roentgenograms in the sitting position and coccygeal discography. *Spine (Phila Pa 1976)* 19:930-934, 1994.
30. Melzack R, Wall PD: Pain mechanisms: a new theory. *Science* 150:971-979, 1965.
31. Shaker H et al: Role of C-afferent fibres in the mechanism of action of sacral nerve root neuromodulation in chronic spinal cord injury. *BJU Int* 85:905-910, 2000.
32. Matharu MS et al: Central neuromodulation in chronic migraine patients with suboccipital stimulators: a PET study. *Brain* 127:220-230, 2004.
33. Chadha S et al: Histopathologic features of vulvar vestibulitis. *Int J Gynecol Pathol* 17:7-11, 1998.

34. Elbadawi AE, Light JK: Distinctive ultrastructural pathology of non-ulcerative interstitial cystitis: new observations and their potential significance in pathogenesis. *Urol Int* 56:137-162, 1996.

35. Elgavish A et al: Evidence for altered proliferative ability of progenitors of urothelial cells in interstitial cystitis. *J Urol* 158:248-252, 1997.

36. Haque R, Winfree CJ: Spinal nerve root stimulation. *Neurosurg Focus* 21:E4, 2006.

37. Aboseif S et al: Sacral neuromodulation as an effective treatment for refractory pelvic floor dysfunction. *Urology* 60:52-56, 2002.

38. Chai TC et al: Percutaneous sacral third nerve root neurostimulation improves symptoms and normalizes urinary HB-EGF levels and anti-proliferative activity in patients with interstitial cystitis. *Urology* 55:643-646, 2000.

39. Jonas U et al: Efficacy of sacral nerve stimulation for urinary retention: results 18 months after implantation. *J Urol* 165:15-19, 2001.

40. Richter EO, Abramova MV, Alò KM: Percutaneous cephalocaudal implantation of epidural stimulation electrodes over sacral nerve root—a technical note on the importance of the lateral approach, Neuromodulation—Technology at the Neural Interface. *Neuromodulation* 14:62-67, 2011.

41. Alò KM: Selective nerve root stimulation: facilitating the cephalocaudal "retrograde" method of electrode insertion. In: Deer T, editor: *Atlas of implantable therapies for pain management*, New York, 2011, Springer, pp 107-114.

42. Alò K, Feler CA: Retrograde peripheral nerve root stimulation for interstitial cystitis: update of clinical results, Worldwide pain conference, San Francisco, California, July 18, 2000.

43. Schmidt RA et al: Sacral nerve stimulation for treatment of refractory urinary urge incontinence: Sacral Nerve Stimulation Study Group. *J Urol* 162:352-357, 1999.

44. Chai TC, Mamo GJ: Modified techniques of S3 foramen localization and lead implantation in S3 neuromodulation. *Urology* 58:786-790, 2001.

45. Fall M, Oberpenning F, Peeker R: Treatment of bladder pain syndrome/interstitial cystitis 2008: can we make evidence-based decisions? *Eur Urol* 54:65-75, 2008.

46. Peters KM, Feber KM, Bennett RC: A prospective, single-blind, randomized crossover trial of sacral vs pudendal nerve stimulation for interstitial cystitis. *BJU Int* 100:835-839, 2007.

47. Alò K, McKay E: Selective Nerve root stimulation (SNRS) for the treatment of intractable pelvic pain and motor dysfunction: case report. *Neuromodulation* 4:19-23, 2001.

48. Comiter CV: Sacral neuromodulation for the symptomatic treatment of refractory interstitial cystitis: a prospective study. *J Urol* 169:1369-1373, 2003.

49. Feler CA WL, Brookoff D, Powell R: Recent advances: sacral nerve root stimulation using a retrograde method of lead insertion for the treatment of pelvic pain due to interstitial cystitis. *Neuromodulation* 2:211-216, 1999.

50. Maher CF et al: Percutaneous sacral nerve root neuromodulation for intractable interstitial cystitis. *J Urol* 165:884-886, 2001.

51. Peters KM: Neuromodulation for the treatment of refractory interstitial cystitis. *Rev Urol* 4(suppl 1):S36-43, 2002.

52. Peters KM, Konstandt D: Sacral neuromodulation decreases narcotic requirements in refractory interstitial cystitis. *BJU Int* 93:777-779, 2004.

53. Whitmore KE et al: Sacral neuromodulation in patients with interstitial cystitis: a multicenter clinical trial. *Int Urogynecol J Pelvic Floor Dysfunct* 14:305-308; discussion 308-309, 2003.

54. Steinberg AC, Oyama IA, Whitmore KE: Bilateral S3 stimulator in patients with interstitial cystitis. *Urology* 69:441-443, 2007.

55. Zabihi N et al: Short-term results of bilateral S2-S4 sacral neuromodulation for the treatment of refractory interstitial cystitis, painful bladder syndrome, and chronic pelvic pain. *Int Urogynecol J Pelvic Floor Dysfunct* 19:553-557, 2008.

56. Aboseif S et al: Sacral neuromodulation in functional urinary retention: an effective way to restore voiding. *BJU Int* 90:662-665, 2002.

57. Alò K, Gohel R, Corey C: Sacral nerve root stimulation for the treatment of urge incontinence and detrusor dysfunction utilizing a cephalocaudal intraspinal method of lead insertion: a case report. *Neuromodulation* 4:53-58, 2001.

58. Alò K et al: A study of electrode placement at the cervical and upper thoracic nerve roots using an anatomic trans-spinal approach. *Neuromodulation* 2:222-227, 1999.

59. Powell CR, Kreder KJ: Long-term outcomes of urgency-frequency syndrome due to painful bladder syndrome treated with sacral neuromodulation and analysis of failures. *J Urol* 183:173-176, 2010.

60. Sutherland SE et al: Sacral nerve stimulation for voiding dysfunction: One institution's 11-year experience. *Neurourol Urodyn* 26:19-28; discussion 36, 2007.

61. Oh MY et al: Peripheral nerve stimulation for the treatment of occipital neuralgia and transformed migraine using a c1-2-3 subcutaneous paddle style electrode: a technical report. *Neuromodulation* 7:103-112, 2004.

62. Alò KM: Technical tips: percutaneous lead anchoring techniques—drain suture technique, *Pain Relief News*. Medtronic Neurological l1(Issue 2):7, 2005.

63. Stojanovic MP: Stimulation methods for neuropathic pain control. *Curr Pain Headache Rep* 5:130-137, 2001.

14 Emerging Indications and Other Applications of Spinal Cord Stimulation

Konstantin V. Slavin

CHAPTER OVERVIEW

Chapter Synopsis: This chapter deals with the emerging indications for electrical stimulation of the spinal cord (SCS). Although primarily used to treat neuropathic pain conditions, SCS has been shown to be effective in other realms. It is important to note that it has been shown to improve the pathophysiology that underlies some conditions. SCS can relieve ischemia caused by vascular insufficiencies, as in chronic refractory angina and peripheral vascular disease. Further study will be required to confirm early results of SCS effects on cerebral blood flow as well, which one could imagine might have far-reaching implications for numerous pathological brain conditions. Improvements have also been documented in motor control, including relief of spasticity, dystonia, and even parkinsonian symptoms. One study documented patients with complete motor spinal cord injury who experienced recovery of motor function in the legs after receiving SCS. Urinary functional improvements have been seen in neuropathic pelvic conditions and in paraplegics, and female sexual function has also been improved. Even cognitive function can be normalized by SCS in some applications. A number of patients have emerged from coma after treatment with SCS. Hopefully the number of FDA-approved indications for SCS will continue to grow in the coming years in order to make use of the technique in these currently "off-label" areas.

Important Points:
- Spinal cord stimulation may be used for many indications other than pain.
- Motor, vasoactive, genitourinary, and even cognitive effects of spinal cord stimulation have been extensively explored since the modality was introduced half a century ago.
- All of these indications are considered "off-label" based on regulatory approval of national device-regulating authorities and by most manufacturing companies.
- In most cases (with the exception of spinal cord stimulation for peripheral vascular disease and intractable angina), more research will be needed in order to get scientific proof of effect and subsequent acceptance by medical community.

Introduction

Spinal cord stimulation (SCS) is an established modality for treatment of chronic pain. Over the years it has become the most common surgical intervention for medically intractable pain and is now used worldwide with full acceptance by the medical community, patients, and third-party payers. The underlying principle appears to involve electrical activation of the dorsal columns of the spinal cord that is delivered through epidurally placed cylindrical or paddle-type electrodes. Production of paresthesias in the region of pain strongly correlates with the pain relief, and the steering of paresthesias is an integral part of SCS trial procedures.

However, in addition to the beneficial effect on chronic pain, SCS has been used successfully in many other conditions. Indications for clinical and laboratory SCS applications other than pain may be divided into several large categories (**Box 14-1**):

- Motor control, including relief of spasticity, dystonia, and, most recently, parkinsonian symptoms
- Vasoactive SCS effects that are used in treatment of peripheral vascular disease and coronary ischemia
- Genitourinary applications ranging from incontinence control in paraplegics to augmentation of female sexual function in anorgasmia

- More esoteric indications such as impaired consciousness caused by various cerebral pathologies, management of autonomic hyperreflexia, prevention and treatment of cerebral arterial vasospasm, and improvement in tissue perfusion in brain tumors aimed at increased radiosensitivity and chemosensitivity

Motor Control

Beneficial effects of SCS on spasticity were discovered early; multiple reports in the 1970s documented usefulness of SCS in improvement of spasticity. Objective evaluation of stretch and H reflexes was used to support clinical results,[1] and the most responsive cause of spasticity was dysfunction of the spinal cord as a result of injury or demyelination.[2] Developed as an alternative to destructive interventions,[3,4] SCS was used in many clinical centers throughout Europe, Asia, and America with impressive long-term results.[5-8] In addition to patients with spinal cord injuries, SCS was tried in patients with multiple sclerosis, poststroke hemiparesis, dystonia, and cerebral palsy. Animal experiments were used to confirm clinical observations and to find an explanation for the SCS effect and putative mechanism of SCS action in these circumstances.[9]

It has been postulated that spasticity may be relieved with electrical inhibition of impulses transmitted through the reticulospinal tract. The anterior location of the reticulospinal tract in the spinal cord does not allow direct stimulation of this structure from the posterior epidural space without impulses traveling through the dorsal columns. This may explain (a) the observed need in higher-than-usual settings for spasticity control, (b) the fact that paresthesia coverage may not correlate with spasticity relief, and (c) that the spasticity control seems to be more pronounced in patients with more advanced stages of demyelination when sensory impairment allows one to use higher electrical stimulation parameters.

Although the initial impression suggested that spasticity of cerebral origin does not respond to SCS,[2] subsequent studies showed sustained benefits of SCS in patients with poststroke weakness,[10,11] dystonia,[12] and posthypoxic encephalopathy.[13] The general enthusiasm was lowered by reports indicating a lack of clinical long-term effectiveness[14,15] or cost-effectiveness of SCS in spasticity,[16] but the main reason for almost complete abandonment of this once popular SCS indication was introduction of intrathecal baclofen administration.[17] However, in countries where intrathecal baclofen is not available because of regulatory barriers, SCS remains a useful tool for treatment of otherwise refractory spasticity through nondestructive intervention.[18,19]

In addition to suppression of spasticity in symptomatic patients, SCS may be effective in recovery of motor function in paraplegic patients. A study of 10 patients with complete motor spinal cord injury indicated that epidural SCS at the lumbosacral spinal cord level recruited leg muscles in a segmental-selective way, generating integrated motor behavior of sustained extension and rhythmic flexion and extension movements.[20] In the case of an incomplete spinal cord injury, a wheelchair-dependent patient was able to walk with a walker essentially in effortless manner after prolonged SCS. The superiority of gait assisted by SCS was particularly impressive in ambulation at longer distances.[21]

The latest surge of interest to SCS in treatment of motor disorders came from an experimental study showing improvement in locomotion in an experimental model of Parkinson disease (PD).[22]

The improvement in mobility and restoration of normal patterns of neuronal activity were observed with dorsal column stimulation in both the acute PD model of pharmacologically dopamine-depleted mice and the chronic PD model of hydroxydopamine lesioned rats.[22]

Vasoactive Applications of Spinal Cord Stimulation

With the primary intent of pain relief, early SCS implanters noticed that in addition to paresthesias and/or sense of vibration, patients described a sensation of warmth in their extremities; along with this subjective sensation there may have been objective vasodilation and blood flow augmentation. As early as 1976, multiple groups described changes in peripheral blood flow in response to SCS, laying a foundation for subsequent widespread clinical applications.[23,24]

This consistent and reproducible effect on autonomic functions became the basis of SCS application for blood flow augmentation and ischemic pain relief in treatment of vascular disorders such as peripheral arterial occlusive disease,[25] coronary ischemia/intractable angina,[26] and vasospastic disease in extremities.[27]

A significant wealth of information for these indications exists in the current literature; in this text there are separate chapters dealing with peripheral vascular disease and intractable angina as indications for SCS.

Genitourinary Effects of Spinal Cord Stimulation

Conus medullaris SCS for micturition control in a paraplegic patient was first performed in 1970; this approach was later used in a group of 10 other paraplegic patients with long-lasting symptomatic improvement.[28] Improved bladder control was one of the major results of SCS in a group of 24 patients with upper motor neuron disease, including multiple sclerosis, traumatic spinal cord injury, and neurodegenerative conditions,[29] and another group of 11 patients with multiple sclerosis.[30]

When SCS was implanted specifically to treat neurogenic bladder, most patients developed complete or almost complete normalization of urination with relief of bladder spasticity, marked increase of bladder capacity, and reduction or abolition of postvoid residual urine volume.[31] The same group of authors noticed no changes in bladder striatal activity or detrusor reflexes in patients who underwent SCS for pain treatment and had intact bladder function.[31]

The urodynamic changes do not occur in all patients undergoing SCS. In a study of patients with spinal cord injury who underwent SCS implantation for control of spasticity, less than 20% (6 of 33) were found to have changes in lower urinary tract function.[32]

In addition to bladder function normalization, SCS appeared to facilitate normalization of bowel regimen and morning erections in a group of patients with posttraumatic paraplegia.[3]

In a somewhat unconventional approach, SCS was used to treat female orgasmic dysfunction.[33] In this series of 11 patients, a single percutaneous SCS electrode was used to produce pleasurable genital stimulation and subsequent orgasm. In 91% of subjects, SCS resulted in increased lubrication, greater frequency in sexual activity, and overall satisfaction. An orgasmic capacity returned in 80% of patients with secondary anorgasmia while using SCS, but anorgasmia returned once the device was removed. Despite pleasurable paresthesias in the genital area, none of the patients with primary anorgasmia (those who never had an orgasm) experienced orgasm during the study, making the researchers speculate on whether the underlying difficulty that prevented orgasm from occurring throughout the patient's life could not be overcome with SCS application. At the same time a possibility of a longer stimulation period (longer than 9 days) resolving primary anorgasmia was also brought up.[33]

Other Areas of Spinal Cord Stimulation Application

Impaired Consciousness

Anecdotal experience exists with use of SCS for treatment of impaired consciousness. Out of eight patients with severe brain dysfunction resulting from head injury, vasospasm, or tumor resection, two regained consciousness and speech after 1 to 2 months of cervical SCS.[34] The patients were implanted with a four-contact paddle electrode at the C2-C4 level, and the stimulation was delivered twice a day for 4 hours. The authors concluded that SCS may accelerate the natural course of recovery in patients after brain injury.

In the treatment of a vegetative state, 8 out of 23 patients who underwent SCS exhibited symptomatic improvement, and 7 of these were able to follow verbal orders.[35] It was noted that onset of improvement varied from the first few weeks to as long as 10 to 12 months after SCS initiation. There was significant improvement in cerebral blood flow (CBF) associated with SCS in some of the patients, but this phenomenon did not correlate with clinical improvement.

As to the mechanism of symptomatic improvement, positron emission tomography revealed changes in glucose consumption in two patients with prolonged posttraumatic unconsciousness.[36] The patient who improved clinically had higher glucose uptake in the brainstem, hypothalamic, thalamic, and certain cortical regions, whereas the other patient whose consciousness did not improve had no or minimal changes in glucose uptake.

SCS was investigated as an early-stage intervention in patients with hypoxic encephalopathy.[37] An SCS electrode was inserted, and therapy was started within a month after a hypoxic event in 12 patients ranging in age from 7 to 72. The improvement was observed in 58% of patients within 2 weeks after start of SCS. Although there was an improvement in ability to communicate with others and express emotions, disturbances of writing, picture drawing, and calculation were not improved by stimulation.

In the most recent update on this topic, it appears that, based on clinical experience with more than 200 patients treated with SCS for impaired consciousness, indications for surgery may include young age, history of brain trauma, evidence of brain atrophy with no other major lesions, and CBF values of 20 mL/100 g/min or higher.[38] It appears that, of 15 patients who satisfied all criteria for surgery, 12 improved with SCS, and 7 of these improved significantly, thereby indicating that SCS was effective in 80% of this selected patient group.[38]

Another direction recently explored in the literature involves a combination of cervical SCS and hyperbaric oxygenation (HBO) in 12 patients whose coma lasted more than 3 months.[39] Six patients (50%) emerged from coma as a result of combined treatment and regained consciousness. SCS was delivered through four-contact paddle electrodes, and the stimulation regimen was set as 15 minutes on/15 minutes off for a duration of 14 hours during the daytime. However, it is unclear whether SCS or HBO was responsible for symptomatic improvement since every patient who emerged from his or her vegetative state did so within the first 6 months of treatment, during or soon after the period when both SCS and HBO were administered, and there were no additional dramatic improvements when SCS was used alone.[40]

Autonomic Hyperreflexia

Autonomic hyperreflexia, a frequent and difficult-to-manage symptom of spinal cord injury, was significantly reduced or eliminated in four of five patients implanted with SCS.[41]

Spinal Cord Stimulation and Cerebral Blood Flow

Although mechanism of vasoregulation appears different between cerebral and peripheral or coronary circulations, the ability of SCS to augment peripheral and coronary blood flow was tested in regard to CBF in the mid-1980s. Similar to other fields of SCS use, human experience preceded animal studies. In 1985 Hosobuchi[42] found that SCS at upper cervical levels can increase CBF. The same result was not found with stimulation of thoracic levels. Later, the same author tested cervical SCS for three patients with symptomatic cerebral ischemia (one with anterior and two with posterior circulation occlusion); although positive results were obtained, further studies were suggested to confirm its clinical application.[43]

Multiple animal experiments in rats, cats, rabbits, and dogs[44-52] have shown augmentation of CBF with cervical SCS. Level of stimulation seemed to have direct effect on the blood flow, with stimulation of upper levels (C1-C3) generating higher flow values.

Using a cat model, a group from Japan showed that CBF augmentation with cervical SCS is no longer observed after sectioning of the dorsal columns at the cervicomedullary junction.[44] Based on this, the authors postulated that CBF is increased from cervical SCS mainly through a central pathway. Later, similar results were obtained using a rat model by a group of American researchers.[48] They also showed lack of changes in CBF after resection of superior cervical ganglion while using SCS.

Researchers from Italy demonstrated that SCS can increase, decrease, or have no effect in CBF.[53] The difference correlated mainly with the stimulated level of the spinal cord. Thoracic stimulation had low effect and sometimes even decreased CBF. Cervical stimulation more frequently produced CBF augmentation (61%). In another study the same group found that vasoconstriction of carotid arteries with sympathetic trunk stimulation was attenuated by cervical SCS.[54] In this experiment they used rabbit models to observe CBF changes with SCS alone, sympathetic trunk stimulation alone, and simultaneous spinal cord and sympathetic trunk stimulation.

The hypothetic treatment for cerebral vasospasm after subarachnoid hemorrhage (SAH) with SCS has been tried in different animal models. Increased blood flow was found in rats with SAH and SCS compared to control groups.[46] Similarly, prevention of early vasospasm was described in rabbits treated with SCS after induced SAH.[55] Recently the vasodilation effect of SCS was shown in the basilar artery of rats 5 days after induction of SAH. Radiotracer studies, laser Doppler flowmetry, and histological photomicrographs were used to prove these changes in the delayed spasm.[51]

Based on the literature data suggesting several possible mechanisms for SCS action in the prevention and treatment of SAH-related vasospasm, we hypothesized that stimulation at different levels of the cervical spinal cord results in different clinical effects.[56] In theory, stimulation of the lower cervical spinal cord may allow one to prevent vasospasm by acting through modulation of sympathetic activity, essentially constituting a functional, temporary sympathectomy and preventing cerebral arteries from vasoconstriction after SAH. But once the vasospasm is present, the patient may receive additional benefit and possibly improve clinical outcome by CBF augmentation and treatment of the vasospasm by stimulation of the upper cervical spinal cord, possibly acting through more central, medullary mechanisms that are responsible for immediate vasospasm after SAH and for subsequent vasodilation needed for vasospasm treatment.[56]

A pioneering study related to the use of SCS for cerebral vasospasm in humans was performed in the late 1990s in Japan.[57] Ten SAH patients with a secured cerebral aneurysm were implanted with percutaneous quadripolar epidural cervical leads. The stimulation was continuous and started on day 5 ($\pm$1) after bleeding for 10 to 15 days. CBF was measured with Xenon computed tomography; it was significantly increased in the distribution of the middle cerebral artery with SCS. Four patients presented with angiographic vasospasm, and three were reported with clinical vasospasm. One patient died, and the overall outcome was good or excellent in seven. No major adverse effect was attributed to the use of SCS. The data analysis correlated an increase in CBF with SCS.

To prove the concept, we recently performed a prospective safety/feasibility study of cervical SCS in the prevention/treatment of cerebral vasospasm after aneurysmal SAH. In our study 12 patients were implanted with percutaneous eight-contact SCS electrodes immediately on completion of the aneurysm-securing procedure, either clipping or coiling, while the patient was still under general anesthesia (**Fig. 14-1**). By the study protocol SCS had to be initiated the following morning and within 72 hours after SAH and then administered continuously for 14 consecutive days. We found that cervical SCS was safe and feasible since there were no complications related to the electrode insertion or the stimulation itself. One patient died during the study from unrelated causes, and two electrodes were pulled out prematurely. Angiographic vasospasm was observed in 6 of 12 patients, and clinical vasospasm in 2 out of 12. Both incidences were smaller than predicted based on Fisher and Hunt and Hess grades, although this incidence reduction did not reach statistical significance. There were no long-term side effects of SCS during 1-year follow up. Subsequent data analysis indicated that preventive effects of cervical SCS on vasospasm may correlate with stimulated level.[58]

In addition to acute ischemia from cerebral vasospasm, SCS has been shown to increase CBF in chronic ischemic conditions. The results were encouraging in the patients with chronic vascular occlusion,[43] and in a case of old cerebral infarction, SCS resulted in a dramatic increase of blood flow velocities measured by transcranial Doppler.[59]

Spinal Cord Stimulation and Brain Tumors

In a novel application of SCS, at cervical level it was shown to increase local blood flow in patients with brain tumors.[60] This phenomenon was then used in a clinical series of 23 patients with high-grade malignant brain tumors.[61] Based on the known association between hypoxia and low perfusion in malignant neoplasms and resistance to radiotherapy and the significant increase in tumor radiosensitivity with increased local tissue oxygenation, the researchers postulated that, with its augmentation of CBF and ability to increase glucose metabolism, SCS may improve treatment outcome in high-grade gliomas. Although clinical outcome data are still pending, the preliminary results were described as promising, and the blood flow and glucose metabolism have been consistently higher in patients with high-grade gliomas undergoing continuous cervical SCS.[61] In this patient group a single four-contact percutaneous SCS electrode was placed over the dorsal surface of the spinal cord at the C2-C4 level; the stimulation was delivered at amplitude of 3 V or less, producing mild paresthesias in upper extremities.

Spinal Cord Stimulation and Radiation-Induced Brain Injury

Since hypoxia and impaired tissue perfusion are hallmarks for the radiation-induced brain injury, cervical SCS was used to improve

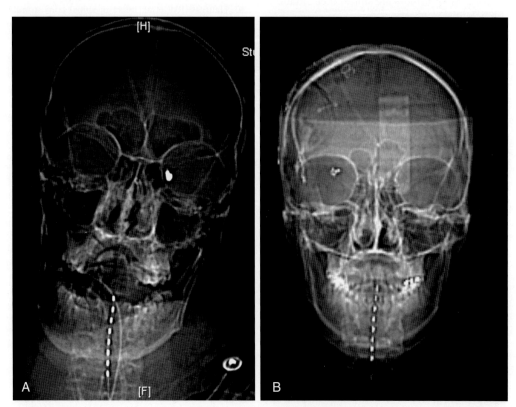

Fig. 14-1 Postoperative radiographs of eight-contact spinal cord stimulation electrode in patient after recent subarachnoid hemorrhage. **A,** Patient with recent endovascular obliteration of ruptured cerebral aneurysm. **B,** Patient after craniotomy for aneurysm clipping.

glucose metabolism in a prospective series of eight patients.[62] As the glucose metabolism increased by about 40% as the result of stimulation, the authors noted a decrease in corticosteroid requirements in patients without concurrent tumor. These results may offer a new avenue for treatment of radiation-induced brain injury, perhaps decreasing or eliminating the need in radical surgical interventions for this frustrating and hard-to-manage pathological condition.

Conclusions

Although SCS is used primarily for control of chronic pain, interest in SCS applications for a variety of other indications continues to grow. In the constantly changing field of neuromodulation, some indications disappear as a result of advancement of competing approaches (as in the case of intrathecal baclofen replacing SCS use for treatment of spasticity), whereas others become more promising. For example, the use of SCS for treatment of PD may be a less invasive alternative to the deep brain stimulation.

Use of SCS for peripheral vascular disease and intractable angina remains extremely common in Europe, but the lack of Food and Drug Administration approval prevents its widespread acceptance in the United States.

SCS for the minimally conscious and vegetative state may be used before considering more invasive approaches such as deep brain stimulation.

In the field of genitourinary conditions, sacral nerve stimulation may be augmented in some patients with SCS, and changes in sexual function may become another common use of this technology if the anecdotal published experience is confirmed by larger clinical series.

The newer and promising indications such as cerebral vasospasm have a potential of significant improvement in morbidity and mortality in a very difficult patient category, whereas other directions such as SCS for brain tumors are still in their infancy with rather uncertain potential implications.

References

1. Siegfried J et al: Electrical spinal cord stimulation for spastic movement disorders. *Appl Neurophysiol* 41:134-141, 1978.
2. Siegfried J: Treatment of spasticity by dorsal cord stimulation. *Int Rehabil Med* 2:31-34, 1980.
3. Richardson RR et al: Percutaneous epidural neurostimulation in modulation of paraplegic spastic: six case reports. *Acta Neurochir (Wien)* 49:235-243, 1979.
4. Barolat G: Surgical management of spasticity and spasms in spinal cord injury: an overview. *J Am Paraplegia Soc* 11:9-13, 1988.
5. Reynolds AF, Oakley JC: High frequency cervical epidural stimulation for spasticity. *Appl Neurophysiol* 45:93-97, 1982.
6. Koulousakis A, Buchhaas U, Nittner K: Application of SCS for movement disorders and spasticity. *Acta Neurochir (Wien)* 39(suppl):112-116, 1987.
7. Barolat G, Myklebust JB, Wenninger W: Effects of spinal cord stimulation on spasticity and spasms secondary to myelopathy. *Appl Neurophysiol* 51(1):29-44, 1988.
8. Kanaka TS, Kumar MM: Neural stimulation for spinal spasticity. *Paraplegia* 28:399-405, 1990.
9. Maiman DJ, Mykleburst JB, Barolat-Romana G: Spinal cord stimulation for amelioration of spasticity: experimental results. *Neurosurgery* 21:331-313, 1987.
10. Nakamura S, Tsubokawa T: Evaluation of spinal cord stimulation for postapoplectic spastic hemiplegia. *Neurosurgery* 17:253-259, 1985.
11. Cioni B, Meglio M: Spinal cord stimulation improves motor performances in hemiplegics: clinical and neurophysiological study. *Acta Neurochir (Wien)* 39(suppl):103-105, 1987.
12. Goetz CG, Penn RD, Tanner CM: Efficacy of cervical cord stimulation in dystonia. *Adv Neurol* 50:645-649, 1988.
13. Terao T et al: Therapeutic effect of spinal cord stimulation for a patient suffering spasticity after hypoxia of the brain. *No Shinkei Geka* 32:613-618, 2004.
14. Gottlieb GL et al: Evaluation of cervical stimulation for chronic treatment of spasticity. *Neurology* 35:699-704, 1985.
15. Hugenholtz H et al: Cervical spinal cord stimulation for spasticity in cerebral palsy. *Neurosurgery* 1988;22:707-714, 1988.
16. Midha M, Schmitt JK: Epidural spinal cord stimulation for the control of spasticity in spinal cord injury patients lacks long-term efficacy and is not cost-effective. *Spinal Cord* 36:190-192, 1998.
17. Lazorthes Y et al: The surgical management of spasticity. *Eur J Neurol* 9(suppl 1):35-41; discussion 53-61, 2002.
18. Shabalov VA et al: The use of chronic epidural electrostimulation of the spinal cord in children with spastic diplegia—a type of infantile cerebral palsy. *Zh Vopr Neirokhir Im N N Burdenko* (3):2-6, 2000.
19. Shabalov VA, Dekopov AV, Troshina EM: Preliminary results of treatment for spastic forms of infantile cerebral paralysis by chronic epidural neurostimulation of lumbar enlargement. *Zh Vopr Neirokhir Im N N Burdenko* 3:10-13, 2006.
20. Minassian K et al: Stepping-like movements in humans with complete spinal cord injury induced by epidural stimulation of the lumbar cord: electromyographic study of compound muscle action potentials. *Spinal Cord* 42:401-416, 2004.
21. Herman R et al: Spinal cord stimulation facilitates functional walking in a chronic, incomplete spinal cord injured. *Spinal Cord* 40:65-68, 2002.
22. Fuentes R et al: Spinal cord stimulation restores locomotion in animal models of Parkinson's disease. *Science* 323:1578-1582, 2009.
23. Dooley DM, Kasprak M: Modification of blood flow to the extremities by electrical stimulation of the nervous system. *South Med J* 69:1309-1311, 1976.
24. Cook AW et al: Vascular disease of extremities: electric stimulation of spinal cord and posterior roots. *NY State J Med* 76:366-368, 1976.
25. Vincenzo S, Kyventidis T: Epidural spinal cord stimulation in lower limb ischemia. *Acta Neurochir* 97(suppl 1):253-258, 2007.
26. Hautvast RW et al: Effect of spinal cord stimulation on myocardial blood flow assessed by positron emission tomography in patients with refractory angina pectoris. *Am J Cardiol* 77:462-467, 1996.
27. Robaina FJ et al: Spinal cord stimulation for relief of chronic pain in vasospastic disorders of the upper limbs. *Neurosurgery* 24:63-67, 1989.
28. Nashold BS, Jr et al: Electrical stimulation of the conus medullaris in the paraplegic: a 5-year review. *Appl Neurophysiol* 40:192-207, 1977.
29. Campos RJ et al: Clinical evaluation of the effect of spinal cord stimulation on motor performance in patients with upper motor neuron lesions. *Appl Neurophysiol* 44:141-151, 1981.
30. Read DJ, Matthews WB, Higson RH: The effect of spinal cord stimulation on function in patients with multiple sclerosis. *Brain* 103:803-833, 1980.
31. Meglio M: Epidural spinal cord stimulation for the treatment of neurogenic bladder. *Acta Neurochir (Wien)* 54:191-199, 1980.
32. Katz PG et al: Effect of implanted epidural stimulator on lower urinary tract function in spinal-cord-injured patients. *Eur Urol* 20:103-106, 1991.
33. Meloy TS, Southern JP: Neurally augmented sexual function in human females: a preliminary investigation. *Neuromodulation* 9:34-40, 2006.
34. Matsui T et al: Beneficial effects of cervical spinal cord stimulation (cSCS) on patients with impaired consciousness: a preliminary report. *Pacing Clin Electrophysiol* 12:718-725, 1989.
35. Kanno T et al: Effects of dorsal column spinal cord stimulation on reversibility of neuronal function: experience of treatment for vegetative states. *Pacing Clin Electrophysiol* 12:733-738, 1989.
36. Yamaguchi N et al: Effects of cervical spinal cord stimulation in glucose consumption in patients with post traumatic prolonged unconsciousness. *Neurol Med Chir (Tokyo)* 35:797-803, 1995.
37. Fujii M et al: Spinal cord stimulation in an early stage for unresponsive patients with hypoxic encephalopathy. *No Shinkei Geka* 26:315-321, 1998.

38. Morita I, Keith MW, Kanno T: Dorsal column stimulation for persistent vegetative state. *Acta Neurochir* (suppl) 97(1):455-459, 1007.

39. Liu JT et al: Neuromodulation on cervical spinal cord combined with hyperbaric oxygen in comatose patients—a preliminary report. *Surg Neurol* 72(S2):28-34, 2009.

40. Slavin KV: Commentary to Liu et al (ref 39). *Surg Neurol* 72(S2):34-35, 2009.

41. Richardson RR, Cerullo LJ, Meyer PR: Autonomic hyper-reflexia modulated by percutaneous epidural neurostimulation: a preliminary report. *Neurosurgery* 4:517-520, 1979.

42. Hosobuchi Y: Electrical stimulation of the cervical spinal cord increases cerebral blood flow in humans. *Appl Neurophysiol* 48:372-376, 1985.

43. Hosobuchi Y: Treatment of cerebral ischemia with electrical stimulation of the cervical spinal cord. *Pacing Clin Electrophysiol* 14:122-126, 1991.

44. Isono M et al: Effect of spinal cord stimulation on cerebral blood flow in cats. *Stereotact Funct Neurosurg* 64:40-46, 1995.

45. Sagher O, Huang DL: Effects of cervical spinal cord stimulation on cerebral blood flow in the rat. *J Neurosurg* 93(suppl 1):71-76, 2000.

46. Ebel H et al: High cervical spinal cord stimulation (CSCS) increases regional cerebral blood flow after induced subarachnoid haemorrhage in rats. *Minim Invasive Neurosurg* 44:167–171, 2001.

47. Patel S, Huang DL, Sagher O: Sympathetic mechanisms in cerebral blood flow alterations induced by spinal cord stimulation. *J Neurosurg* 99:754-761, 2003.

48. Patel S, Huang DL, Sagher O: Evidence for a central pathway in the cerebrovascular effects of spinal cord stimulation. *Neurosurgery* 55:201-206, 2004.

49. Gurelik M et al: Cervical spinal cord stimulation improves neurological dysfunction induced by cerebral vasospasm. *Neuroscience* 134:827-332, 2005.

50. Karadağ Ö et al: Cervical spinal cord stimulation increases cerebral cortical blood flow in an experimental vasospasm model. *Acta Neurochir (Wien)* 147:79-84, 2005.

51. Lee JY et al: Effect of electrical stimulation of the cervical spinal cord on blood flow following subarachnoid hemorrhage. *J Neurosurg* 109:1148-1154, 2008.

52. Yang X et al: Roles of dorsal column pathway and transient receptor potential vanilloid type 1 in augmentation of cerebral blood flow by upper cervical spinal cord stimulation in rats. *Neuroscience* 152:950-958, 2008.

53. Visocchi M: Spinal cord stimulation and cerebral haemodynamics. *Acta Neurochir* 2006;99(suppl):111-116, 2006.

54. Visocchi M et al: Spinal cord stimulation and cerebral blood flow: an experimental study. *Stereotact Funct Neurosurg* 62:186-190, 1994.

55. Visocchi M et al: Spinal cord stimulation and early experimental cerebral spasm: the "functional monitoring" and the "preventing effect." *Acta Neurochir (Wien)* 143:177-185, 2001.

56. Goellner E, Slavin KV: Cervical spinal cord stimulation may prevent cerebral vasospasm by modulating sympathetic activity of the superior cervical ganglion at lower cervical spinal level. *Med Hypotheses* 73:410-413, 2009.

57. Takanashi Y, Shinonaga M: Spinal cord stimulation for cerebral vasospasm as prophylaxis. *Neurol Med Chir (Tokyo)* 40:352-356, 2000.

58. Slavin KV et al: Cervical spinal cord stimulation for prevention of cerebral vasospasm in aneurysmal subarachnoid haemorrhage: preliminary results of first North American study. *J Cerebr Blood Flow Metabolism* 29:S308, 2009.

59. Visocchi M et al: Increase of cerebral blood flow and improvement of brain motor control following spinal cord stimulation in ischemic spastic hemiparesis. *Stereotact Funct Neurosurg* 62:103-107, 1994.

60. Clavo B et al: Increased locoregional blood flow in brain tumors after cervical spinal cord stimulation. *J Neurosurg* 98:1263-1270, 2003.

61. Robaina F, Clavo B: The role of spinal cord stimulation in the management of patients with brain tumors. *Acta Neurochir* 97(suppl 1):445-453, 2007.

62. Clavo B et al: Modification of glucose metabolism in radiation-induced brain injury areas using cervical spinal cord stimulation. *Acta Neurochir (Wien)* 151:1419-1425, 2009.

15 Complications of Spinal Cord Stimulation

Patrick J. McIntyre and Marshall D. Bedder

CHAPTER OVERVIEW

Chapter Synopsis: Electrical stimulation of the spinal cord (SCS) is generally a safe and effective treatment for neuropathic pain and other conditions. However, it requires implantation of an electrode array and its associated power source. This minimally invasive surgical procedure is subject to complications, which can be avoided with awareness and vigilance. This chapter addresses these potential pitfalls in successful SCS implantation, which can arise at any phase of treatment from patient selection to stable use of an implanted device. One reported mean complication rate is 36%, with complications classified as technical, biological, and other types. Device-related complications can include lead migration, generator migration, or damage to the leads and generally require surgery to repair or replace the device. Risks can increase with repeated surgeries. Loss of paresthesia or unpleasant paresthesias can indicate these technical complications. Implantations in the cervical spine are apparently more subject to migration because of the increased mobility relative to lumbar implantations. Biological complications generally consist of infection or wound breakdown but can also include pain at the site. Intravenous antibiotics before surgery can reduce this risk, but infection can arise even months or years after implantation when organisms lurk inside a device. Allergic reaction to the device has also been documented. Most complications with SCS can be successfully treated or surgically revised when recognized early and given proper attention.

Important Points:
- Spinal cord stimulation is typically a safe and effective treatment for appropriate patients with chronic intractable pain.
- Awareness of potential complications is an important key to avoiding such events.
- Practitioners must remain vigilant throughout the entire SCS process, including patient selection, surgical preparation, and implantation procedure.
- Recognition of the signs and symptoms of a complication can decrease untoward effects on the patient.
- Instituting the appropriate treatment for the particular complication may improve the outcome.

Clinical Pearls:
- Patient selection is an important tool in improving outcomes.
- Surgical technique directly affects outcomes.
- Expeditious recognition and treatment of complications improves outcomes.

Clinical Pitfalls:
- Ignoring changes in neurologic status may lead to poor outcomes.
- If suspicion of a complication arises, avoidance of a permanent complication can often be achieved by explantation of the SCS device.

Introduction

Spinal cord stimulation (SCS) is a treatment for chronic intractable pain that was introduced by Shealy in 1967.[1] With technological advances, SCS has become an increasingly effective treatment for those with many types of chronic pain conditions. In 2007 it is estimated that a total of 27,484 SCS implants occurred over all major payer types in the United States.[2] The majority of patients have a positive outcome involving a reduction of pain with no untoward events. Unfortunately complications of SCS occur just as complications occur with all other interventional procedures. The goal of this chapter is provide information regarding the types and prevalence of complications and trends noted. Anecdotal information can also be useful as a way to increase awareness. Increased awareness of potential contributors of untoward events may help to decrease the likelihood of complications.[3] When appropriate, recommendations will be proffered.

In an epidemiological report published in 1999, more than 1 million injuries and nearly 100,000 deaths occur annually as a result of errors in medical care.[4] According to the systematic review by Turner and associates[5] of 22 studies involving patients with diagnoses, including failed back surgery syndrome or complex regional pain syndrome (Table 15-1), complication rates associated with SCS are noted to be 34%.

Cameron[6] reported a mean complication rate of 36% in her review of the literature involving 68 studies and 3679 patients. She divided the complications into the categories of technical (27.2%), biological (4%), and others (5%). Different case series report that between one quarter[5] and one third[7] of patients undergo at least one SCS revision surgery to reverse a complication.[8] The majority of complications associated with SCS are treatable conditions that may require simple treatments or minor surgical revisions. Timely recognition and treatment of complications reduce the likelihood that the condition progresses into an untreatable or permanent complication.

Prospective studies regarding complications of interventional procedures are rare. A summary of device-related complications from three prospective randomized SCS studies is presented in **Table 15-2**.

Kumar and associates[9] published a prospective study regarding SCS in 2007. They compared conventional medical management

Table 15-1: Complication Rates Associated with Spinal Cord Stimulation

	Mean across studies* (%)	Mean across studies (%)	Range across studies (%)	No. of studies reporting complication†
Any complication	34.3	40.0	0-81	18
Superficial infection	4.5	4.0	0-12	20
Deep infection	0.1	0	0-1	20
Pain in region of stimulator components	5.8	0	0-40	20
Biological complication other than infection or local pain	2.5	0	0-13	19
Equipment failure	10.2	6.5	0-40	20
Stimulator revision (additional operation) reasons other than battery change	23.1	21.5	0-81	16
Stimulator removal	11.0	6.0	0-47	19

From Turner JA et al: *Pain* 108:137-147, 2004.
*Weighted by study sample size.
†Of 22 studies.

Table 15-2: Device-Related Complications from Three Prospective Randomized Spinal Cord Stimulation Studies

Trial	Indication	Follow-up	Number of participants given SCS	Number of patients with device-related event	Total device-related complications (some patients more than one event)	Surgery required to resolve	Removal of SCS required
PROCESS	FBSS	12 months	84	27	40	20 (24%)	
North	FBSS	6 months	17	4	—	4 (24%)	One removed and replaced (because of infection)
Kemler	CRPS	6 months	24	6	13 (11 + 2 dural puncture)	6 (5 + 1 removed) (28%)	One removed and replaced (because of infection)
Kemler	CRPS	24 months	24	—	76 (67 + 9 surgery)	9 (38%)	

CRPS, Complex regional pain syndrome; *FBSS*, failed back surgery syndrome; *SCS*, spinal cord stimulation.

(CMM) to SCS for patients with failed back surgery syndrome resulting in residual predominant leg pain. One hundred patients were randomized to SCS or CMM, and cross over was permitted. Ultimately 84 patients received an electrode during the 12 months of the study. A total of 27 (32%) patients experienced a total of 40 device-related complications. Surgery was required to resolve the issues of 20 (24%) patients. Hardware-related issues, including lead migration, damage to the leads, and generator migration, accounted for 13 of the events. Six patients had loss of therapeutic effect, loss of paresthesia, or unpleasant paresthesia. Biological complications totaled 16 events and included infection or wound breakdown, pain at the incision site, and fluid collection in the pocket. Iatrogenic issues related to technique numbered five events: dural tear during implant, lead damage during implant, anterior migration of lead during implantation, suboptimal connection of the extension to the generator, and a cap not installed on the generator when one lead was implanted. This prospective study demonstrates the effectiveness of SCS while illustrating the point that complications can be a significant limiting aspect of the modality and must be factored into the decision-making process by both physician and patient when SCS is being considered as a treatment.

Complication rates are often extrapolated from observations in prospective studies, case reports, retrospective reviews, and closed claim studies.[10] Avoidance of complications requires awareness and vigilance. Strict adherence to evidence-based surgical techniques is also mandatory to give the patient the best opportunity for a suc-

cessful outcome.[11] Most complications of SCS are not life threatening and can be resolved by explantation of the system.[6]

Revisions of SCS systems are minimally invasive procedures that are rarely done on an emergent basis, and such procedures are associated with little permanent morbidity.[12] However, repeated procedures expose patients to further risk and continuing disability and increase costs to the health care system. In the retrospective analysis by Rosenow and associates,[12] the authors reviewed the charts of 289 patients who underwent 577 procedures. Hardware revision was required in 46% of patients, and nearly half (48.9%) of those patients underwent more than one revision.

In the 2-year follow up to the randomized controlled trial of effect of SCS on chronic reflex sympathetic dystrophy, Kemler[13] reported that complications occurred in 38% of patients. However, he also states that, because SCS is a lifelong therapy, it is recognized that the incidence of complications is reduced after the first year. He concludes by asserting that SCS is safe and effective if there is careful patient selection and test stimulation.

Furthermore, Kumar[14] reported that biological complications are more prevalent within the first 3 months after implantation, whereas hardware-related complications are likely to occur in the first 2 years after implantation. Despite an overall complication rate of 35%, incidence of life-threatening complications has been shown to be very rare in two large retrospective studies.[5,6,8]

Complications to be discussed include those related to the technology itself, biological complications, and other complications.

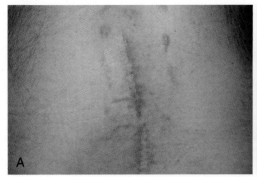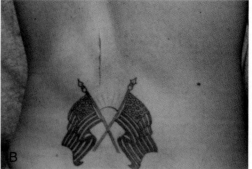

Fig. 15-1 **A,** One-incision technique above a laminectomy surgical incision. **B,** One-incision technique.

Technical complications include electrode migration, electrode breakage, hardware malfunction, and other complications related to the hardware. Biologic complications include infection, seroma, headache, neurological sequelae, gastroenterological effects, urologic effects, pain at the implantation site, and allergic reaction. Other complications include undesirable stimulation, changes in stimulation with position changes, system tolerance, and skin erosion.

Technical Complications

Technical complications are typically issues related to the hardware itself. The complications may occur because of operator error or negligence, but they also may occur as a result of limitations inherent in the SCS systems that are available at the time of implantation. Technological improvements are capable of reducing the incidence of complications. Van Buyten[15] discussed the effect of technological improvements and their effect on the overall complication rate. Devulder and associates[16] published a report of 69 patients with implanted SCS systems who were followed for up to 8 years. Of these 69 patients, there were 174 revision surgeries. Battery replacements accounted for 67 of the surgeries. Electrode migration, insufficient stimulation paresthesias in the painful area, technical failure, and electrode breakage made up the remaining 107 surgeries. Most cases of migration of the electrodes occurred in cases in which the electrodes were implanted in the cervical spine. During revision surgeries for lead migration, attempts at anchoring the leads to bony or ligamentous elements helped to ensure that the lead would not migrate again. Epidural fibrosis tended to respond to lead revision as well.

Andersen reviewed the complications associated with 60 patients with intractable angina who had SCS systems implanted.[17] The first 22 patients had unipolar electrodes implanted, whereas the remaining 38 had quadripolar systems. The most frequent complication was electrode migration. The unipolar systems migrated in 10 patients; 11 of the quadripolar electrodes migrated. This difference is not statistically significant. All of the unipolar lead migrations required reoperation, but only 4 of the 11 patients with quadripolar electrode migrations underwent reoperation. By increasing the number of contacts, the area that is covered by stimulation increases; thus the placement of the electrode is more forgiving if there is a minor migration. The technological advance of progressing from unipolar to quadripolar electrodes reduces the number of reoperations, which in turn decreases the risk of further surgical complications as a larger area of the spinal cord is covered.

In Cameron's literature review of 2972 patients treated with SCS,[6] the most common complication was electrode migration. Kumar and associates[18] noted that electrodes in the cervical spine were twice as likely to migrate as electrodes in the lumbar spine. This occurs because of the increased mobility of the cervical spine compared to the lumbar spine. Directional forces on the lead determine the direction of the displacement, whether laterally or longitudinally. Displacement occurs when the tensile load on the electrode exceeds the capacity of the anchor to stabilize it.[18] Tensile load changes with range of motion of the spine, the position of the generator, and the elasticity of the electrode and the surrounding tissues. When the generator was implanted in the gluteal region (3 [21%] of 14), the electrodes were more likely to move than when the generator was implanted in the abdominal wall (15 [10%] of 146). The authors postulate that there is more traction on the electrode with lumbar range of motion if the generator is in the gluteal region.

In 2006 Pyles[19] presented the notion of a single incision for the implantation of the SCS device in the lumbar spine. Kumar[18] suggested that the traditional placement of the generator in the buttock pocket might lead to increased strain and fulcrum effect on the leads and anchors. Having only one incision may decrease the amount of postoperative pain that patients experience[11] (**Fig. 15-1**). There is also reduced operating time that may reduce the likelihood of time-sensitive complications such as infection. A potential complication that is unique to this technique is that revision surgery may be more difficult if the generator is enveloped in the same planes of scar tissue as the electrodes and the anchors.

Another technique to avoid electrode migration was described by Kumar.[8] He warns that migration is more likely if the nose of the anchor is not pushed through the deep fascia layer and the anchor is secured to that layer. Adding a strain relief loop may also decrease the likelihood of lead migration by reducing tension on the electrode when the patient is moving.

In his review of 10 years of experience at a single center in Belgium, Van Buyten[20] found that most complications were of a technical nature.[20] Fracture of the electrode occurred in 5% of the patients; fracture of the extension cable also occurred in 5%. Almost 8% of patients had a fracture in the temporary wires, and just over 8% had a dislocation of the electrode. Eleven percent experienced pain at the site of the electrode-extension connection. One of 24 patients in the Kemler and associates' study of chronic reflex sympathetic dystrophy had a defective lead implanted that was corrected with a revision surgery.[21] In his review of problems encountered with SCS devices published in 1974, Fox[21a] noted that lead breakage is more likely to occur during revision surgery since the lead is less likely to be identified among scar tissue.

Heidecke[22] published a retrospective analysis of a group of 42 failed back surgery syndrome patients using a single percutaneous lead.[22] The patients were followed for 6 to 74 months, and 12 of the 42 patients had systems that experienced hardware failures. Eight of the leads broke. The other four hardware issues included two broken extension cables and two cases of receiver insulation failure at the plug connector site. Electrode breakage or a disruption in stimulation should be suspected when a sudden disappearance of stimulation occurs. Six of the cases of electrode breakage were caused by disrupted insulation, and the other two cases of electrode dysfunction were without known cause. One of the eight cases was caused by trauma, whereas the other seven were spontaneous.[22]

There were two cases of receiver failure because of short circuiting caused by leaks in the insulation at the plug connection.[22] Special attention must be paid to all connections. Heidecke[22] recommends securing connections with screws while still under pressure. In the cases of the disconnected extension cable at the junction of the lead and cable, the loosening was likely secondary to insufficient tightening of the connector screws that were in use at the time. Another possible problem with that scenario could have been increased traction on the extension cable that could be averted by forming a loop in the course of the electrode. Inadequate connections may be avoided by careful and diligent handling during implantation.

In his retrospective analysis of 160 SCS patients, Kumar and associates[18] discovered nine patients whose electrodes were fractured. Of these patients, one had a paddle electrode; the remaining eight patients had percutaneous electrodes. In this series there were a total of 28 paddle electrodes and 132 percutaneous electrodes. The likelihood of an electrode fracture is higher in the percutaneous implants. The fracture developed in the percutaneous electrodes cephalad to where the lead is affixed to the deep fascia at the point at which the electrode enters the spinal canal.

However, in their article reviewing the charts and operative reports of 289 patients who had undergone SCS implantation between 1998 and 2002, Rosenow and associates[12] reported that the rate of breakage of electrodes was twofold higher in laminotomy electrodes as compared to the percutaneous variety. They also reported that electrode migration was marginally higher in the laminotomy electrodes.

Many of the technical complications are avoidable by careful handling of the hardware during implantation. Many of the reports regarding complications resulting from technical issues related to hardware were older studies involving patients whose SCS systems were older and less technologically advanced.

Eisenberg and Waisbrod[23] reported a case in which a patient experienced an electrical injury to the central nervous system as a result of the cervical SCS becoming activated uncontrollably by an antitheft device. Six months after implantation the patient entered a store that was protected by an antitheft device. The patient requested the store representative to deactivate the deterrent system. The patient entered the store at the direction of the representative. The patient recalls a shocklike sensation at the back of his skull before losing consciousness. The patient regained consciousness in the emergency room where he demonstrated moderate confusion, dysarthric speech, gait ataxia, bilateral upper-extremity intention tremor, and weakness of the left upper extremity. Brain computed tomography (CT) and electroencephalography were normal. After 6 months the patient's condition improved; however, dysarthria, impaired memory, tremor of the right hand, and gait ataxia were still present. CT of the brain revealed an old infarction in the left basal ganglia.

Given the low voltage that the battery is able to generate, it is assumed that the antitheft device induced a sudden burst of electrical current. The low voltage was strong enough to cause neurological injury because of its proximity to the delicate structures and the low electrical resistance of the meninges. External electrocution is less likely to cause such damage at this voltage level because of the relatively high resistance of skin. Radiofrequency transmission is the likely mechanism that activated the SCS in an uncontrollable manner.

Biological Complications

Infection

Implanting hardware in patients bears a potential risk of infection. Infection in the spinal canal is rare, but superficial infections at the site of the generator or the connector between the generator and the electrode occur more frequently.[5] The typical rate of infection is approximately 5%.[24] According to Barolat,[25] patients may present at any time with an infected device, whether it is within a few days of implantation or a few years. Risk factors for infections of implanted hardware include tobacco and alcohol use and immunosuppressive therapy.[26] Co-morbidities such as diabetes mellitus and rheumatoid arthritis may also increase the risk.[27]

Another risk factor for infection that was illustrated by Barolat[28] is multiple surgeries. He reported that 3.4% of patients and 3.7% of implanted electrodes developed infection. In his review of his experience with 509 implanted plate electrodes, 12 patients developed infection involving a total of 19 plate electrodes. In four patients the infection presented after multiple revisions of the electrodes. He adds that two of the four patients had a history of infections in the course of previous surgical interventions.

According to Follett and associates,[29] the most commonly reported organism cultured in infected SCS systems is *Staphylococcus* at 48%, followed by *Pseudomonas* at 3%. Of the remaining organisms, 24% were unknown or not reported, 18% demonstrated no growth, and 6% of cultures grew multiple organisms. They also found that the location of the infection is most likely to be the generator pocket at 54%, followed by the SCS electrodes at 17% and the lumbar incision site at 8%. Multiple sites were infected in 14%, and 8% were not reported.

In a study of 84 patients receiving a total of 92 dorsal column stimulators, Pineda[30] reported that only one patient experienced an infection. The patient presented $2\frac{1}{2}$ years after implantation with an infection at the site of the generator. *S. aureus* was isolated from the wound. According to the author, it was likely that the bacteria were sequestered in the hardware. The infection was treated with antibiotics, and the hardware was explanted. Pineda also reported the case of a patient whose electrode extruded through the skin at the site of the generator $1\frac{1}{2}$ years after the implantation surgery. The extruded electrode ultimately became infected with *Staphylococcus*, and the system was removed.

Kemler and associates[21] reported one infected SCS system out of 24 (4%) patients receiving SCS, and the system was explanted. The infection was not confirmed by culture. After the infection had resolved, the patient underwent a successful reimplantation. Devulder and colleagues[16] reported that 2 of 69 (3%) patients had infected SCS devices. One of the patients had a successful reimplantation procedure. SCS was abandoned for the other patient since the infection was recurrent.

In Kay and associates' review of 70 patients who were treated with SCS,[31] six patients were diagnosed with an infection. Three of those patients had their SCS system explanted; the others were treated successfully with antibiotics. Prophylactic antibiotics were not administered to these patients, which the authors assert may have contributed to the infection rate of 9%. Three of the infected patients had previously undergone revision surgery. The additional surgical procedures exposed these patients to added risk and increased the likelihood of complications for these patients.

Meglio, Cioni, and Rossi[32] reported a 9-year experience in their institution with SCS. Of the 109 patients treated with SCS, seven patients developed an infection related to the implanted hardware. One of the patients became paraplegic within a few days of the explantation of the SCS device. A myelographic block was noted at the level where the electrode had been implanted. A bacterial epidural and intradural abscess was discovered and drained. The recovery of this patient was not complete.

Prophylactic antibiotic administration during implantation procedures is an important step in reducing the likelihood of an infection.[11] Optimal prophylaxis takes into consideration the appropriate choice of antibiotic, proper timing of administration, and limiting the duration of antibiosis. In the case of spinal cord stimulator implantation, a single dose of a cephalosporin is generally adequate unless there is history of an allergy to that class of antibiotic agent. To ensure maximal effect, adequate tissue levels must be attained before incision. The usual recommendation is that the drug should be administered between 30 minutes and 2 hours before incision. There is no advantage to prescribing post-implantation antibiotics,[33] although this has not been prospectively tested for SCS implantation procedures.

Recommendations to reduce the likelihood of infection also include vigilance when preparing and draping the surgical area and gentle treatment of tissue.[34] Electrocautery near the superficial tissues should be limited, and there should be a two- or three-layer closure to carefully approximate the edges of the incision.[34] The implanting physician must maintain a low threshold for suspicion with new complaints of increased pain, new neurological deficits, and constitutional signs and symptoms. A significant increase in pain over the baseline level and new neurological deficits in patients with an implanted SCS device are harbingers of infection. Any suspicion of infection should initiate a complete work-up. Useful laboratory studies include a complete blood count with differential, erythrocyte sedimentation rate, C-reactive protein, a gram stain and cultures with sensitivities. A CT scan of the areas in which the hardware is implanted is also indicated. [31]

If the infection is superficial, successful treatment is possible with oral or intravenous antibiotics.[34] Explantation should not be delayed if there is lack of improvement or if the infection is neuraxial. A consultation from an infectious disease expert is recommended. Typically the device may be reimplanted after a period of 12 weeks. An approach that has been suggested in reducing the risk of infection is to soak the electrode in gentamicin solution before implantation[30] (**Figs. 15-2** and **15-3**).

Seroma

Seroma should be part of the differential diagnosis if a patient presents with erythema and edema in the area of the generator incision.[34] A seroma is a noninfectious process resulting in a collection of serosanguineous fluid in the pocket of the generator. Patients typically do not present with constitutional signs or symptoms. Culture of a sample does not demonstrate growth. Pineda reports that 10 out of 84 patients who received 92 implants developed a seroma. The seromas were treated successfully with aspiration,[30] although this procedure bears the risk of introducing infection into the pocket. Fox[21a] reported that 5% of patients developed a seroma; these accumulations were treated with one or two aspirations. Open incision and drainage is another treatment option, together with pressure dressings or abdominal binder, depending on the location of the generator (**Fig. 15-4**).

Postdural Puncture Headache

The most common neurological complication in SCS implantation procedures is inadvertent dural puncture.[34] Sundaraj and associates[35] report an incidence of 0.46%. In their review of 153 patients in a single center in Belgium, van Buyten[20] reported that 9 of 153 (6%) had dural puncture. Kemler and associates[21] reported that dural puncture occurred in 2 of the 24 SCS systems implanted for patients with chronic reflex sympathetic dystrophy. One these patients developed a postdural puncture headache, whereas the other did not.

Risk factors for dural puncture are previous surgery at the site of needle placement, obesity, spinal stenosis, calcified ligamentum flavum, and patient movement.[34] Risk factors for developing a

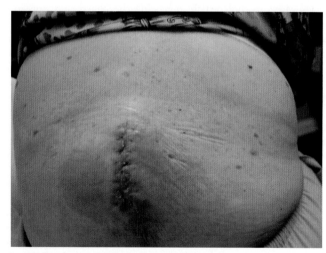

Fig. 15-3 Signs of infection, including erythema and edema of the implantable pulse generator incision site.

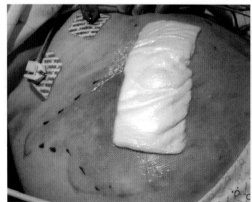
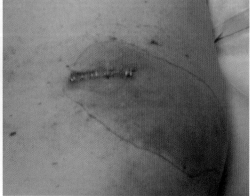

Fig. 15-2 Infected spinal cord stimulation hardware. Photos courtesy Hammam Akbik, MD, FIPP.

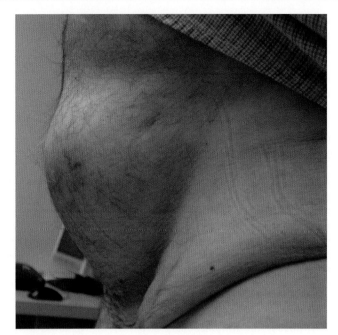

Fig. 15-4 Seroma in the pocket of an implantable pulse generator. Photo courtesy Hammam Akbik, MD, FIPP.

postdural puncture headache include female gender, young age, pregnancy, and use of a large-bore needle.[36]

Eldrige and associates[36] reported two cases of postdural puncture headache during SCS procedures in which the successful treatment of the headaches was different.[36] The first patient was treated successfully with conservative measures, including intravenous caffeine sodium benzoate, placement of abdominal binder, opioids, and hydration. Conservative measures failed to treat the headache of the second patient; so the patient was offered an epidural blood patch. Since the dural puncture occurred during the permanent implantation, particular care had to be taken to avoid interrupting the stimulation. Fluoroscopy was used to guide the needle to the epidural space while the patient was awake, and the SCS remained activated to monitor changes in the stimulation pattern throughout the procedure. The authors were concerned about the mechanical stress that the injected blood may have on the implanted leads and the possibility that the electrodes may be displaced by the volume of the injectate. Other considerations include the risk of infection since blood is a rich bacterial growth medium.[34]

Kumar and associates[18] recommended that an autologous blood patch be administered as soon as a dural puncture is identified. The authors of this analysis also recommend terminating the procedure and rescheduling 3 weeks later to allow the dura enough time to heal from the insult from a large-bore Tuohy needle. This recommendation is made to avoid bathing the electrodes in cerebrospinal fluid (CSF) and increasing the risk of an electrical short circuit.[18] If there is no increased risk to the procedure, other authors may continue the procedure at a cephalad level since long-term outcomes have not been affected.[34]

Wolfensberger and Borruat[37] reported a case of sixth nerve palsy after SCS implantation in a 56-year-old male with scleroderma and peripheral limb ischemia. A few days after implantation the patient complained of tinnitus and headache. On postoperative day 5 the patient developed diplopia, especially when looking to the left. Examination revealed a sixth nerve palsy but no other neuroophthalmological abnormalities. The patient was treated conservatively and was free of symptoms at the 3-month follow-up visit.

The authors postulate that the likely etiology of the headache and abducens palsy is secondary to CSF leak at the site of epidural fixation of the electrode. Sixth nerve palsy is a known complication of lumbar puncture.[38] A sixth nerve palsy may ensue after a drop in CSF because the sagging of the intracranial contents may induce mechanical pressure on the sixth cranial nerve as it passes over the petrous bone.[39]

Headache

Ward and Levin[40] reported a case in which a patient developed headaches during the use of SCS. The electrodes were placed in the upper cervical spine to treat a bilateral brachial neuritis causing bilateral shoulder pain. The cephalad electrode was placed at the level of C3. Before placement, CT of the brain and magnetic resonance imaging (MRI) of the cervical spine were obtained and read as normal. The patient reported a good response to his shoulder pain with the SCS; however, within 1 week of implantation the patient complained of headaches. He developed a constant mild headache that would occasionally become severe and persist for hours to days before reverting to the baseline headache. The headaches did not respond adequately to acetaminophen. Sumatriptan (Imitrex) gave inadequate relief.

The patient did not have a history of headaches, and his neurological examination did not demonstrate any deficits. The patient was eventually treated with a variety of medications, including verapamil, divalproex sodium, desipramine, dihydroergotamine, and gabapentin (Neurontin). The headaches subsided for a few weeks before returning. Several months later the headaches improved dramatically after much bending and stretching of his neck. Plain films of his cervical spine demonstrated that the cephalad electrode had descended to the C5 level. Eventually the patient discontinued his headache medications while the SCS still controlled his shoulder pain. The authors postulate that the electrode at the level of C3 was stimulating the spinal nucleus or a tract of the trigeminal nerve, leading to alteration of the trigeminovascular activity. This aberrant stimulation resulted in the patient's headache. When the electrode descended to the level of C5, these neurovascular structures were no longer in the field of stimulation, and the headaches ceased.

Other Neurological Sequelae

There are a multitude of different types of neurological sequelae that may occur as a result of SCS hardware implantation. Direct needle or hardware trauma and epidural or intraspinal hematomas may occur. Increased neuropathic pain, quadriparesis, and seizures have also been reported.

Epidural hematoma is a rare complication in SCS. In a review of 509 consecutive surgical plate electrodes implanted, Barolat[28] reported one epidural hematoma. This hematoma was located at the surgical site and resulted in postoperative paraplegia. Pineda[30] reported 1 subdural hematoma in 84 patients who received a total of 92 dorsal column stimulator systems.

In 2005 Franzini and colleagues[41] published a report of a huge epidural hematoma after implantation of a laminectomy lead at the level of the L1 vertebra. The patient had failed conservative treatment for chronic low back and leg pain and was not a candidate for a surgical intervention. SCS was offered in an attempt to treat the patient's pain. Immediately after the implantation, the patient had progressive loss of lower-extremity strength that became complete flaccid paraplegia within 2 hours. CT and MRI of the thoracic and lumbar spine demonstrated an epidural hematoma. An 11-level laminectomy successfully decompressed the spinal canal. No coagulopathies were discovered before or after the SCS implantation.

The authors recommend that patients at risk for epidural hematomas should have periodical assessment of motor and sensory function for the first 36 hours after surgery.[41] Delays in recovery from anesthesia should prompt a full neurological examination and possibly imaging in the form of a CT or MRI. There is a bimodal age distribution with peaks in childhood and fifth and sixth decades of life. By a ratio of 4:1 male gender is more likely to develop an epidural hematoma, as are patients who have had multilevel laminectomies.[42]

Chiravuri and associates[43] described a case of a subdural hematoma following SCS device implantation. The SCS system was implanted to treat chronic intractable angina in a 49-year-old male. An inadvertent dural puncture occurred during placement of the Tuohy needle. During a postprocedure follow-up phone call, the patient complained of a positional headache. The patient was advised to present to emergency room because of a change in the character of his headache. On physical examination there were nonfocal neurological findings and an absence of meningeal signs. Stat CT of the head revealed a subdural hematoma.

The patient underwent an emergency craniotomy. On postoperative day 3 the patient recalled having a fall in which he struck his head but did not lose consciousness in the day preceding the implantation procedure. This patient experienced a blunt head trauma and a dural puncture within 24 hours. The authors propose that the cause of the subdural hematoma may be solely secondary to the drop in intracranial pressure because of the dural puncture or the subdural hematoma may have been subclinical until after the dural puncture. An epidural blood patch is a common treatment for postdural puncture headaches. However, in the setting of a subdural hematoma, an epidural blood patch can cause rebound intracranial hypertension. Increased volume in the epidural space may cause increased intracranial pressure.[44]

Because epidural hematomas can result in devastating complications, avoidance is imperative. Recommendations to avoid complications associated with hematomas include awareness of anticoagulant medications and potential coagulopathies. A consultation from a hematologist should be requested if there is a lack of familiarity or experience with relevant anticoagulant medications or coagulopathies.

Grillo, Yu, and Patterson[45] reported a case of delayed intraspinal hemorrhage 18 months after implantation of a dorsal column stimulator. The patient had a dorsal column stimulator implanted in the subarachnoid space at the C4-C5 level in an attempt to treat her low back and leg pain after the failure of more conservative treatments. The patient used the stimulator for the first 6 months after implantation, but then the pain returned spontaneously. At this point the patient stopped using the stimulator. She woke up with a sudden sharp pain in the right side of her body associated with paralysis of the right upper and lower extremities. She also lost control of her bladder and developed Horner syndrome. Lumbar puncture revealed bloody, xanthochromic cerebral spinal fluid. Myelography demonstrated widening of the spinal cord between C3 and C6 associated with the electrode. The patient underwent surgical exploration, and a 2-mL hematoma beneath the electrode was evacuated. Her neurological status improved with the exception of residual right-hand weakness. The authors suspect that the ultimate cause of the hematoma was a mechanical trauma of the SCS device on a neurovascular structure likely secondary to neck motion that lacerated a pial vessel.[45] Electrical damage to the vasculature is unlikely since the device had not been used in approximately 1 year preceding the hemorrhage.

Pineda[30] reported that two patients of 84 with 92 systems developed progressive paraparesis with no evidence of arachnoiditis and with no indication of the original pathology that is the source of the pain.[30] The patients were advised to stop using their systems. Both continued to use the stimulators because of the relief, despite one relying on a walker for ambulation and the other using a wheelchair. The author stated that it is unclear if the system was responsible for the paraparesis in these patients.

Meyer, Swartz, and Johnson[46] reported a case in which the SCS electrode was placed inadvertently in the spinal cord, which resulted in quadriparesis. A 25-year-old female with complex regional pain syndrome in the left upper extremity had improvement in her pain and function after the initial SCS implantation procedure. Six months after the implant she required a revision of the generator for technical reasons. General anesthesia was induced. Intraoperatively it was discovered that the lead connectors also needed to be revised, which required placement of new epidural electrodes. The original electrodes were removed. The new leads were placed through a Tuohy needle by the standard approach. In the postanesthesia care unit the patient exhibited profound weakness in all four extremities. An immediate postoperative CT of the cervical and thoracic spine demonstrated an intramedullary lead with the tip at the level of C2.

Ultimately the intramedullary electrode was removed in an open surgical procedure that resulted in further neurological deterioration. The authors note that, had the electrode been left in the spinal cord, use of SCS and MRI would not be possible. They mention that consideration should be given to performing revision procedures in an open manner rather than through the percutaneous approach. At the least, percutaneous electrodes should not be placed while a patient is rendered unconscious to protect against such catastrophic outcomes.

A case of severe pain and pseudotabes was reported in the *Journal of Neurology, Neurosurgery & Psychiatry* in 1987.[47] The patient afflicted was a 65-year-old male with failed back surgery syndrome. He experienced severe pain in his back and legs and saddle anesthesia. In 1986 he had an electrode implanted through the T10-T11 interspace and positioned at the level of T7-T8. Radiographic imaging confirmed that the electrode was in the extradural space. Initially extreme pain was felt at the site of the laminectomy, but the patient also developed pain in his legs and the area of his penis and scrotum. The pain was eliminated when the stimulation ceased, and it was reproducible. Despite attempts to adjust the current, the pain persisted, and the system was explanted. The authors described the pain as pseudotabetic because of the location of the pain and the relationship of tabes dorsalis to nerve root or dorsal horn ganglion damage. They suggested that the pain was a result of antidromic conduction of the dorsal tracts of the spinal cord involving neurologically damaged segmental cells that resulted in an altered response.

Devulder and associates[16] reported several neurological complications in their experience with 69 SCS patients.[16] One patient developed torticollis when the electrode was implanted at the level of T2 until the electrode was revised and placed at T9. The torticollis resolved while the SCS was still effective for the patient's pain. Two patients experienced cooling in the leg that was confirmed by thermography. The patients perceived the paresthesias in the appropriate areas, but the SCS did not provide relief. In both patients, revising the electrode and implanting the electrode one thoracic segment lower resolved this issue. One patient developed Horner syndrome with the electrode implanted at the paramedian C5 level, which resolved when the electrode was moved to the midline. Five patients had gait problems. Four of these patients had anesthetized legs that resolved immediately with reprogramming the SCS device. One patient had gait difficulties that were improved with reprogramming the SCS device at the expense of relief. The gait problem completely resolved after 3 years without explanation.

In his review of implantation of 509 plate electrodes, Barolat[28] reported that four patients complained of radicular-like symptoms following implantation. In three of the patients, the etiology of the pain was spinal stenosis on postoperative CT imaging. The stenosis was in part created by the space occupied by the electrode. The symptoms resolved with limited laminotomies over the site of the electrode. An electrode in the epidural space may result in spinal stenosis even if no stenotic lesion was present before implantation. An MRI of the cervical spine is recommended before implantation of an electrode in the cervical spine.[34] Thoracolumbar imaging is not necessary before implantation of electrodes into those areas unless there is suspicion of a potential neurological mass effect secondary to the presence of the electrode.

Epidural fibrosis has been identified as another complication for several reasons. As a space-occupying lesion, the fibrosis may result in stenosis, thereby displacing the neural structures. The fibrosis may also affect the ability of the electrodes to deliver current.[34] Surgical revision may be necessary to reinstate stimulation if reprogramming is unsuccessful. Painful stimulation may also occur with fibrosis since the direction of the current may be redirected to nerve roots or other neuraxial structures.[34]

Turner and colleagues[48] published a prospective, population-based controlled cohort study regarding SCS as treatment for failed back surgery syndrome in a workers' compensation setting.[48] Eventually 28 patients underwent a permanent SCS implantation. One patient developed seizures after the SCS implantation. The seizures subsided when the system was turned off and resumed after the stimulator was activated. The SCS system was explanted after 8 months because of the seizure activity and lack of pain relief.

Gastroenterological

Kemler, Barendse, and van Kleef[49] reported a case involving the relapse of ulcerative colitis in a patient. The theory that the SCS device was the cause of the relapse of the symptoms was tested twice before attributing SCS to this condition. The symptoms of ulcerative colitis began when the patient was 23 years old. He had two relapses at ages 37 and at 43. At age 46 he developed complex regional pain syndrome in the right upper extremity after a Colles' fracture. After conservative treatments failed to relieve his pain, the patient underwent a successful SCS trial over 4 days. The SCS system was implanted with a quadripolar lead placed at the level of C4. The pulse generator was implanted in the left anterior abdominal wall.

After $1\frac{1}{2}$ months of continuous stimulation, the ulcerative colitis relapsed. After the patient's gastroenterologist suggested that there might be an association between the SCS and the ulcerative colitis, the SCS device was turned off. Shortly thereafter the ulcerative colitis went into remission. The SCS was attempted again, but within 2 weeks the ulcerative colitis returned. Placing the battery elsewhere was not attempted.

There were no confounding factors discovered. Possible causes of the relapse of the ulcerative colitis as it related to SCS include the effect that an electromagnetic field may have on the colon. The effect of electricity on colonic circulation was also considered together with effect of SCS on the brain-gut axis through electricity or γ-aminobutyric acid (GABA). It was proposed that the cause might be neurogenic inflammation in a separate article.[50]

In 2003 Thakkar, Connelly, and Vierira[51] published a report of two cases of women developing gastrointestinal symptoms after spinal cord stimulators were implanted. The symptoms ceased after discontinuation of use of the stimulator. The first patient developed nausea and diarrhea 1 month after implantation. The second patient complained of worsened gastroesophageal reflux, flatulence, and diarrhea. The authors propose that a sympathectomy resulting in an unopposed parasympathetic state is the cause of the symptoms that these two patients experienced.

Urologic

In 2008 Larkin, Dragovich, and Cohen published the first case report of acute renal failure occurring during an SCS trial.[52] The patient was a 48-year-old male with failed back surgery syndrome resulting in neuropathic leg pain. His past medical history also included hypertension and hepatitis B. He was offered a spinal cord stimulator trial since conservative treatments for his pain had failed. After an uneventful SCS trial procedure, the patient experienced a syncopal episode. He requested that the electrode be removed on the second postoperative day. He did not recall urinating for 2 days. He complained of light-headedness when he was sitting or standing. The electrode was removed, and the patient was referred to the emergency department. He was hypotensive, and his blood urea nitrogen (BUN) and creatinine were 83 mg/dL and 8.1 mg/dL, respectively. The patient was admitted to the medical intensive care unit, where he was monitored and hydrated. His BUN and creatinine normalized within the next few days.

Given the rapid normalization of the laboratory values, the authors surmise that the renal failure was not chronic. They hypothesize that the sympathectomy caused by the SCS may have decreased renal blood flow through peripheral shunting, decreased renal perfusion pressure, and produced an attenuated cardiovascular response.[52]

Loubser[53] reported a case in which a patient with chronic pain secondary to spinal cord injury underwent implantation of a SCS system. The patient was a 41-year-old male with an incomplete injury at T12-L1 that resulted in severe cauda equina syndrome. After failing conservative approaches to treat his pain, the patient underwent a successful SCS trial. Within a few months of the implantation of the SCS system, the patient required higher amplitudes to effectively address his pain. At amplitudes such as 6.5 V, the patient was no longer able to self-catheterize because of urethral sphincter spasm. The episodes of urethral sphincter spasm persisted for 3 hours after deactivation of the SCS system. Ultimately the patient's SCS system was explanted. The urinary retention and recurrent urinary tract infections that ensued were attributed to the SCS system. The author proposed that patients with spinal cord injury should have urodynamic function testing incorporated into the SCS trial.

Allergic Reactions

Allergic reactions to cardiac pacemakers have been documented in the literature.[54] A few cases of allergic reactions to components of SCS systems are reported. In his series of 198 patients with SCS systems implanted, Burton[55] reported that one patient developed an allergic reaction to the silicone component of the hardware. McKenna and McCleane[56] reported a case of a 53-year-old male with intractable angina who was offered an SCS system in an attempt to treat his pain. One month after implantation, the patient developed eczema on the skin of the left lateral chest over the receiver. The receiver circuitry was encased in epoxy resin, with a polyurethane connector block where an insulated stimulating electrode was attached by four titanium screws in silicone rubber grommets. A transmitter was attached to the patient's belt with a lead that was secured to the patient's skin by adhesive. The patient had a previous history of rashes from contact with cheap metal. Patch testing revealed a reaction to nickel.

The authors contend that the nickel allergy did not play a role in the dermatitis. They believe that the patient had an isomorphic response to expansion of the underlying tissues by the hard device as has been seen after placement of cardiac pacemakers.[57]

The Long and Erickson study reviewing the experiences of 69 patients with SCS systems implanted from 1969 to 1973 reported that one patient had the device explanted because of an allergic reaction.[58] They did not expound on the nature or circumstances of the allergy except to state that the patient had phantom limb pain that was relieved by the stimulator. Meglio, Cioni, and Rossi[32] reported that 2 of 109 patients with SCS devices (1.8%) experienced a rejection phenomenon in which the electrodes were involved. The SCS systems were explanted; no other details were offered.

Ochani and associates[59] published a report of an allergic reaction to a spinal cord stimulator in 2000. The patient was a 41-year-old female with a diagnosis of complex regional pain syndrome of the left upper and lower extremities. The patient underwent implantation of electrodes in the cervical and lumbar epidural space. Two weeks after the implantation procedure, she complained of burning and erythema along the tunneled leads that worsened when the stimulator was activated. The SCS device provided relief to the patient and allowed her to improve her function. There were no systemic signs, symptoms, or studies compatible with infection.

Four weeks after implantation, the patient presented with generalized hives and edema, which resolved with steroids. Two weeks later the rash recurred. A dermatology consultation was requested. Patch testing to elements of the device, including platinum, silicone, and polyurethane, was positive. Conservative treatment was not successful, so the SCS system was explanted. The patient's erythema and edema resolved, but the pain returned.

The ability to recognize contact sensitivity is important for implanters of SCS devices.[59] A level of suspicion must be maintained for contact sensitivity since it may mimic infection. Unnecessary antibiosis and reimplantation would be poor treatment approaches for patients who have contact dermatitis (**Fig. 15-5**).

Pain at Site of Spinal Cord Stimulation

Alò[60] reported outcomes of patients with SCS devices implanted at 24, 30, and 48 months. He found that the most common reason for device explantation was pain at the site of the generator.[60] At the 48-month time point, only 30% of patients responded that they would undergo the implantation again; the most common reason for not wanting to repeat the procedure was pain at the site of the

generator. On the other hand, Kemler and associates[21] reported that 2 of 24 patients had pain at the site of the generator. The generator pockets of these two patients were modified successfully.

Pineda[30] encountered patients with pain at the site of the generator or at the site of the lumbar incision. Usually the pain was transitory and treated successfully with lidocaine (Xylocaine) in 12 of 84 patients who had received 92 SCS implants. Pineda reported that three SCS systems were explanted for intractable pain at the site of the generator. One of the patients had intractable pain at the site of the electrode; this system was also explanted. The patients in Pineda's report underwent dorsal column stimulation that involved an incision into the dura. The dural incision was closed with minimal overlap of edges over the plate electrode to lower the risk of iatrogenic stenosis. The closure itself, with possible predisposing spinal pathology, and not the electrode conceivably could have been the etiology of this patient's pain.

Pineda[30] reported that 1 patient in 84 with 92 implants developed an ulcerative dermatosis that resolved after the patient stopped using the stimulation. A relationship between stimulation and trophic changes of the skin could not be identified.

Other Complications

Long and Erickson[58] published a case series involving 69 patients with chronic intractable pain who underwent SCS implantation between December 1969 and January 1973. The authors commented that the major serious complication limiting evaluation of the effectiveness of the device for pain control was failure of stimulation into a painful part. Fox's 1974 article[21a] recounting the experience of ten neurosurgeons who had implanted a total of 600 dorsal column stimulators claimed that 20% of patients had stimulation of the incorrect dorsal fibers and 15% had irritating thoracic dermatome stimulation. Most of these patients underwent reoperation. Reoperation exposes patients to increased risk of further complications such as infection or dural puncture. Kemler and associates[21] reported that 5 of 24 patients had unsatisfactory positioning of their electrodes. A single operation was successful in four patients; a second revision was required for the other patient. Pineda reported that inappropriate distribution of stimulation occurred in 6 of 84 patients with 92 SCS systems implanted.[30] He also reported that eight of these patients had paresthesias in the wrong area. The electrodes were repositioned so these patients had appropriate coverage of their painful areas.

Change of patient position or posture is another factor that may affect stimulation. With the unipolar or bipolar electrodes of dorsal column stimulation, Fox[21a] wrote that 60% of patients experienced a change in current strength to the dorsal columns with change of position. He adds that most patients adjusted well to the necessity of adjusting the voltage in certain positions. Van Buyten[20] reported that 11% of patients had changed perception of paresthesias or changed distribution of paresthesias with changes in position. Kemler[13] reported that 19 of 22 patients complained that the paresthesias created by SCS changed with their position, resulting in troublesome amplitude changes.[13]

Barolat[61] reported a case of a patient with positional changes in paresthesias. The patient perceived paresthesias while supine but had reduced paresthesias while standing or sitting. Cameron and Alò[62] reported that changes in position may cause spinal cord movement that result in changes of perception threshold of stimulation.[62] There are postural effects of SCS for percutaneous electrodes that may or may not exist for plate electrodes that are fixed in place. The mean threshold for paresthesia is lowest in the recumbent position. Another consideration is that the layer of CSF changes in different levels of the spinal cord. Typically the least

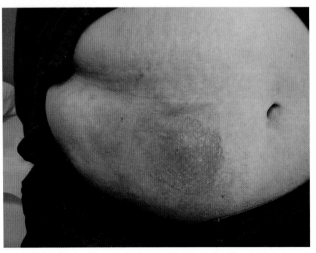

Fig. 15-5 Signs of an allergic reaction to an implantable pulse generator. Photo courtesy Hammam Akbik, MD, FIPP.

amount of CSF is present in the thoracic spine. Newer SCS devices that are programmable may allow adjustments in stimulation in response to position changes.

Kay and associates[31] reported the experience of 70 patients with SCS systems implanted for a variety of pain states over a 13-year period from 1984 to 1997. There were 72 surgical revisions, including electrode revisions or replacement, generator replacement, cable failure, and explantation. Other than battery replacement because of depletion, the most common reason for a revision surgery was inappropriate area of paresthesias. Ten patients underwent reoperation for revision of the placement of the electrode in an attempt to place the electrode in the correct location. Inadequate paresthesias caused by migration, fibrosis, and unknown causes accounted for a total of 21 patients.

The success of SCS as a treatment depends on multiple factors, but success relies on patients not having an unpleasant response to the paresthesias created by the device. A small percentage of patients find the paresthesias to be unpleasant. The 10 neurosurgeons who responded to Fox's survey reported that 1% of patients found the paresthesias to be more unpleasant than their pain.[21a] Pineda[30] added that 34% of patients had insufficient relief because no paresthesias were perceived or the paresthesias were unpleasant. Turner and colleagues[5] published their systematic review of the effectiveness and complications associated with SCS in 2004. The authors discussed the potential loss of effectiveness over time of SCS to treat the patient's pain. Alò and associates[60] reported the outcomes of patients at 24 months, 30 months, and 48 months. Median pain ratings were higher at 30 and 48 months than at 24 months. The pain ratings at 30 and 48 months were lower than the pre-SCS implantation pain. At 30 months 72% of patients were still using their stimulators, but at 48 months only 37% were still using their device.

Kumar and associates[18] describe this phenomenon as system tolerance and define it as progressive loss of pain control despite the presence of a fully functioning stimulating system. There is no specific time at which such tolerance may occur. The etiology may be related to plasticity of pain pathways of the central nervous system.[9] Thus far attempts at treatment of system tolerance have failed. Fibrosis at the site of the electrode has also been considered but not proven,[18] although Sundaraj and associates[35] reported that the electrode of a patient who lost stimulation was surrounded by dense, fibrous tissue. That tissue was presumed to be epidural fibrosis that resulted from a foreign body reaction.

SCS and other implantable devices have eroded through skin. With SCS devices specifically, patients typically have less pain and are able to be more active with activities and exercise. As patients become more active, they may lose weight. The weight loss may change the positioning of the generator relative to body mass, which may result in decreases in subcutaneous tissue between the generator and the surface of the skin. Ohnmeiss, Rashbaum, and Bogdanffy[63] reported one patient with pain secondary to diabetic peripheral neuropathy who developed local skin erosion over the SCS device. The SCS system was explanted, and the erosion healed. Another SCS system was eventually reimplanted.

The importance of decreasing or lack of effectiveness over time in relation to complications is that these patients underwent the SCS implantation procedure without benefit. These patients exposed themselves to myriad and potentially significant risk to obtain little or diminishing gain.

Conclusion

The treatment of chronic pain can be challenging. SCS is a powerful tool in a physician's armamentarium. SCS has improved the lives of many patients. However, any intervention—no matter how conservative—is associated with risk. The implantation and maintenance of SCS devices are no exception.

Complications that are unique to SCS include migration, breakage, and malfunction of the implanted hardware and undesirable stimulation and tolerance to the stimulation. Because of the hardware, there is a substantial risk of seroma, infection, and rejection. As the electrodes reside in the epidural space, neurological sequelae have been reported. Two large systematic reviews have demonstrated the overall risk to be 34% and 36%.[5,6] The complications of SCS are largely treatable or reversible. If a complication cannot be treated successfully while maintaining the device, the device can be explanted in an attempt to reverse the untoward effect. Direct injuries to neural structures are difficult to treat and often not reversible.

The signs and symptoms of SCS complications typically manifest themselves early. Awareness of the potential complications is an important key to avoidance. Vigilance in preparation and technique aids in averting complications. Recognition of the signs and symptoms of complications can decrease the risk of permanent and catastrophic results by instituting the correct treatment plan.

Despite the potential pitfalls associated with SCS, many patients suffering with chronic intractable pain have responded well to this modality. The complications of SCS can typically be avoided by careful selection, implantation, and maintenance of the device. Overall SCS is a safe and effective treatment for patients with chronic intractable pain.

References

1. Shealy CN, Mortimer JT, Reswick JB: Electrical inhibition of pain by stimulation of the dorsal columns: a preliminary clinical report. *Anesth Analg* 46:489-491, 1967.
2. Prager J: Estimates of annual spinal cord stimulator implant rises in the United States. *Neuromodulation* 13:68-69, 2010.
3. Hayek SM: Complication: a painful entity for patient and physician. *Techniques Regional Anesth Pain Manage* 11:121, 2007.
4. Kohn LT, Corrigan JM, Donaldson MS, editors: *To err is human: building a safer health system.* Institute of Medicine, 1999, Committee on Quality of Health Care in America. Washington, DC, National Academy Press.
5. Turner JA et al: Spinal cord stimulation for patients with failed back surgery syndrome or complex regional pain syndrome: a systematic review of effectiveness and complications. *Pain* 108:137-147, 2004.
6. Cameron T: Safety and efficacy of spinal cord stimulation for the treatment of chronic pain: a 20-year literature review. *J Neurosurg* 100:254-267, 2004.
7. Quigley DG et al: Long-term outcome of spinal cord stimulation and hardware complications. *Stereotact Funct Neurosurg* 81:50-56, 2003.
8. Kumar K: Avoiding complications from spinal cord stimulation: practical recommendations from an international panel of expert. *Neuromodulation* 10:24-33, 2007.
9. Kumar K et al: Spinal cord stimulation versus conventional medical management for neuropathic pain: a multicentre randomised controlled trial in patients with failed back surgery syndrome. *Pain* 132:179-188, 2007.
10. Fitzgibbon DR et al: Chronic pain management: American Society of Anesthesiologists Closed Claim Project. *Anesthesiology* 100:98-105, 2004.
11. Bedder MD, Bedder HF: Spinal cord stimulation surgical technique for the nonsurgically trained. *Neuromodulation* 12:1-19, 2009.
12. Rosenow JM et al: Failure modes of spinal cord stimulation hardware. *J Neurosurg Spine* 5:183-190, 2006.
13. Kemler MA et al: The effect of spinal cord stimulation in patients with chronic reflex sympathetic dystrophy: two years' follow-up of the randomized controlled trial. *Ann Neurol* 55:13-18, 2004.

14. Kemler MA et al: Avoiding complications from spinal cord stimulation: practical recommendations from an international panel of experts. *Neuromodulation* 10:24-33, 2007.

15. Van Buyten JP: The performance and safety of an implantable spinal cord stimulation system in patients with chronic pain: a 5-year study. *Neuromodulation* 6:79-87, 2003.

16. Devulder J et al: Spinal cord stimulation in chronic pain: evaluation of results, complications, and technical considerations in sixty-nine patients. *Clin J Pain* 7:21-28, 1991.

17. Andersen C: Complications in spinal cord stimulation for treatment of angina pectoris. Differences in unipolar and multipolar percutaneous inserted electrodes. *Acta Cardiol* 52:325-333, 1997.

18. Kumar K et al: Complications of spinal cord stimulation, suggestions to improve outcome, and financial impact. *J Neurosurg Spine* 5:191-203, 2006.

19. Pyles ST, Khodavirdi A: Placement of a spinal cord stimulation system using a single incision: a novel surgical technique. Poster Presentation at the North American Neuromodulation Society Annual Meeting, 2006. Florida Pain Clinic, Ocala, FL.

20. Van Buyten JP et al: Efficacy of spinal cord stimulation: 10 years of experience in a pain centre in Belgium. *European J Pain* 5:299-307, 2001.

21. Kemler MA et al: Spinal cord stimulation in patients with chronic reflex sympathetic dystrophy. *N Engl J Med* 343:618-624, 2000.

21a. Fox JL: Dorsal column stimulation for relief of intractable pain: problems encountered with neuropacemakers. *Surg Neurol* 2:59-64, 1974.

22. Heidecke V et al: Hardware failures in spinal cord stimulation for failed back surgery syndrome. *Neuromodulation* 3:27-30, 2000.

23. Eisenberg E, Waisbrod H: Spinal cord stimulator activation by an antitheft device: case report. *J Neurosurg* 87:961-962, 1997.

24. Woods DM et al: Complications of neurostimulation. *Techniques in Regional Anesthesia and Pain Management* 11:178-182, 2007.

25. Barolat G: Spinal cord stimulation for chronic pain management. *Arch Med Res* 31:258-262, 2000.

26. Temel Y et al: Management of hardware infections following deep brain stimulation. *Acta Neurochir (Wien)* 146:355-361, 2004.

27. Torrens JK et al: Risk of infection with electrical spinal-cord stimulation. *Lancet* 349:729, 1997.

28. Barolat G: Experience with 509 plate electrodes implanted epidurally from C1 to L1. *Stereotact Funct Neurosurg* 61:60-79, 1993.

29. Follett KA et al: Prevention and management of intrathecal drug delivery and spinal cord stimulation system infections. *Anesthesiology* 100:1582-1594, 2004.

30. Pineda A: Complications of dorsal column stimulation. *J Neurosurg* 48:64-68, 1978.

31. Kay AD: Spinal cord stimulation—a long-term evaluation in patients with chronic pain. *Br J Neurosurg* 15:335-341, 2001.

32. Meglio M, Cioni B, Rossi GF: Spinal cord stimulation in management of chronic pain: a 9-year experience. *J Neurosurg* 70:519-524, 1989.

33. McDonald M et al: Single versus multiple dose antimicrobial prophylaxis for major surgery: a systematic review. *Aust NZ J Surg* 68:388-396, 1999.

34. Deer TR: Complications of spinal cord stimulation: identification, treatment, and prevention. *Pain Med* 9: S93-S101, 2008.

35. Sundaraj SR et al: Spinal cord stimulation: a seven-year audit. *J Clin Neurosci* 12:264-270, 2005.

36. Eldrige JS, Weingarten TN, Rho RH: Management of cerebral spinal fluid leak complicating spinal cord stimulator implantation. *Pain Pract* 6:285-288, 2006.

37. Wolfensberger TJ, Borruat FX: Sixth nerve palsy following epidural spinal cord stimulation for lower limb ischaemia. *Eye (Lond)* 14(Pt 5):811-812, 2000.

38. Insel TR et al: Abducens palsy after lumbar puncture. *N Engl J Med* 303:703, 1980.

39. Fairclough WA: Sixth nerve paralysis after spinal analgesia. *Br Med J* 11:801-803, 1945.

40. Ward TN, Levin M: Case reports: headache caused by a spinal cord stimulator in the upper cervical spine. *Headache* 40:689-691, 2000.

41. Franzini A et al: Huge epidural hematoma after surgery for spinal cord stimulation. *Acta Neurochir (Wien)* 147:565-567; discussion 567, 2005.

42. Kou J et al: Risk factors for spinal epidural hematoma after spinal surgery. *Spine (Phila Pa 1976)* 27:1670-1673, 2002.

43. Chiravuri S et al: Subdural hematoma following spinal cord stimulator implant. *Pain Physician* 11:97-101, 2008.

44. Kardash K, Morrow F, Beique F: Seizures after epidural blood patch with undiagnosed subdural hematoma. *Reg Anesth Pain Med* 27:433-436, 2002.

45. Grillo PJ, Yu HC, Patterson RH, Jr: Delayed intraspinal hemorrhage after dorsal column stimulation for pain. *Arch Neurol* 30:105-106, 1974.

46. Meyer SC, Swartz K, Johnson JP: Quadriparesis and spinal cord stimulation: case report. *Spine (Phila Pa 1976)* 32:E565-568, 2007.

47. Cole JD, Illis LS, Sedgwick EM: Pain produced by spinal cord stimulation in a patient with allodynia and pseudo-tabes. *J Neurol Neurosurg Psychiatry* 50:1083-1084, 1987.

48. Turner JA et al: Spinal cord stimulation for failed back surgery syndrome: outcomes in a workers' compensation setting. *Pain* 148:14-25, 2009.

49. Kemler MA, Barendse GA, Van Kleef M: Relapsing ulcerative colitis associated with spinal cord stimulation. *Gastroenterology* 117:215-217, 1999.

50. Barbara G et al: Relapsing ulcerative colitis after spinal cord stimulation: a case of intestinal neurogenic inflammation? *Gastroenterology* 117:1256-1257, 1999.

51. Thakkar N, Connelly NR, Vieira P: Gastrointestinal symptoms secondary to implanted spinal cord stimulators. *Anesth Analg* 97:547-549, table of contents, 2003.

52. Larkin TM, Dragovich A, Cohen SP: Acute renal failure during a trial of spinal cord stimulation: theories as to a possible connection. *Pain Physician* 11:681-686, 2008.

53. Loubser PG: Adverse effects of epidural spinal cord stimulation on bladder function in a patient with chronic spinal cord injury pain. *J Pain Symptom Manage* 13:251-252, 1997.

54. Virbow J: Pacemaker contact sensitivity. *Contact Dermatitis* 3:173, 1985.

55. Burton CV: Safety and clinical efficacy. *Neurosurgery* 1:214-215, 1977.

56. McKenna KE, McCleane G: Dermatitis induced by a spinal cord stimulator implant. *Contact Dermatitis* 41:229, 1999.

57. Wilkerson MG, Jordan WP, Jr: Pressure dermatitis from an implanted pacemaker. *Dermatol Clin* 8:189-192, 1990.

58. Long DM, Erickson DE: Stimulation of the posterior columns of the spinal cord for relief of intractable pain. *Surg Neurol* 4:134-141, 1975.

59. Ochani TD et al: Allergic reaction to spinal cord stimulator. *Clin J Pain* 16:178-180, 2000.

60. Alò KM et al: Four-year follow-up of dual electrode spinal cord stimulation for chronic pain. *Neuromodulation* 5:79-88, 2002.

61. Barolat G: Epidural spinal cord stimulation in the management of reflex sympathetic dystrophy. *Stereotactic Functional Neurosurg* 53:29-39, 1989.

62. Cameron T, Alò KM: Effects of posture on stimulation parameters in SCS. *Neuromodulation* 1:177-183, 1998.

63. Ohnmeiss DD, Rashbaum RF, Bogdanffy GM: Prospective outcome evaluation of spinal cord stimulation in patients with intractable leg pain. *Spine (Phila Pa 1976)* 21:1344-1350; discussion 1351, 1996.

III Peripheral Nerve Stimulation

16 Peripheral Nerve Stimulation

Ashwin Viswanathan, Diaa Bahgat, Jonathan Miller, and Kim J. Burchiel

CHAPTER OVERVIEW

Chapter Synopsis: Electrical stimulation of a peripheral nerve (PNS) can be used to treat neuropathic pain, ideally that arises from a single nerve and often follows peripheral nerve damage. This chapter considers the issues relevant to successful PNS. The conditions most amenable to PNS include occipital neuralgia, peripheral neuropathic pain, and trigeminal branch pain. With a more regional subcutaneous stimulation, PNS can affect lower back pain and migraine headache. Similar to spinal cord stimulation, our understanding of the mechanism behind PNS is rooted in Melzack and Wall's gate control theory of pain: stimulation of large-diameter fibers decreases the pain signaling from small-fiber neurons. Other hypotheses suggest that PNS may result in peripheral nerve block or other peripheral changes in action potential kinetics to suppress pain. PNS was traditionally delivered with a cuff electrode wrapped around the target nerve, but this can lead to perineural fibrosis. Today, plate or wire electrodes are more commonly implanted, either surgically or percutaneously. An implantable pulse generator is commonly implanted in the abdominal wall or gluteal region. With surgical implantation, a piece of fascia may be implanted between the electrode and the nerve itself, fulfilling a role analogous to the dura mater in implantation of a spinal cord stimulator. Percutaneous implantation carries its own set of considerations. More recently, the leadless bionic neuron (BION) system has been developed with an eye toward PNS.

Important Points:
- PNS is most effective for neuropathic pain attributable to a single peripheral nerve.
- Some sensory preservation should be present in the region of pain.
- Implantation of PNS should be preceded by a successful trial of stimulation.
- Outcome evidence for subcutaneous and regional field stimulation is in progress.

Clinical Pearls:
- Lack of improvement with TENS is not a contraindication to a trial of PNS.
- Fascial cuff can be placed between peripheral nerve and plate electrode during surgical implantation (serves an analogous to role to the dura in spinal cord stimulation).
- Percutaneous trial of stimulation for occipital neuralgia and trigeminal branch neuralgia can be successfully performed under general anesthesia.

Clinical Pitfalls:
- Risk of infection is significant; use of local antibiotics may reduce risk.
- Incidence of lead migration can be minimized through careful anchoring and tunneling of leads.
- Cuff electrodes should not be placed around peripheral nerves because of risk of perineural fibrosis.

Introduction

Peripheral nerve stimulation (PNS) has been recognized as a treatment modality for peripheral neuropathic pain beginning with Wall and Sweet's original description in 1967.[1] By inserting percutaneous needle electrodes into their own infraorbital regions, these authors were able to test the effects of stimulation on peripheral nerves. Through stimulation with square-wave pulses at 100 Hz and with a pulse width of 100 msec, they were able to induce diminished sensation to pin prick in the area of the stimulation. This led the way to investigations of PNS as a modality for treating neuropathic pain.

The last two decades have seen an increased interest in the use of PNS with application to occipital neuralgia, facial pain, and complex regional pain syndrome.[2] In addition to targeting defined peripheral nerves, clinicians are also applying the techniques of PNS to subcutaneous and regional stimulation.[3,4] This has led to a number of trials assessing the efficacy of PNS for a wide array of conditions, including lower back pain, postherniorrhaphy inguinal pain, sacral pain, and migraine headaches.[5]

Basic Science

Our understanding of the mechanism underlying PNS is still being developed. One hypothesis for achieving pain control with PNS involves the gate control theory of pain management proposed by Melzack and Wall in 1965.[6] In their initial description of the gate theory, the authors postulated that large- and small-diameter fibers both send input to inhibitory neurons within the substantia gelatinosa. They theorized that small-diameter fibers provided inhibitory input to the substantia gelatinosa and the large-diameter fibers provided excitatory input. The summation of these inputs modulated the overall inhibitory connections from the substantia gelatinosa neurons to the dorsal horn transmission (T) cells, the projections of which formed the anterolateral system. In accordance with this theory, an increase in large-diameter afferent input

147

would lead to increased inhibitory output from the substantia gelatinosa and consequently decreased transmission of nociceptive input to suprasegmental centers. Thus neurostimulation of peripheral nerves through its effect on the lowest threshold large-diameter fibers would act to "close the gate," effectively inhibiting the transmission of small-diameter pain fibers. Although the gate control theory provides a framework for understanding the mechanism of PNS, the specifics have been challenged.[7]

Other investigators have shown additional mechanisms that may contribute to the potential efficacy of PNS. Campbell and Taub[8] explored the mechanism of PNS through transcutaneous nerve stimulation of the median nerve. The authors stimulated the median nerve proximally with a 100-Hz, 1-msec stimulus. They found that the response elicited depended on the stimulus amplitude. At 10 V to 12 V touch threshold was elevated. With increased voltage pain thresholds were also elevated, and at intensities of 50 V analgesia was elicited. In addition, the development of analgesia was correlated with the loss of the Aδ portion of the compound action potential, suggesting that peripheral nerve transmission block may underlie the suppression of pain by PNS.

Ignelzi and Nyquist[9] further explored the mechanism of PNS by placing cuff PNS electrodes around the sural and superficial radial nerves of cats. They found that, with stimulation, all of the components of the compound action potential were affected, although the Aδ fiber peak was more affected following neurostimulation than were the Aα or Aβ peaks. The changes were represented by either a reduction in amplitude or an increase in the latency of these waves. These findings also support the involvement of a more peripheral mechanism underlying the analgesic effect of PNS.

Indications/Contraindications

Indications

PNS is usually indicated for patients with peripheral neuropathic pain that can be attributed to a single peripheral nerve.[10] Candidates for PNS should have undergone multimodal therapy, including medical management, anesthetic blockade, and physical therapy. As with patients who are being evaluated for spinal cord stimulation, neuropsychological testing can be valuable. In addition, before permanent implantation of the internal pulse generator, patients should have undergone a successful trial of stimulation with a predetermined therapeutic benefit.

More recent studies of subcutaneous target stimulation (STS) and regional stimulation have broadened the traditional inclusion criteria of neuropathic pain attributable to a single peripheral nerve.[11] Retrospective case series of subcutaneous stimulation applied to painful areas has demonstrated therapeutic benefit for lower back pain, neck pain, inguinal pain, and others. However, the longer-term efficacy for this application is unknown.

Contraindications

PNS is a well-tolerated procedure. Consequently the contraindications to implantation are generally those related to the patient's ability to undergo a surgical procedure. Specifically the patient should not be coagulopathic and should be able to tolerate the stress of general anesthesia. Since the procedure involves the implantation of a medical device, the patient should not have an active infection, and the surgical area should be free of infection.

Equipment

The system for PNS includes the electrode through which stimulation is applied to the target nerve and the implantable pulse generator (IPG). Initial electrode designs were cuff electrodes, which were wrapped around the target nerves. This electrode design was found to lead to an increase in perineural fibrosis with some association of peripheral nerve injury. Newer electrode designs are either plate electrodes, which are surgically implanted, or wire electrodes, which may be implanted percutaneously.[12]

Both types of electrodes may be used for a trial of PNS. If the plate electrodes are used during the trial, an extension cable is externalized during the trial and is removed should the trial prove successful. If a percutaneous trial is conducted, the trial wire is removed before the implantation of the permanent system.

The IPG may be implanted in various sites, depending on the site of the stimulation electrode. Locations for the IPG include infraclavicular region, abdominal wall, gluteal region, or lateral thigh. The life span of the IPG varies, depending on the level of stimulation required for clinical efficacy, but 3 to 5 years is a reasonable estimate with current generators.

There has been significant recent research on BION (bionic neuron) technology, which is being applied to the field of PNS.[13] BION is an implantable stimulator that can be used to target nerves and muscles. The design is quite unique from currently used technologies since it is a leadless system, in which the generator and electrode are incorporated into a single miniature apparatus. Technology is being developed to percutaneously implant these devices to be used as peripheral nerve stimulators.[14] Reports have been published with this technique targeting the occipital and pudendal nerves, among others.

Technique

Peripheral nerve stimulators can be implanted through either an open surgical or a percutaneous approach. **Box 16-1** lists nerves that are commonly targeted for PNS. If using a surgical approach, the first step is the exposure of the target nerve. An approximate 4-cm distance of the nerve is dissected free from the surrounding tissues. Care is taken not to excessively disrupt the vascularity of the nerve. Once the nerve has been dissected free, the next step is placing the electrode under the nerve so the electrode contacts lie in proximity to the nerve. The electrode can then be sutured to the surrounding tissues to prevent migration. Some authors have advocated placing a piece of fascia between the stimulating electrodes and the nerve.[12] This is thought to be analogous to the dura in spinal cord stimulation, which separates the spinal cord–stimulating electrode from the underlying spinal cord. **Fig. 16-1** illustrates the surgical technique for placement of an ulnar nerve stimulator.

The techniques for percutaneous implantation of peripheral nerve stimulators to specific target nerves are discussed in the following paragraphs. A recent report by Huntoon and Burgher[15]

Box 16-1: Nerves Targeted for Peripheral Nerve Stimulation

Craniofacial
- Trigeminal branch nerves (supraorbital, infraorbital)
- Occipital nerves

Extremities
- Ulnar, median, radial
- Sciatic, peroneal, posterior tibial

Other Targets
- Inguinal pain (ilioinguinal, iliohypogastric)
- Chest wall (intercostal)

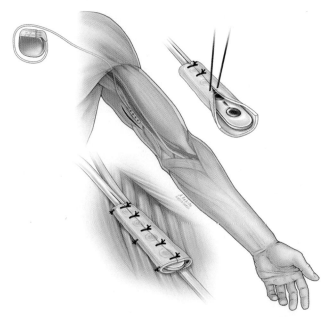

Fig. 16-1 Illustration of the surgical technique used during implantation of a paddle electrode for ulnar nerve stimulation. The electrode may be implanted either above or below the target nerve. A fascial cuff can be secured around the paddle electrode and to the underlying tissues to prevent migration. The lead can then be tunneled to the infraclavicular region for generator implantation. Created by Andy Rekito, MS, and published with permission from Oregon Health & Science University.

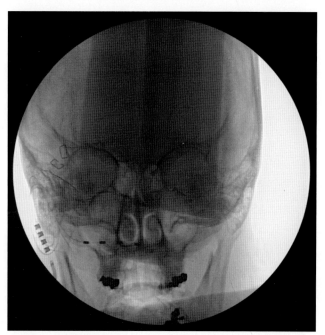

Fig. 16-2 Anteroposterior radiograph of the skull demonstrating a four-contact occipital nerve stimulator. From an entry point medial to the mastoid tip, the electrode is aimed toward the tip of the odontoid process.

describes an ultrasound-guided technique for percutaneously implanting PNS in close proximity to the target peripheral nerve. They have used this technique to implant PNS around the median, radial, ulnar, peroneal, and posterior tibial nerves with efficacy similar to surgically implanted leads.

Occipital Nerve Stimulation

A trial of occipital nerve stimulation may be performed under local or general anesthesia. The senior author (KJB) has found radiographic targeting effective and thus performs the trial under general anesthesia to aid in patient comfort. For a unilateral trial the patient may be positioned supine on the operating table with head turned contralateral to the side of implantation. If a bilateral trial is to be performed, the patient may be positioned either in the lateral position or prone on the operating room table. Anteroposterior (AP) fluoroscopy is used to guide the positioning of the electrode. A Tuohy needle can be gently curved to approximate the curvature of the suboccipital region, and an entry point is chosen slightly medial to the mastoid tip. The needle can then be advanced subcutaneously with the beveled edge down radiographically angled toward the tip of the odontoid as a guide to the superior/inferior plane (**Fig. 16-2**). The electrode is then passed to the midline through the Tuohy needle. Alternatively some authors[12,16] prefer to aim the electrode along the posterior arch of C1. Care is taken so the Tuohy needle does not penetrate the scalp as it passes medially.

Following a successful trial, permanent implantation can be performed under general anesthesia with the IPG placed in the infraclavicular region. During the permanent implantation a small 2-cm vertical incision is made in the retromastoid incision to allow anchoring of the lead to the underlying fascia (**Fig. 16-3**).

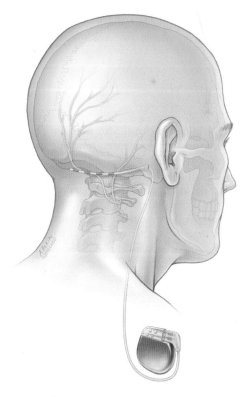

Fig. 16-3 Technique for occipital nerve stimulator placement. Through a 2-cm retromastoid incision, the Tuohy needle and electrode can be passed toward the midline aimed toward the tip of the odontoid. The distal electrode can then be tunneled to the infraclavicular region where the generator is implanted. Created by Andy Rekito, MS, and published with permission from Oregon Health & Science University.

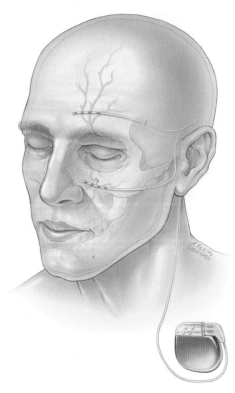

Fig. 16-4 Technique for infraorbital and supraorbital electrode placement. Through a small stab incision either superolateral to orbital roof (supraorbital stimulation) or inferolateral to orbital floor (infraorbital stimulation), the percutaneous electrode can be advanced to span the affected territory. The electrode is then anchored in the retromastoid region and tunneled to the infraclavicular region where the generator is implanted. Created by Andy Rekito, MS, and published with permission from Oregon Health & Science University.

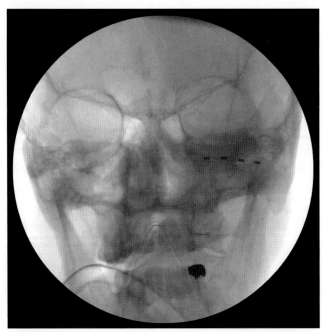

Fig. 16-5 Anteroposterior radiograph of the skull with an infraorbital stimulator aimed to span the infraorbital foramen.

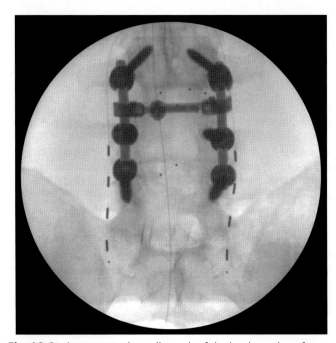

Fig. 16-6 Anteroposterior radiograph of the lumbar spine after implantation of two paramedian subcutaneous electrodes for field stimulation in the treatment of lower back pain.

Supraorbital and Infraorbital Stimulation

Implantation of supraorbital and infraorbital stimulator electrodes may be performed with the patient awake or under general anesthesia. Similarly to occipital nerve stimulation, we prefer to implant the trial electrode using radiographic guidance under general anesthesia for patient comfort. For supraorbital stimulation, a small stab incision is made in the anterior portion of the temple above the orbital ridge. A gently curved Tuohy needle is advanced subcutaneously toward the midline, and the electrode is passed through the needle with the goal of spanning the supraorbital foramen. For permanent implantation the trial electrode is removed, and a new percutaneous electrode is inserted as described. This electrode is then tunneled to the ipsilateral retromastoid region, where it can be anchored to the underlying fascia through a small 2-cm incision. The electrode and extension cable can then be tunneled and connected to the IPG through an infraclavicular incision (**Fig. 16-4**).

For infraorbital stimulation, an entry point is chosen lateral and inferior to the orbital floor, and the electrode is advanced so it spans the infraorbital foramen (**Fig. 16-5**). During permanent lead implantation, a 2-cm incision is made approximately 1 cm in front of the tragus, and the electrode is tunneled to this incision where it is anchored to the fascia. The electrode and extension cable can then be tunneled to an infraclavicular incision where the IPG will be implanted.

Subcutaneous Stimulation

Trial and implantation of electrodes for subcutaneous stimulation is a newer technique. Technically, however, the implantation of the electrode and pulse generator is identical as for other percutaneously placed peripheral nerve stimulators. For subcutaneous stimulation, leads are implanted with the goal of placing the active contacts in the center of the painful area.[11]

Some authors have advocated peripheral nerve field stimulation techniques by subcutaneously placing two parallel electrodes on either side of the painful region (**Fig. 16-6**). In applying regional stimulation, one lead can serve as the anode, and the other parallel lead can serve as the cathode.[3]

Outcomes Evidence

Peripheral Nerve Stimulation

In 1976 Campbell and Long[17] reported their series of 23 patients who had been treated with PNS for a variety of conditions, including peripheral nerve injuries, sciatica, and lower back pain. The authors used a bipolar electrode that was wrapped around the affected peripheral nerve. At an average follow-up of 12 months, 14 of the 23 patients were found to have failed treatment. Four patients in the series had excellent outcomes, and five patients had intermediate results. In reviewing the patient characteristics and clinical outcomes, the authors found that the patient's diagnosis was the factor most correlated with their outcome. None of the patients who were implanted with a sciatic nerve stimulator for lower back pain had good outcomes. Conversely, patients implanted with PNS for chronic peripheral nerve injury had the best outcomes and the highest chance for success.

Reports of PNS applied to patients with peripheral nerve injury have been very favorable. Law, Swett, and Kirsch[18] reported their results with 22 patients who had been treated with PNS for chronic posttraumatic neuropathy. At a mean follow-up of 25 months, 13 (59%) patients reported benefit from their stimulators and continued to use them.[18] Similarly Waisbrod and associates[19] reported their experience using a cuff electrode from Avery in the treatment of 19 patients with traumatic peripheral nerve injuries. Their series incorporated a range of targets, including the sciatic, femoral, median, posterior tibial, and other nerves. At a mean follow-up of 11.5 months, the authors report complete pain relief in 11 patients (58%) and significant pain relief in four other patients (21%). Poor pain relief was seen in the remaining four (21%) patients.

Van Calenbergh and associates[20] reported long-term outcomes of a small group of patients who had been implanted with PNS in the treatment of neuropathic pain after nerve injury. The authors used a circumferential Avery electrode that was surgically implanted around the injured nerve proximally. Of the 10 patients available for follow-up, four were not using the device because of hardware complications or infection. The remaining five patients were found to have excellent pain relief from the PNS at a mean follow-up of 22 months.

Occipital Nerve Stimulation

Slavin, Nersesyan, and Wess[16] and Slavin and associates[21] reported their experience with unilateral and bilateral occipital nerve stimulation for occipital neuralgia. In their series five patients underwent a trial of unilateral stimulation, and nine patients had a bilateral electrode trial. A successful trial was determined by a 50% reduction in pain by the visual analog pain scale. On the basis of this criterion, 10 patients (71%) underwent permanent implantation. In a mean follow-up of 22 months, 70% of patients who were implanted were found to have beneficial effects of stimulation.

In a series of patients who underwent implantation of an occipital nerve stimulator following a successful trial, Weiner[12] reported excellent pain relief in 55%, good relief in 27%, and fair relief in 15%.

Trigeminal Branch Stimulation

Amin and associates[22] reported their experience with 16 patients who underwent a trial of PNS in the treatment of supraorbital neuralgia. Ten patients experienced a greater than 50% reduction in the visual analog score and consequently were implanted with the IPG. In the 30-week follow-up after implantation, patients were found to have a significantly decreased pain score and a significantly reduced requirement for morphine equivalents.

In a longer-term follow-up study, Johnson and Burchiel[23] reported a series of 10 patients who had undergone implantation of supraorbital or infraorbital nerve stimulators for trigeminal neuropathic pain following facial trauma or herpes zoster infection. At a mean follow-up of 26 months, 70% of patients were found to have continued benefit from the stimulation and experienced greater than 50% reduction in their pain compared with preimplantation. All of the patients with posttraumatic neuropathic pain had greater than 50% pain reduction and reduced their intake of medications.

Slavin and associates[21] shared their follow-up of 12 patients who had undergone a trial of PNS to the trigeminal branches for facial pain, reporting that 9 patients had a successful trial warranting implantation. Over a mean follow-up of 44 months, five of these nine patients maintained greater than 50% pain relief. One patient underwent explantation because of infection, another was explanted as his pain improved, and the remaining two patients did not maintain benefit.

Subcutaneous Target Stimulation

Subcutaneous stimulation of painful areas of the body without targeting a specific peripheral nerve is a newer technique that has been applied since the late 1990s. In 2006 Goroszeniuk, Kothari, and Mamann[4] reported their technique and outcomes with a series of three patients who suffered from chronic pain that had been unresponsive to multimodal therapy. During a subcutaneous trial of stimulation using slow frequency stimulation at 2 Hz for 2 minutes, the authors were able to achieve several hours of pain control in each of the patients. The patients went on to permanent implantation with positive results. Of note, the authors found that each of these patients did not receive significant benefit with a transcutaneous electrical nerve stimulation (TENS) unit.

In 2010 Sator-Katzenschlager and associates[11] reported a multicenter retrospective series of 119 patients who underwent a trial of STS between 1999 and 2007. The indications for STS included low back pain, failed back surgery syndrome, neck pain, and postherpetic neuralgia. Of the 119 patients, 111 reported a more than 50% reduction in the numerical rating scale (NRS) for pain with the trial of stimulation and underwent permanent implantation. In short-term follow-up of 3 months, the average reduction in the NRS was from 8.2 before surgery to 4.0 after surgery. As the authors conclude, prospective long-term studies will be needed to fully assess the efficacy of this treatment modality.

Risk and Complication Avoidance

Risks associated with PNS are generally related to those of any implantable device. The most notable risks include infection, lead breakage, migration of the stimulating electrode, and nerve injury. The rates of complications range from 5% to 43% in published series, with infection remaining the major risk.[10] As a means for limiting the risk of device explantation, the present authors have found local injection of antibiotics before skin closure to be effective in reducing the risk of surgical site infections. Miller, Acar, and Burchiel[24] found a 5.7% risk of infection associated with implantation of neurostimulation and intrathecal devices with prophylaxis by intravenous antibiotics before surgery. When a local injection of neomycin/polymyxin before skin closure was used in addition to intravenous antibiotics, the infection rate dropped to 1.2%.

Conclusion

Peripheral nerve stimulation can be an effective technique for patients in whom multimodal therapy has not been efficacious. The most well-established indications for this therapy include peripheral neuropathic pain, occipital neuralgia, and trigeminal branch pain. Increasingly, peripheral nerve stimulators are being applied subcutaneously to painful regions. Initial reports show promise, but the longer benefit still needs to be demonstrated before they become standard techniques in our armamentarium.

References

1. Wall PD, Sweet WH: Temporary abolition of pain in man. *Science* 155:108-109, 1967.
2. Hassenbusch S: Peripheral nerve stimulation. In Follett K, editor: *Neurosurgical pain management*, Philadelphia, 2004, Elsevier, pp 144-149.
3. Falco FJE et al: Cross talk: a new method for peripheral nerve stimulation: an observational report with cadaveric verification. *Pain physician* 12:965-983, 2009.
4. Goroszeniuk T, Kothari S, Hamann W: Subcutaneous neuromodulating implant targeted at the site of pain. *Reg Anesth Pain Med* 31:168-171, 2006.
5. Slavin KV: Peripheral nerve stimulation for neuropathic pain. *Neurotherapy* 5:100-106, 2008.
6. Melzack R, Wall PD: Pain mechanisms: a new theory. *Science* 150:971-979, 1965.
7. Nathan PW: The gate-control theory of pain: a critical review. *Brain* 99:123-158, 1976.
8. Campbell JN, Taub A: Local analgesia from percutaneous electrical stimulation: a peripheral mechanism. *Arch Neurol* 28:347-350, 1973.
9. Ignelzi RJ, Nyquist JK: Direct effect of electrical stimulation on peripheral nerve evoked activity: implications in pain relief. *J Neurosurg* 45:159-165, 1976.
10. Gybels J, Nuttin B: Peripheral nerve stimulation. In Loeser J, editor: *Bonica's management of pain*, ed 3, Philadelphia, 2000, Lippincott, pp 1851-1855.
11. Sator-Katzenschlager S et al: Subcutaneous target stimulation (STS) in chronic noncancer pain: a nationwide retrospective study. *Pain Pract* 10(4):279-286, 2010.
12. Weiner RL: Peripheral nerve stimulation. In Burchiel K, editor: *Surgical management of pain*, New York, 2002, Thieme Medical Publishers, pp 498-504.
13. Loeb GE, Richmond FJR, Baker LL: The BION devices: injectable interfaces with peripheral nerves and muscles. *Neurosurgery* 20:E2, 2006.
14. Kaplan HM, Loeb GE: Design and fabrication of an injection tool for neuromuscular microstimulators. *Ann Biomed Eng* 37:1858-1870, 2009.
15. Huntoon MA, Burgher AH: Ultrasound-guided permanent implantation of peripheral nerve stimulation (PNS) system for neuropathic pain of the extremities: original cases and outcomes. *Pain Med* 10:1369-1377, 2009.
16. Slavin KV, Nersesyan H, Wess C: Peripheral neurostimulation for treatment of intractable occipital neuralgia. *Neurosurgery* 58:112-119; discussion 112-119, 2006.
17. Campbell JN, Long DM: Peripheral nerve stimulation in the treatment of intractable pain. *J Neurosurg* 45:692-699, 1976.
18. Law JD, Swett J, Kirsch WM: Retrospective analysis of 22 patients with chronic pain treated by peripheral nerve stimulation. *J Neurosurg* 52:482-485, 1980.
19. Waisbrod H et al: Direct nerve stimulation for painful peripheral neuropathies. *J Bone Joint Surg Br* 67:470-472, 1985.
20. Van Calenbergh F et al: Long term clinical outcome of peripheral nerve stimulation in patients with chronic peripheral neuropathic pain. *Surg Neurol* 72:330-335; discussion 335, 2009.
21. Slavin KV et al: Trigeminal and occipital peripheral nerve stimulation for craniofacial pain: a single-institution experience and review of the literature. *Neurosurgery* 21:E5, 2006.
22. Amin S et al: Peripheral nerve stimulator for the treatment of supraorbital neuralgia: a retrospective case series. *Cephalalgia* 28:355-359, 2008.
23. Johnson MD, Burchiel KJ: Peripheral stimulation for treatment of trigeminal postherpetic neuralgia and trigeminal posttraumatic neuropathic pain: a pilot study. *Neurosurgery* 55:135-141; discussion 141-132, 2004.
24. Miller JP, Acar F, Burchiel KJ: Significant reduction in stereotactic and functional neurosurgical hardware infection after local neomycin/polymyxin application. *J Neurosurgery* 110:247-250, 2009.

17 Peripheral Nerve Stimulation: Open Technique

Michael Stanton-Hicks

CHAPTER OVERVIEW

Chapter Synopsis: Although peripheral nerve stimulation (PNS) has been shown to be effective in the treatment of many neuropathic pain indications, it has been underused in the clinic. This chapter considers some of the hurdles to more widespread use of the open surgical implantation of PNS stimulators. Some hurdles are regulatory: the U.S. Food and Drug Administration (FDA) has not approved most implantable pulse generators for use with PNS; therefore they are considered off label. Neuropathic pain may be treated with PNS when it does not respond to other modalities. As in any neurostimulatory modality, the success of PNS rides on proper patient selection, including psychological evaluation and possibly a trial period. In contrast to spinal cord stimulation, PNS affects the first-order afferent neurons affected by neuropathy. Peripheral nerve anatomy and histology present significant considerations in successful use of PNS, particularly in "mixed" nerves that carry both sensory and motor information. The chapter also covers technical details of implantation—many of which are location-specific—that should be considered for optimum PNS success. Development of site-specific electrodes for PNS, perhaps including the new leadless BION device, will advance this modality in the coming years.

Important Points:
- Scope of PNS is unlimited
- Unmet need to address neuropathic pain
- Utilizes minimally invasive surgical techniques
- Either single nerve or multiple (plexus) nerve applications are possible
- Compatible with high-impact activities

Clinical Pearls:
- Allows selective fascicular stimulation
- Uses smallest therapeutic current
- Assures optimal target nerve/electrode interface
- Facilitates surgical stabilization of electrode

Clinical Pitfalls:
- Potential for severe nerve damage with trauma
- Therapeutic stimulation might not result from implantation
- Might require removal if mandatory MRI testing is needed

Background

For almost 40 years stimulation of peripheral nerves has been used for the control of neuropathic pain. Like spinal cord stimulation (SCS), the mechanism of peripheral nerve stimulation (PNS) is believed to have its basis in the gate control theory of pain.[1] Although PNS and SCS have been accepted techniques for the treatment of neuropathic pain, SCS has become more widely used. A number of factors have prevented the evolution of PNS, not least of which is a perception that PNS is an orphan modality. This has resulted in PNS never receiving the medical attention that it deserves from either manufacturers of implantable devices or implanting surgeons. Unfortunately, appropriate investigation of its scope and application remains latent.

Open surgical implantation of PNS electrodes, which was described between the early 1970s and 1990s, presaged the ongoing interest at selected centers in the United States and elsewhere to manage peripheral neuropathic pain by PNS.[2-13]

Another handicap for the development of PNS is the lack of any coordinated effort by the implanting physicians who have a vested interest in furthering the scope of PNS to engage in a dialog with the U.S. Food and Drug Administration (FDA). For example, a dialog to extend the current approval for the radiofrequency (RF) interface to include approval for an implantable power source implantable pulse generator (IPG) is wanting. Only one manufacturer, Medtronic (Minneapolis, Minn), has FDA approval to provide an electrode in conjunction with an RF external generator for PNS. All IPGs, whether Medtronic, Advanced Neuromodulation Systems (ANS, Plano, Tex), or Boston Scientific (Valencia, Calif), that are used in conjunction with PNS are considered "off-label" indications. The PNS (On-Point) electrode itself was originally developed as a quadripolar electrode for use in SCS. Recently PNS has received a boost through the efforts to develop occipital nerve stimulation.[14,15]

Definition

"Neuropathic pain is pain initiated or caused by a primary lesion, dysfunction, or transitory perturbation in the central or peripheral nervous system."[16]

Indications

PNS is indicated for the treatment of neuropathic pain in the distribution of a peripheral nerve or nerve trunk that is chronic and unresponsive to conventional medical management (CMM). Loss of function, an inability to participate in exercise therapy, and the nonresponse to local anesthetic or sympathetic blocks are considerations for PNS. Cases of neuropathic pain arising from a plexus injury or mononeuropathies from various causes may have in addition a partial or complete sensory loss that is within a particular nerve distribution. Common indications for open PNS are shown in **Table 17-1**.

A number of conditions amenable to PNS are as follows: occipital neuralgia;[17,18] postherpetic neuralgia;[19,20] postherniorrhaphy pain;[21] complex regional pain syndrome (CRPS);[22] cluster headache;[23-26] chronic daily headache;[18,27] coccygodynia;[28] fibromyalgia;[29] cervicogenic pain;[30,31] and migraine.[32] Neurogenic pain following surgery for tarsal or carpel tunnel and postherpetic pain in a peripheral nerve distribution on the face, trunk, or limb are obvious indications for PNS. As a consequence of the foregoing indications, the contemporary unavailability of dedicated electrode designs should stimulate the engineering of nerve-specific electrode interfaces. Other potential sites for PNS are the sphenopalatine ganglion (SPG)[26] and other autonomic nervous system targets.

As is customary in every prospective case of SCS, it is essential to obtain a psychological evaluation for all potential PNS patients. This has been summarized by Doleys.[33]

Although a trial of neurostimulation always precedes implantation of an SCS, in the case of open PNS the success and stability of this technique in most cases does not warrant the risk of infection from having an externalized connection to a pulse generator for 48 to 72 hours. In addition, the high success rate of the modality precludes this initial step. This approach does not apply to percutaneous applications, in which case a trial is always mandated.

Contraindications

PNS is not associated with many contraindications other than the aspects that apply to all surgeries. Patients with bleeding diatheses or those in whom the discontinuation of anticoagulants is contraindicated are obviously excluded from PNS. Active infection, particularly in cases in which the possibility of bacteremia is high, and patients whose medical condition or malignancy may require serial magnetic resonance imaging (MRI) studies would preclude PNS at the present time.

Neuroanatomy

The axon is the functional unit of a peripheral nerve. Both afferent and efferent axons with their Schwann cells are enclosed in a delicate layer of endoneurial tissue (endoneurium). This is connective tissue that allows the free diffusion of fluids to and from neural structures. Each bundle of axons is enclosed by the perineurium. Cell bodies in the dorsal root ganglion are the source of an axon with a long branch that extends to its peripheral functional source and a shorter branch that passes from its cell body to the spinal cord. Sensory axons are unipolar and transmit sensory information from receptors in the periphery to second-order neurons in the spinal cord. On the other hand, motor neurons arise from the cell bodies in the ventral horn of the spinal cord and in contrast are multipolar with many dendrites. In addition, an axon carries impulses peripherally to activate their specific effector organs. Both dendrites and cell bodies of these neurons are highly specialized to integrate postsynaptic currents that modulate effector organs.

Myelinated nerve fibers have many concentric laminae that form from a single Schwann cell. The nodes of Ranvier are interruptions in the myelin sheath where the inward currents during depolarization are regenerated. An axon of a sensory neuron varies in diameter from as little as 2 µm to 11.75 µm.[34,35] To facilitate regional distribution and therefore sensory coverage, nerve fibers divide into many branches, thereby allowing the innervation of a significant tissue mass by a single neuron. Clinically this results in referred pain that may originate in a single neuron being transmitted by branches to other tissues in the same region. The axon reflex is another mechanism that allows pain to be felt in undisturbed tissue. In this case antidromic transmission passes to other adjacent tissue, causing an expansion of the painful area. **Table 17-2** lists the diameters of nerve fibers and their conduction velocities and function. The fascicular anatomy within nerve trunks is shown in **Fig. 17-1. Figs. 17-1** and **17-2** show nerve fibers grouped within a thin laminated sheet (epineurium) that covers the axons.

Table 17-1: Indications for Open (Surgical) PNS Implant Using the FDA-Approved On-Point (Paddle) Electrode		
Brachial plexopathy		
Mononeuropathy	**Upper limb**	
	Radial nerve	
	Median nerve	
	Ulnar nerve	
	Lower limb	
	Sciatic nerve	
	Peroneal nerve	
	Anterior tibial nerve	
	Posterior tibial nerve	

FDA, Food and Drug Administration; *PNS,* Peripheral nerve stimulation.

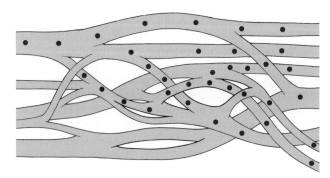

Fig. 17-1 Plexiform pattern of fascicular anatomy in a peripheral nerve. The dots demonstrate the expanding distribution of nerve fibers with distal projection.

Table 17-2: Classification and Physiological Characteristics of Peripheral Nerve Fibers

Class	Aα	Aβ	Aγ	Aδ	B	C
Function	Motor	Touch/pressure	Proprioception/motor tone	Pain/temperature	Preganglionic autonomic	Pain/temperature
Myelin	+ + +	+ + +	+ +	+ +	+	–
Diameter (μm)	12-20	5-12	1-4	1-4	1-3	0.5-1
Conduction speed (m/sec)	70-120	30-70	10-30	12-30	10-15	0.5-1.2
Local anesthetic sensitivity	‡‡	‡‡	‡‡‡	‡‡‡	‡‡	‡

+ + +, Heavily myelinated; + +, moderately myelinated; +, lightly myelinated; –, nonmyelinated; ‡‡‡, most susceptible to impulse blockade; ‡‡, moderately susceptible; and ‡ least susceptible
Adapted from Strichartz, Pastijn, and Sugimoto: Neural physiology and local anesthetic action. In Cousins MI et al, editors: *Cousins & Bridenbaugh's neural blockade in clinical anesthesia and pain medicine*, ed 4, Philadelphia, 2008, Lippincott, Williams & Wilkins, pp 35.

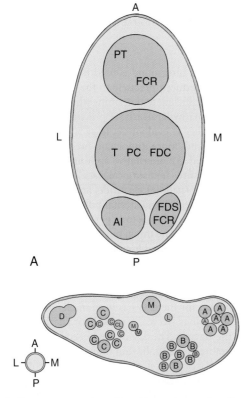

Fig. 17-2 **A,** Transverse section of median nerve at the elbow. **B,** Groups of fasciculi are shown as circles. Letters AMPL reflect orientation. The letters within each fascicle are abbreviations of the distal motor and sensory nerves in the arm and forearm.

A collection of nerve fibers (axon bundles) are known as *fascicles*. Each fascicle containing many axons is encased by a connective tissue layer and perineurium. The entire nerve is contained within a loose outer covering, the epineurium. Although fascicles vary in size from 0.04 to 4 mm, the majority are found between 0.04 and 2 mm in diameter. As nerves proceed distally, their fascicles begin to divide into smaller and smaller units and become more numerous. In addition, this organization takes on a topographically discrete nature, particularly in mixed (motor and sensory) nerves, and is responsible for providing an intimate view of the fascicular architecture.[36-39] For example, in the ulnar nerve behind the medial epicondyle many nerve fibers are grouped into a single fascicle. A similar arrangement is found in the radial nerve in the spinal

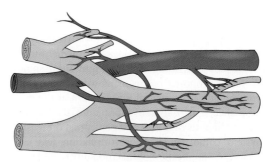

Fig. 17-3 Dissection of the axilla showing collateral blood supply from the axillary artery supplying several adjacent nerves.

groove, the axillary nerve behind the humerus, and the common peroneal nerve in the lower thigh.

The histology of nerve fibers has considerable bearing on the ability to selectively stimulate the sensory or motor nerve fibers. The cross sectional area of a nerve trunk is comprised of 25% to 75% epineurial tissue, the highest amount being in the sciatic nerve in the gluteal region and the lowest in the ulnar nerve at the medial epicondyle. This characteristic influences the effect of neurostimulation. The greater the thickness (higher impedance), the greater is the attenuation of the electric field. In a similar manner, this effects the diffusion of local anesthetics and therefore the amount necessary to achieve their mechanism of action at the axon.

Blood Supply

The vasa nervorum provide nutrition to peripheral nerves derived from collateral vessels, which are branches of adjacent veins and arteries (**Fig. 17-3**). Because of the dynamic nature of tissues and the translational movement of nerves, the vasa nervorum are quite tortuous. The magnitude of this movement increases in the vicinity of joints. There is considerable variation of the collateral blood supply throughout the length of each nerve. This has the effect of creating various watershed zones in each nerve between collateral sources. These zones of relatively poor nutrition may jeopardize the integrity of the nerve and cause increased stress such that extraneous compression or handling may compromise nerve function. In spite of the foregoing hazards, Ogata and Naito 1996[40] and Smith[41] report that a reduced interneural blood flow during and/or after, for example, surgical resection of a nerve, is generally reestablished within 3 days.

Many of the complications that resulted from nerve stimulation during its evolution can be largely attributed to the morbidity induced at the time of electrode placement, implanter inexperience, and the overall slow technical development of PNS systems. Some of the blame can be laid at the feet of electrode-neural interface, an aspect that has been largely resolved.

Certainly compression injury or contusion to a nerve is a greatly diminished factor underlying contemporary PNS morbidity. Preexisting trauma caused by congenital, occupational, or incidental trauma is now largely responsible for any associated PNS morbidity.

Physics and Physiology Underlying Neurostimulation

The mechanism by which PNS achieves it effect is the activation of peripheral low threshold Aβ fibers, which in turn inhibit activity of small-diameter nociceptor Aδ and C fibers. Modulation of this nociceptor input is either direct through the selective activation of Aβ fibers, giving rise to inhibitory postsynaptic potentials or indirect via inhibitory spinal interneurons.[42] Peripheral Aβ fiber activity most likely engages the medial lemniscal pathways, which in turn provide input to the ventral posterior medial nucleus of the thalamus, thereby overriding afferent input from spinothalamic tracts.[43-45] These proposed mechanisms would have the effect of modulating activity from central sensitization at the dorsal horn. As a consequence, sensitization of supratentorial structures such as those involved in both cognitive and perceptual dimensions in the limbic system could render neurostimulation less effective or absent. Thus early application of this modality would be crucial to achieving its maximum effective potential. In contrast to SCS, PNS electrodes are placed on nerves affected by whatever is the ongoing neuropathic process; the primary action of peripheral neurostimulation tends to be direct inhibition of the first-order nociceptor and not second-order or higher neurons. It is clear that both allodynia and hyperalgesia, if present, are frequently reduced or eliminated by PNS. This suggests that sensitization can be subverted by suppressing peripheral nociceptor activity in the spinal cord and overriding nociceptor input at the thalamus. Given the constraints of slowing any temporal attempt on the progression of nociception, PNS may be more effective than SCS in providing inhibition at an interneuronal level.

Equipment

Only the On-Point and Quad Plus electrodes manufactured by Medtronic (Minneapolis Minn) are approved by the FDA for open PNS (**Fig. 17-4**). Other electrodes such as the Resume, Resume II, or Resume TL from Medtronic; the Artisan from Boston Scientific (Valencia, Calif); and the Quattrode and Axxess 6 from St. Jude Systems (Plano, Tex) are also used off label. For percutaneous PNS applications and trial, cylindrical wire type leads such as the Quad, Quad Plus, or Quad Compact from Medtronic and the Quattrode, Octrode, or Axxess from St. Jude, and Artisan from Boston Scientific are also used in an off-label basis.

Although the RF-coupled transmitter receiver made by Medtronic is approved by the FDA as a power supply for PNS, IPGs made by St. Jude Systems and Boston Scientific and Medtronic are used as power sources for PNS as off-label indications.

Surgical Technique

This description is confined to the open surgical approach to a peripheral nerve. If a trial of PNS is desired, this may be undertaken using a percutaneous lead that is passed through a needle to the

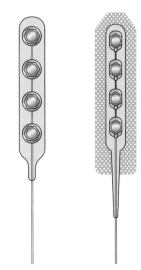

Fig. 17-4 Two electrodes, Quad and On-Point, approved by the Food and Drug Administration for use in peripheral nerve stimulation.

selected nerve. If ultrasound is used for guidance, a percutaneous lead can be introduced precisely to the target nerve. A 2- to 3-day trial would be sufficient to determine whether function is improved or that allodynia/hyperalgesia, if present, is reduced and to what degree pain relief is evident. At least 50% or more symptomatic improvement and, more important, functional restoration should be demonstrated. An alternative approach to a percutaneous trial is surgical exposure (first surgical stage) of the affected nerve; fixation of the plate (paddle) electrode; and passage of the extension, which is connected to an external pulse generator. This will allow the patient to try the device for a period of 2 to 3 days. Demonstration of pain relief is one thing; but more important, the restoration of function in the affected limb is the measure that should be used to determine a successful outcome. At second-stage surgery the wound is reopened; the extension is removed from the skin site; and, after creating a tunnel, the lead extension is passed to a site where a pocket for the IPG has been made. For PNS of the radial, median, and ulnar nerves, a pocket for the IPG is usually made beneath the clavicle. The device can be secured to the fascia overlying the pectoralis major. In thin individuals the IPG can be placed beneath the fascia, but it must not exceed the depth that allows interrogation of a rechargeable generator. Nonrechargeable IPGs can be sutured to the fascia overlying the ribs beneath the pectoralis major muscle. Because of the current limitations of electrode design, the only nerves in the lower extremity amenable to PNS are the femoral, sciatic, common peroneal, and tibial.

Access to the sciatic nerve is by an incision in the lateral thigh posterior to the iliotibial band. Dissection is carried down to the hamstring compartment, where the sciatic nerve lies between the adductor magnus and long head of biceps. Once identified, the sciatic nerve is carefully dissected from its bed while retaining its vasa nervorum and protecting any related muscular branches for a length sufficient to accommodate two On-Point electrodes (**Figs. 17-5** and **17-6**). Each electrode is placed adjacent to the tibial and peroneal components. To stabilize the two On-Point electrodes, their adjacent Gore-Tex skirts are sutured together using 4.0 nylon sutures. The two electrodes are then wrapped around the nerve as a "sandwich," making sure that each bank of contacts is adjacent to the peroneal and tibial divisions, respectively. The free Gore-Tex edges are then tacked to the epineurium using 4.0 to 5.0 nylon sutures, taking care not to constrict the nerve. A pocket can be

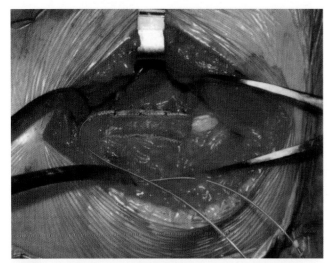

Fig. 17-5 Shown are two On-Point electrodes placed so the contacts are in opposition to the tibial and common peroneal components of the sciatic nerve.

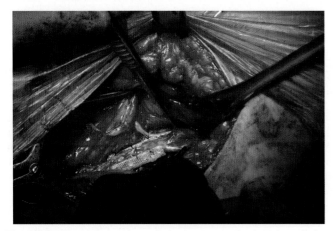

Fig. 17-6 A prototype electrode is shown attached to the sciatic nerve.

made either deep to the iliotibial band or under the deep fascia, whichever seems most appropriate at the time. The IPG can be retained in situ using 2.0 braided nylon or silk sutures to the fascia. This position has the advantage of avoiding the need to pass a long extension from the midthigh to a pocket in the buttock.

Because of the small current requirements of PNS, it is common to implant a nonrechargeable IPG. For most purposes a life of 9 to 12 years can be expected. Depending on the surgeon's preference, pockets for the IPGs can be made in the gluteal area[30] and abdominal wall.[46]

Irrespective of where the IPG is implanted, the pocket should be deep enough to prevent erosion through the skin. It should not be too deep to interfere with programming (if it is a programmable IPG), and its location should be in an area where there is minimal mobility. Likewise, to minimize mechanical damage the extension should pass, at the most, around only one joint.

For PNS in the upper limb, both the ulnar and median nerves are found superficial and medial to the biceps brachii and medial head of the triceps (**Fig. 17-7**). The best surgical site for the radial nerve is in the spiral groove between the lateral and medial heads at the triceps and is found by dissecting the intermuscular septum. In each case, while protecting the collateral blood supply and preserving the motor branches to the triceps, a length of nerve sufficient to accommodate the On-Point electrode is dissected free. This is retained using 4.0 nylon sutures to the epineurium.

Patient Management and Evaluation

To allow for healing and stabilization of the neural electrode interface, exercise therapy is withheld for a period of 6 weeks. Rehabilitation of the affected extremity together with general physical therapy should then be undertaken. Therapy should be continued until optimal function is established. It may be necessary to reprogram the neurostimulator immediately and subsequently following implant, particularly in patients who may have required significant medication, including opioids, for the management of their neuropathic pain. With the anticipated improvement of function during exercise therapy, it should be possible to gradually decrease

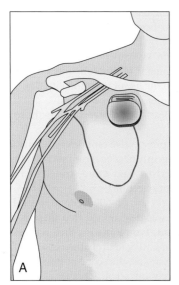
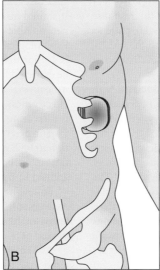
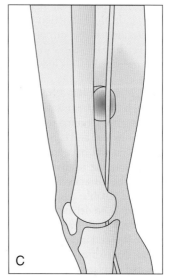

Fig. 17-7 Common implant sites on the torso and thigh for sourcing power of the implantable pulse generator for peripheral nerve stimulation (PNS) of nerves in the upper and lower extremities. **A,** Median/ulnar nerve PNS generator placement. **B,** Femoral nerve PNS generator placement. **C,** Sciatic nerve PNS generator placement.

this dependence. However, in some cases weaning from opioids may require a significant investment of time.

Because most nerves that are currently amenable to neurostimulation are mixed nerves and because fascicular selective electrodes are not available, the plexuslike fascicular arrangement significantly influences sensory thresholds. Therefore only a small window between sensory and motor stimulation is available. Under ideal circumstances provision of a bipole to a number of sensory fascicles would not only reduce collateral stimulation of motor fascicles but could also allow for the smallest possible current to achieve a sensory threshold for paresthesia in the nerves involved in neuropathic pain. Stimulation currents used for PNS are significantly less than those required for SCS. Under most circumstances the amplitude required to achieve therapeutic stimulation is 0.5 to 7 mA, a pulse width of 120 to 180 msec, and a frequency that varies between 40 and 90 Hz.

Outcomes Evidence

No prospective studies of PNS are currently available. A few case series and clinical reports provide an insight into the value of PNS. The most important from a functional point of view are described here. Hassenbusch and associates[11] described 30 patients with CRPS II in whom symptoms had been present, in some cases for many years. Although 35% noted a decrement in analgesia over the first 2 years after implant, residual analgesia persisted at 15 years. Also noteworthy is the fact that 23% of these patients went back to work full or part time. Of the eight most recently published studies,[47,48] a study of 17 patients by Novak and Mackinnon in 2000[49] described 60% (10 patients) having good to excellent pain relief, 4 with fair pain relief, and 3 with no adequate change in their symptoms at 21 months. However, a third of their patients returned to work. Eisenberg, Waisbrod, and Gerbershagen[50] looked at data from three institutions: the Red Cross Center, Mainz; the Institute for Back Care, Bad Kreuznach; and the Linn Medical Center, Haifa. Earlier data (1985 to 1986) were compared with recent (1993 to 1995) data at the Red Cross, Mainz. Seventy-eight percent of the patients were regarded as good, and 22% as poor out of 46 total. It is also important to realize that these patients had failed CMM.

Mobbs, Nair, and Blum[51] published data on 38 patients (M = F). Assessment was based on pain relief, narcotic use, function, and activities of daily living. Sixty percent had significant improvement in pain and return to work. No distinction between the response from workers' compensation patients or noncompensable patients was found (p >0.05). Verbal pain scores were 5.1 with SD = 2.73, a figure that was acknowledged by an independent evaluation at 31 months.

From the foregoing, it is clear that PNS can be associated with good outcomes. Although the current indications for PNS include neuropathic pain resulting from trauma, surgical injury, and CRPS, new indications such as migraine and cluster headaches, trigeminal neuralgia, and fibromyalgia will have to await the development-specific electrodes. Certainly the relatively low invasive nature of open PNS will increase the attractiveness of this modality. The technique is reversible and testable; and, in comparison with ablative surgical options, there is no debate over its duration of effect. It has become an important clinical alternative. Complications associated with PNS are low and include local infection, hardware erosion, technical failure due to breakage or disconnection, fracture of current electrodes, and displacement.[52-54]

The almost complete absence of site-specific PNS electrode development has seriously handicapped progress of this modality. New electrodes with special arrays are in stark contrast to the level

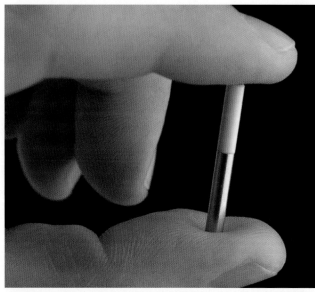

Fig. 17-8 BION peripheral nerve stimulation. This BION microstimulator image is the property of Boston Scientific and was provided by Boston Scientific in response to an unsolicited request. The BION received CE Mark; however the company no longer markets the device in Europe. It was never approved by the Food and Drug Administration for general medical use but was granted an exemption for clinical trials, which have since been discontinued.

of sophistication now reached by functional electrical stimulation. Alternative spacing and lower profile need research if PNS is to be optimized. One completely new concept, an electrode termed BION,[55-57] has the capability of enlarging the scope and indications for PNS (**Fig. 17-8**).

Continuation of these developments, in particular obtaining approval from the FDA with specific research proposals, will ultimately enable a pallet of neural electrode interfaces that will place PNS at the forefront of neuromodulation of neuropathic pain.

Cost-effectiveness and Future of Peripheral Nerve Stimulation

It should be clear from the foregoing that the results of managing neuropathic pain by PNS can be very effective. Unfortunately, the Psychological Pain Assessment Scale (PPAS) as a subjective measure is a poor determinant of any functional improvement that could be expected from the use of this modality. The use of quality-of-life measures is a better and more objective determination of device effectiveness. At least the debate regarding the role of pain measures is increasing.[58,59]

The need for prospective randomized controlled studies in relation to PNS is urgently needed. From such studies cost-effectiveness ratios can be derived, and more stringent characteristics can be applied to patient selection.

Following a review of 6000 citations by Health Technology Assessment,[60] it was determined that there is significant value in terms of function, symptomatic relief, and cost-effectiveness for the use of SCS for CRPS, neuropathic, ischemic, and low back pain.

As already discussed, the scope of PNS remains largely unchartered and will rely on a considerable effort in the development and evolution of neural electrode interfaces. As already mentioned, the introduction of a self-contained electrode power source, the BION (Advanced Bionics, Valencia, Calif) is remarkable.[55-57] Being without a lead or a separate implantable neurostimulator, it can be introduced through a small incision and easily directed to its target nerve. The device is small (3.3 mL, 27-mL length) with cathode and anode at each end. This device can be recharged externally and reprogrammed by telemetry. It is capable of a wide range of stimulation parameters—pulse width 1000 msec, a rate up to 1000 Hz, and an amplitude 12 mA. This is but a foretaste of the type of technical innovation that could propel PNS into the future. Although the scope of PNS has recently broadened by the use of percutaneous and subcutaneous leads, the need for dedicated electrodes on specific cranial nerves and other mixed peripheral nerves requires selective stimulation of afferent fibers with minimal effect on the motor and vasomotor components. Because of the highly selective distribution of PNS, in cases of SCS that lack a more regional topographical effect, PNS can be added to SCS to significantly improve the overall analgesia in the affected region.

Summary

In summary, the stability and low current requirements of PNS systems, particularly in the light of future technological developments, will place PNS at the forefront of neuromodulation technology that will effectively modulate neuropathic pain not otherwise achievable by CMM.

References

1. Melzack RA, Wall PD: Pain mechanisms: a new theory. *Science* 150:971-979, 1965.
2. Cauthen JC, Renner EJ: Transcutaneous and peripheral nerve stimulation for chronic pain states. *Surg Neurol* 4:102-104, 1975.
3. Kirsch WM, Lewis JA, Simon RH: Experience with electrical stimulation devices for the control of chronic pain. *Med Instr* 9:217-220, 1975.
4. Picazza JA et al: Pain suppression by peripheral nerve stimulation. Part II. Observations with implanted devices. *Surg Neurol* 4:115-126, 1975.
5. Campbell N, Long DM: Peripheral nerve stimulation in the treatment of intractable pain. *J Neurosurg* 45:692-699, 1976.
6. Nashold BS, Jr, Mullen JB, Avery R: Peripheral nerve stimulation for pain relief using a multi-contact electrode system. *J Neurosurg* 51:872-873, 1979.
7. Law JD, Swett J, Kirsch WM: Retrospective analysis of 22 patients with chronic pain treated by peripheral nerve stimulation. *J Neurosurg* 52:482-485, 1980.
8. Nashold BS, Jr et al: Long-term pain control by direct peripheral nerve stimulation. *J Bone Joint Surg* 64:1-10, 1982.
9. Waisbrod H et al: Direct nerve stimulation for painful peripheral neuropathies. *J Bone Joint Surg* 67B:470-472, 1985.
10. Iacano RP, Linford J, Sandyke R: Pain management after lower extremity amputation. *Neurosurgery* 20:496-500, 1987.
11. Hassenbusch SJ et al: Long term peripheral nerve stimulation for reflex sympathetic dystrophy. *J Neurosurg* 84:415-423, 1996.
12. Stanton-Hicks M, Salamon J: Stimulation of the central and peripheral nervous system for the control of pain. *J Clin Neurophysiol* 14:46-62, 1997.
13. Shetter AG, Racz G: Peripheral nerve stimulation. In North RB: *Management of pain*, New York, 1997, Springer-Verlag.
14. Weiner RL, Reed KL: Peripheral neurostimulation for control of intractable occipital neuralgia. *Neuromodulation* 2:217-221, 1999.
15. Slavin KV, Burchiel KJ: Peripheral nerve stimulation for painful nerve injuries. *Contemp Neurosurg* 21(19):1-6, 1999.
16. Merskey H, Bogduk N: *Classification of chronic pain: descriptions of chronic pain syndromes and definitions of pain terms*, ed 2, Seattle, Wash, 1994, IASP Press.
17. Weiner RL: Peripheral nerve neurostimulation. *Neurosurg Clin North Am* 14:401-408, 2003.
18. Weiner RL: Occipital neurostimulation for treatment of intractable headache syndromes. *Acta Neurochir* 97(suppl):129-133, 2007.
19. Dunteman E: Peripheral nerve stimulation for unremitting ophthalmic postherpetic neuralgia. *Neuromodulation* 5:32-37, 2002.
20. Johnson MD, Burchiel KH: Peripheral stimulation for treatment of trigeminal postherpetic neuralgia and trigeminal posttraumatic neuropathic pain: a pilot study. *Neurosurgery* 55:135-142, 2004.
21. Stinson LW, Jr: Peripheral subcutaneous electrostimulation for control of intractable postoperative inguinal pain: a case report series. *Neuromodulation* 4:99-104, 2001.
22. Monti E: Peripheral nerve stimulation: a percutaneous minimally invasive approach. *Neuromodulation* 7:193-196, 2004.
23. Schwedt TJ et al: Occipital nerve stimulation for chronic cluster headache and hemicrania continua: pain relief and persistence of autonomic features. *Cephalalgia* 26:1025-1027, 2006.
24. Magis D et al: Occipital nerve stimulation for drug-resistant chronic cluster headache: a prospective pilot study. *Lancet Neurol* 6:314 321, 2007.
25. Leone M et al: Stimulation for occipital nerve for drug-resistant cluster headache. *Lancet Neurol* 6:289-291, 2007.
26. Machado A et al: A 12-month prospective study of gasserian ganglion stimulation for trigeminal neuropathic pain. *Stereotact Funct Neurosurg* 85:216-224, 2007.
27. Schwedt TJ et al: Occipital nerve stimulation for chronic headache: long-term safety and efficacy. *Cephalalgia* 27:153-157, 2007.
28. Kothari S: Neuromodulation approaches to chronic pelvic pain and coccygodynia. *Acta Neurochir* 97(suppl) (Pt 1):365-371, 2007.
29. Slavin KV: Peripheral neurostimulation in fibromyalgia: a new frontier? *Pain Med* 8:621-622, 2007.
30. Kapural L, Mekhail N, Hayek SM et al: Occipital nerve electrical stimulation via the midline approach and subcutaneous surgical leads for treatment of severe occipital neuralgia: a pilot study. *Anesth Analg* 1001:171-174, 2005.
31. Oh MY et al: Peripheral nerve stimulation for the treatment of occipital neuralgia and transformed migraine using a C1-2-3 subcutaneous paddle style electrode: a technical report. *Neuromodulation* 7:103-112, 2004.
32. Rogers LL, Swidan S: Stimulation of the occipital nerve for the treatment of migraine: current state and future prospects. *Acta Neurochir* 97(suppl) (Pt 1):121-128, 2007.
33. Doleys DM: Psychological factors in spinal cord stimulation therapy: brief review and discussion. *Neurosurg Focus* 21(6):E1, 2006.
34. Peters A, Palay S, Webster H: *The fine defined structure of the nervous system: the neuron and supporting cells*, Philadelphia, 1976, Saunders.
35. Hubbard JI, editor: *The peripheral nervous system*, New York, 1974, Plenum Press.
36. Sunderland S: The intraneural topography of the radial, median and ulnar nerves. *Brain* 68:243-298, 1945.
37. Sunderland S: *Nerves and nerve injuries*, ed 2, Edinburgh, 1978, Churchill Livingston.
38. Sunderland S: *Nerve injuries and their repair: a critical appraisal*, Edinburgh, 1991, Churchill Livingston, pp 31-45.
39. DiRosa F, Giuzzi P, Battiston B: Radial nerve anatomy and vesicular arrangement. In Brunelli G, editor: *Textbook of microsurgery*, 1988, Millan, Masson, pp 571.
40. Ogata K, Naito M: Blood flow of peripheral nerve effects of dissection, stretching and compression. *J Hand Surg (BC)* 11:10-14, 1986.
41. Smith JW: Factors influencing nerve repair. I. Blood supply of peripheral nerves. II Collateral circulation of peripheral nerves. *Arch Surg* 93:335, 433, 1966.
42. DeLisa J, editor: *Rehabilitation medicine: principles and practice*, ed 2, Philadelphia, 1993, Lippincott.
43. Giordano J: The neuroscience of pain and analgesia. In Boswell MV, Cole BE, editors: *Weiner's pain management: a guide for clinicians*, ed 7, Boca Raton, Fla, 2005, CRC, pp 15-34.
44. Giordano J: Techniques, technology and tekne: the ethical use of guidelines in the practice of interventional pain management, commentary. *Pain Physician* 10:1-5, 2007.

45. Giordano J: Neurobiology of nociceptive and anti-nociceptive system. *Pain Physician* 277-290, 2005.

46. Hammer M, Doleys DM: Perineuromal stimulation in the treatment of occipital neuralgia: a case study. *Neuromodulation* 4:47-51, 2001.

47. Cooney WP: Chronic pain treatment of direct electrical nerve stimulation. In Gelberman RH, editor: Operative nerve repair and reconstruction, vol II, Philadelphia, 1991, Lippincott, pp 1151-1161.

48. Strege W et al: Chronic peripheral nerve pain treated with direct electrical nerve stimulation. *J Hand Surg (Am)* 19:931-939, 1994.

49. Novak CV, Mackinnon SD: Outcome following implantation of peripheral nerve stimulator in patients with chronic pain. *Plast Reconstr Surg* 105:1967-1972, 2000.

50. Eisenberg E, Waisbrod H, Gerbershagen HU: Lon-term peripheral nerve stimulation for painful nerve injuries. *Clin J Pain* 20:143-146, 2004.

51. Mobbs RJ, Nair S, Blum XP: Peripheral nerve stimulation for the treatment of chronic pain. *J Clin Neurosci* 14:216-221, 2007.

52. Shetter AG et al: Peripheral nerve stimulation. In North RB, Levy RM, editors: *Management of pain*, New York, 1997, Springer-Verlag.

53. Slavin KV, Wess C: Trigeminal branch stimulation for intractable neuropathic pain: a technical note. *Neuromodulation* 8:7-13, 2005.

54. Slavin KV, Nersesyan H, Wess C: Peripheral neurostimulation for treatment of intractable occipital neuralgia. *Neurosurgery* 58:112-119, 2006.

55. Loeb GE et al: BION system for distributed neural prosthetic interfaces. *Med Eng Physics* 23:9-18, 2001.

56. Carbunaru R et al: Rechargeable battery-powered BION microstimulators for neuromodulation. *Conf Proc IEEE Eng Med Biol Soc* 6:4193-4196, 2004.

57. Groen J, Amiel C, Bosch JL: Chronic pudendal nerve neuromodulation in women with idiopathic refractory detrusor overactivity incontinence: results of a pilot study with a novel minimally invasive implantable mini-stimulator. *Neurol Urodyn* 24:226-230, 2005.

58. Turk DC, Rudy TE, Stieg RL: The disability of determination dilemma: toward a multiaxial solution. *Pain* 34:217-229, 1988.

59. Birchiel KJ, Anderson VC, Brown FD: Prospective, multicenter study of spinal cord stimulation for relief of chronic back and extremity pain. *Spine* 21:2786-2794, 1996.

60. Simpson EL et al: Spinal cord stimulation for chronic pain of neuropathic or ischemic origin: systematic and economic evaluation. *Health Technology Assess* 13(17):1-154, 2009.

18 Peripheral Nerve Stimulation: Percutaneous Technique

Marc A. Huntoon

CHAPTER OVERVIEW

Chapter Synopsis: Peripheral nerve stimulation (PNS) directly stimulates peripheral nerves for the treatment of various indications of neuropathic pain. Although the stimulating electrode is usually implanted directly in an open surgical technique, leads can also be implanted percutaneously in a less-invasive procedure that avoids open dissection of the nerve itself. Ultrasound imaging can provide guidance in placement of the electrodes. This technique has some advantages over open surgical implantation, including reduced risk of potential nerve trauma during dissection. Percutaneous implantation also avoids the need for an insulating fascial transplant between the electrode and the nerve because the epineural fat is preserved. Further, a percutaneous trial can identify inappropriate subjects, avoiding unnecessary surgical implants that might fail. The data supporting success of PNS as a treatment for neuropathic pain are somewhat limited, mainly because of experimental confounds inherent in the technique, but they clearly show that PNS can provide pain relief. Anatomical and fascicular details should be considered in advance of percutaneous electrode implantation. As in any neurostimulatory technique, proper patient selection is key to successful treatment, and steps should be taken to prevent migration of the implanted lead.

Important Points:
- Minimally invasive PNS is a novel technique that may allow a trial of peripheral nerve stimulation before permanent placement and potentially allow long-term implantation.
- Percutaneous leads were engineered for spinal cord stimulation indications; thus long-term safety studies of these leads near target nerves have not been performed.
- The operator should be familiar with ultrasound-guided nerve blocks and have a strong working knowledge of cross-sectional anatomy to maximize the safety of these techniques.
- One must understand that discrete fascicles within the peripheral nerve may be targeted differentially based on the location of the electrode relative to the internal configuration of the fascicles.
- A narrow therapeutic window for stimulation (unwanted motor stimulation) is the result of the internal fascicular arrangement relative to the location of the external lead.
- Over time epineurial fibrosis occurs, which may change the impedance and stimulation energy requirements significantly.
- More than one lead may help mitigate the occurrence of lead migration.
- Further research will help define the appropriate role of minimally invasive techniques for clinical applications.

Clinical Pearls:
- Preimplantation nerve block is extremely useful in patient selection, particularly if the patient receives complete relief of pain in a single nerve distribution.
- A transverse (axial) view of the nerve with an in-line approach to lead placement is technically easiest.
- Intraoperative testing allows more precise placements and optimal stimulation parameter selection.
- Similar to spinal cord stimulation, PNS patients should limit activity in the relevant extremity for 4 to 6 weeks.

Clinical Pitfalls:
- Transmuscular placement is undesirable and with muscular movement may cause a ratcheting effect and promote migration.
- When placing leads and generators permanently using this technique, avoiding crossing joint lines and keeping the parts of the system closer together are important considerations.
- One must scan the area of interest thoroughly to stage the anatomy and prevent injury to vascular structures.
- A limited amount of fascia to anchor these leads makes permanent viability of currently available systems less than optimal.

Introduction

Peripheral nerve stimulation (PNS) is a technique of direct electrical stimulation of peripheral nerve(s) to relieve pain or to assist with the functional restoration of patients with severe neurological injuries, including those to the spinal cord. The term *PNS* has also been used to describe the superficial placement of electrical leads in areas of the body such as the back, thorax, or abdomen where no discrete named nerves exist but small nerve fibers near the dermis can be targeted to produce local analgesia. This type of stimulation is mechanistically poorly understood and will be referred to as *peripheral field stimulation* (not the subject of this chapter). PNS became conceptually possible after the development of the gate control theory.[1] Wall and Sweet's experiments with PNS tested the concept of electrical stimulation–produced analgesia, initially of the authors' infraorbital nerves and subsequently in eight patients.[2] Soon many neurological and orthopedic surgeons became interested in the technique, and several case series of these peripheral nerve surgeries were described.[3-6] The early history of the development of these techniques is chronicled by Michael Stanton-Hicks and colleagues,[6] who describe the indications, outcomes, and complications of a series of 91 patients at the Cleveland Clinic. Despite early investigator interest and the development of novel lead and battery technology, innovations in programmability, and other technical improvements for stimulation of the peripheral nerves, the application and study of PNS has been less vigorous in scope than that for spinal cord stimulation. The absence of a comparable minimally invasive trial system that became available with the introduction of percutaneous spinal cord stimulation electrodes in the 1980s may be one reason that peripheral nerve surgeries have not advanced as rapidly. Other potential reasons for decreased interest in PNS may be frequent complications such as lead migration (requiring revision surgery), neurological damage to the axons from mechanical or stimulation-induced nerve injury, and poor patient selection leading to poor outcomes. PNS has always been an open technique since its inception more than 40 years ago, but recently minimally invasive techniques were described.[7-9] Possible advantages to peripheral nerve stimulator placement via a minimally invasive technique might include: (1) minimal nerve trunk dissection and manipulation (potential trauma); (2) the omission of the need for a fascial graft or fat pad interposed between the electrode and the nerve (the fat around the epineurium in situ is minimally perturbed by the percutaneous electrode); (3) a true percutaneous trial avoiding dissection and open surgery; and (4) the ability to perform intraoperative electrical stimulation testing in an awake patient with minimal sedation compared to a patient under general anesthesia. Cadaver feasibility studies were performed in 2008,[7,8] suggesting that ultrasound (US) image guidance might allow safe placement of peripheral nerve stimulating electrodes near target peripheral nerves, similar to nerve catheter placement. Following these feasibility studies, a case series of nine patients who received PNS placements using US was published, based on the principles described in the cadaver studies.[9] In two of the nine cases, patients with good paresthesia coverage did not achieve analgesia and were not implanted, thus avoiding an unnecessary surgical dissection. Most cases produced durable analgesia beyond 1 year. The programming of multiple different stimulation parameters intraoperatively allowed the additional placement of second electrodes parallel to the first or on either side of a nerve trunk to more optimally stimulate the desired fascicles in some cases (**Fig. 18-1**).[9] Others have described a stimulus router concept that eliminates the need for an implanted generator. A surgeon places a passive implant delivery terminal near the target nerve. Current is passed between a surface cathodal electrode and a pick-up terminal, a small fraction of which (10% to15%) is passed to the delivery terminal. This results in PNS at threshold. It is unclear at this time if this type of implant would be less prone to migration without additional study (**Fig. 18-2**).[10]

Currently the only commercial U.S. Food and Drug Administration (FDA)–approved electrodes for PNS are four-contact flat paddle arrays, which must be placed via an open surgical dissection, often with an interposed fascial graft, which is thought to protect the nerve. Neurological surgeons usually place the electrodes longitudinally to maximize the number of contacts in direct apposition to the nerve. Since ideal electrode availability and long-term safety testing is minimal, neurosurgical open procedures with the paddle electrodes are likely to remain the preferred method of placement of these devices in the near term. Whether the use of percutaneous

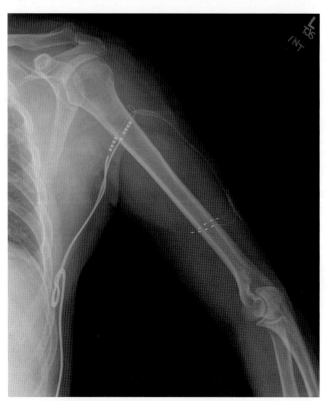

Fig. 18-1 An upper-extremity radiograph after placement of dual four-contact electrodes parallel to the radial nerve. The electrodes can be seen in horizontal orientation to the humerus. In addition, tension loops at the site of anchoring and in the flank are noted.

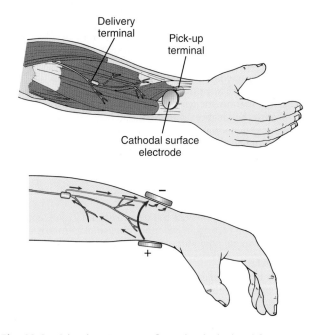

Fig. 18-2 Stimulus router configuration is depicted from reference 10. Both the passive delivery terminal and nerve implant are shown.

techniques might allow future patients to undergo trial placements without significant investment in an open procedure or whether percutaneous permanent placements will become a reality will depend on the pace of new electrode design, future studies of PNS outcomes, and FDA approval of novel leads or other devices.

Current Evidence

At this juncture no prospective randomized and blinded studies have been performed. A recent paper by Bittar and Teddy[11] reviewed the current evidence for PNS. Unfortunately the greatest need for evidence at this time is from prospective, randomized controlled, and blinded studies. Until now these studies have been difficult if not impossible to perform because of patient perception of a physical sensation (paresthesia), which hampers blinding, and the lack of minimally invasive, ethical controls. In an editorial on the subject of peripheral neuromodulation, Davis[12] discussed some of the factors that may make interpretation of currently available studies difficult. Questions regarding the role of external neurolysis (the removal of external scarring around the nerve) on the analgesia seen after PNS, unclear placebo effects, the unequal application of physical therapy in some patient groups, lack of standardization of potentially analgesic drugs (including neuromodulators and opioids), or the increased attention to the patient needs during study protocols are all possible confounding factors. Long-term studies are difficult, but some studies seem to suggest an extremely long-standing effect of PNS, with the possibility of nerve healing over time.[13] Van Calenbergh and colleagues[13] looked back at a group of 11 patients who had been chronically implanted with radiofrequency-coupled peripheral nerve stimulators over an average period of 22 years! Of these 11, four had been explanted, one had died of unrelated causes to his or her stimulator, and one could not participate because of distance from the study center. The remaining five patients had long-term circumferential electrode arrays. These patients demonstrated a durable improvement in their pain, level of function, and use of analgesics when comparing stimulation off to stimulation on. They had sustained minimal complications. Remarkably, benefits persisted despite the passage of over two decades on average. One patient had even demonstrated gradual resolution of his neuropathic pain in the face of neural stimulation. The largest clinical series in print to date are those from Eisenberg, Waisbrod, and Gerbershagen[14] and the Cleveland Clinic.[6] In Eisenberg, Waisbrod, and Gerbershagen's series, 46 patients with isolated peripheral nerve syndromes were treated. Positive results were noted in 78% of patients, whereas 22% had poor results. Decreases in visual analog pain scores from 69 ± 12 before surgery to 24 ± 28 after surgery were seen.[12] The major pathologies treated in the PNS protocols were for the following: (1) nerve lesions incurred from surgeries around the hip or knee, (2) nerve entrapments, (3) persistent pain after nerve graft surgeries, or (4) postaccidental nerve injection injuries.[14] In the previously unpublished Cleveland Clinic series,[6] results on average were positive, with a frequency of revision surgery of 1.6 per patient, not including battery replacements.

Patient Selection

In general patients with neuropathic pain syndromes involving the periphery may qualify for these procedures when they have failed to improve with more conventional and conservative therapies. Patients should be evaluated thoroughly, with the medical history concentrating on previous diagnostic studies, previous failed medication trials, any previous surgical procedures, electrodiagnostic results, and results of any previous nerve block procedures. In the physical examination the physician should concentrate on the neurological, musculoskeletal, and skin examinations. Presence of any motor deficits, sensory deficits, specific dermatomal or peripheral nerve distributions, presence or absence of allodynia, hyperesthesia, hypesthesia, or hyperalgesia should be noted. Vasomotor,

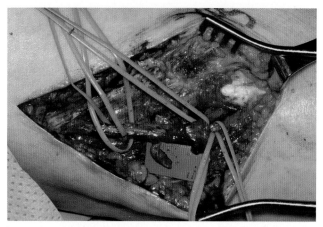

Fig. 18-3 A large neuroma on the common peroneal nerve (bulbous area of nerve to right of picture near the dual blue loops is shown). A cut muscular branch is also shown projecting its stump over the green marker.

sudomotor, or trophic changes should be noted since they may point to a complex regional pain syndrome. Electrodiagnostic studies are extremely important but may be normal in primary pain syndromes. Electromyography (EMG) and nerve conduction studies (NCSs) are also important to the classification, grading, and prognostication of many injuries. In some cases serial evaluations of patients with EMG/NCS can show important trends in reinnervation or ongoing denervation of specific areas. Nerve blocks are an important modality in preoperative patient selection as well. Blocking the suspected nerve proximal to the site of injury helps confirm the involvement of that nerve in the pathophysiology of the pain. One protocol has evolved with the use of local anesthetic coupled with clonidine (Catapres) for neural blockade. In addition to its ability to prolong the effects of the local anesthetic in many cases, clonidine may be important in the inflammatory pain response by blocking production of cytokines involved in hyperalgesia. Indeed, Lavand'homme and Eisenbach[15] have demonstrated prolonged relief of some neuropathic pain states with clonidine. Whether the nerve block is performed with US or electrical stimulation and surface landmarks is perhaps not of paramount importance. However, one advantage of US guidance is the ability to fully scan the patient's area of interest. In some cases one might diagnose a specific underlying cause such as a neuroma (**Fig. 18-3**), a constriction caused by mechanical factors, a foreign body, or an anatomical variant that might pose problems with the technique. Other imaging modalities such as magnetic resonance studies are increasingly sophisticated and capable of influencing treatment decisions.

Safety

It seems intuitively obvious that objects placed in close proximity to a peripheral nerve or abutting against the nerve might potentially cause neural injury. Indeed, previous studies have demonstrated the possibility of neural damage from the surgical procedure itself but also from friction on the epineurium by normal nerve movement (translocation) in an extremity. There have been only minimal studies with respect to a purely mechanical effect. Agnew and colleagues[16] have studied the effects of perineurial electrodes relative to both mechanical and stimulation effects on nerve function long term. These studies were done with helical electrode arrays with three to seven circumferential twists. In one experiment a control side was used to evaluate whether the mechanical or stimulation effects were responsible for adverse changes in histology. Prolonged stimulation with higher frequencies and continuous application of bipolar current have both been shown to cause neurological injury. Interestingly the use of local anesthetics seems to be protective against the development of peripheral nerve injuries from the stimulation.[17] The local anesthetic protective effect suggests that the conduction of long-term high-frequency electrical charge is causative for global axonal changes seen in histological specimens. Other studies of long-term application of stimulation to the other nerves (e.g., phrenic nerves) have shown inconsistent effects. Although significant changes were noted in some, many patients had no histological changes.[18] However, since the phrenic is a motor nerve, any major axonal injury might be more clinically evident. In the initial case series of PNS patients with US-guided placements, stimulation frequencies have been low. Subthreshold stimulation (amplitudes below the perception of a physical paresthesia) at frequencies below 100 Hz and with more narrow pulse widths was frequently used.[9] There were no episodes of neural injury caused by US-guided PNS, despite three episodes of lead migration. In addition, there is a long history of PNS implant surgery over the last four decades, with rare reports of permanent nerve damage from the stimulation implant.

Anatomical Considerations: Nerve Fascicular Arrangement

One issue that complicates any peripheral nerve electrode placement in the four extremities is that nerves must freely glide within fascial/muscle planes along with their vascular supply as the extremity moves. Nerves can be entrapped by scar tissue, and the rough edges of an external electrode could cause constriction and scarring over time. Mixed peripheral nerves are also characterized by a complex internal fascicular arrangement. Briefly, nerve trunks may have sensory, motor, and mixed axons at various locations within the peripheral nerve. This complex cross-sectional anatomical configuration means that optimal stimulation of the desired sensory fascicle might, for example, be at the medial aspect of the ulnar nerve in a supracondylar placement but change location within a matter of a few millimeters to a posterior location. If the amplitude of stimulation is too high above sensory threshold, motor fascicles deeper within the trunk may easily be activated, causing muscle cramping and/or pain. Sunderlund[19] studied the complex fascicular arrangements in the upper-extremity nerves more than 60 years ago. Very little additional work has been done on this topic. Major findings from his work are that even intraindividual (side-to-side) differences, branch points, and number of fascicles at a given anatomical location may vary. Thus stimulation intraoperatively could be useful to determine the potential for good-to-excellent results of PNS. A recent study looked at issues of cross-sectional anatomy more closely; specifically the effects of the fascicle perineurial thickness, diameter, and position within the nerve trunk on axonal excitation thresholds and neural recruitment. A model of human femoral nerve within a nerve circumferential cuff electrode was studied. The study showed that stimulation of target fascicles depends strongly on the cross-sectional anatomy of the nerve being stimulated. The mean thickness of perineurium was $3\% \pm 1\%$ of the fascicle diameter. Increased thickness of the human perineurium or larger fascicle diameter increases the threshold for electrical activation. If a large neighbor fascicle were present, it could also affect stimulation activation of the target fascicle by as much as $80\% \pm 11\%$.[20]

Common Approaches to Ultrasound-Guided Peripheral Nerve Stimulation

Radial Nerve Stimulation

The radial nerve lies close to the lateral surface of the lower third of the humerus at a point 10 to 14 cm proximal to the lateral epicondyle. The nerve is somewhat elliptical in shape, and US scanning is reasonably clear in most cases with a high-frequency probe. An in-plane approach, in which the nerve is viewed in cross section (transverse scan) while the needle is slowly advanced in plane with the transducer is easier, but longitudinal scans are also possible. It is important to prescan the area around the nerve and humerus to define the anatomy. The lateral head of the triceps muscle is overlying the nerve here; and, although one would desire to avoid transgression of large amounts of muscular tissue, there is no more optimal approach to the nerve in a superficial location above the humerus. The profunda brachii artery and recurrent radial artery branch are often seen when scanning by using color Doppler features on the US machine.[7] Electrode migration is prevented by anchoring firmly to muscle fascia and creating a tension loop of the lead. Placing the pulse generator close to the lead is also desirable to prevent migration.[9] Intraoperative stimulation testing can define potential early motor axon recruitment and allow alternate locations of the lead to be attempted.

Ulnar Nerve Stimulation

US scanning with the probe in a transverse orientation to the ulnar nerve is facile in the medial epicondylar groove (cubital tunnel). From this location the nerve can be scanned more proximally in the arm approximately 9 to 13 cm above the condyle. The nerve lies superior to the medial triceps muscle here. In cases of previous transposition surgery, one can target the area just proximal to the patient's scar to begin scanning the nerve, moving from presumed normal areas of nerve to areas of potential pathology such as scarring or neuroma formation. The needle may be advanced, using an in-plane approach with a high-frequency transducer from posterior to anterior on the medial aspect of the arm (**Fig. 18-4**). Anatomically the nerve passes into the cubital tunnel in the ulnar groove behind the medial epicondyle. The cubital tunnel is a

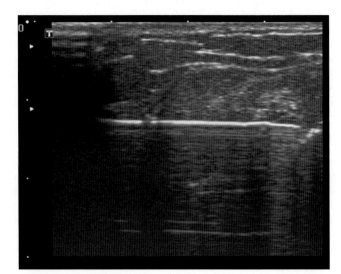

Fig. 18-4 A stimulator electrode introducer needle is shown approaching the ulnar nerve. The nerve is just above the more inferior tip of the needle.

vulnerable area for the nerve, particularly in males, and also a potential area of intraoperative compression.

Median Nerve Stimulation

The most common pathological condition of the median nerve is compression in the carpal tunnel. Scanning proximal to the area of involvement is desirable to target an area of nerve proximal to the pathological area. In the elbow region the median nerve enters the antecubital fossa medial to the biceps muscle and its tendon next to the brachial artery. The artery serves as a good visual aid to help identify the neurovascular bundle. In the upper forearm at a point approximately 4 to 6 cm distal to the antecubital crease, the nerve passes between the two heads of the pronator teres muscle and then under the sublimis bridge of the two heads of the flexor digitorum superficialis. Median nerve stimulation may be accomplished either superior or inferior to the elbow.

Sciatic Nerve Stimulation at Popliteal Bifurcation

The sciatic nerve can be visualized between the greater trochanter and ischium in the subgluteal area, but it is often targeted for PNS in the upper popliteal fossa. US scanning of the area can be initiated at the popliteal crease and, with the probe in a transverse orientation to the leg, continued proximally until the bifurcation of the sciatic nerve is seen. Transverse (axial) US scanning for electrode placement perpendicular to the axis of the nerve is more technically forgiving to avoid loss of capture due to nerve movement (migration). However, longitudinal placement following the nerve's course would allow more electrode contacts to be in proximity to the nerve. The common peroneal, tibial, or sural branches can be seen in this area. The location of the popliteal artery, which lies deep or anterior to the nerves, is noted. The needle is usually advanced from posterolateral to anteromedial in a slightly oblique plane, attempting to avoid passing through the biceps femoris muscle or pushing the muscle down with the needle to achieve a straighter angle at the nerve. Usually anchoring of the lead(s) is to the fascia; often the biceps femoris fascia is easily accessible. The fibular head area would seem to be a reasonable entry point for approaching the common peroneal nerve; but anatomically this area is compacted, and the conventional leads are too large to place with US guidance.

Posterior Tibial Nerve Stimulation

The posterior tibial nerve can stimulated more distally in the leg superior to the medial malleolus. The tarsal tunnel is a common area of potential compression; however, the tissue immediately superior to the tarsal tunnel is very compact and not easily approached with a US-guided approach. Moving a bit more superior to the malleolus (e.g., 10 to 14 cm superior) was found to be a reasonable approach in feasibility testing.[8] The tibialis posterior muscle, the digitorum profundus, one or two large veins, the flexor hallucis longus, and the tibial bone surface are surrounding structures in this location (**Fig. 18-5**). US scanning of the ankle near the medial malleolus, with transverse probe orientation, is continued proximally until an adequate exposure of the nerve is realized. Location of the posterior tibial artery is often not an obstacle but should be noted during electrode placement. When approaching the posterior tibial nerve in the lower leg, the needles may be passed on either side to "sandwich" the nerve, providing stimulation of both sides; or, conversely, the electrodes may be placed parallel to each other if two leads are required (**Fig. 18-6**). The pulse generator may be placed in the upper leg, superficial to the fascia of the quadriceps, or on the fascia of medial gastrocnemius muscle in the lower leg if adequate soft tissue is noted.

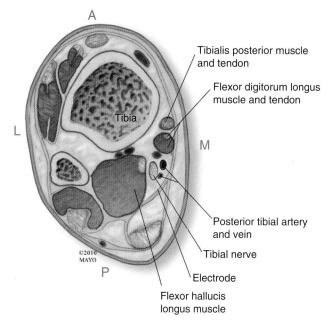

Fig. 18-5 Anatomical cross section showing the structures in the vicinity of the posterior tibial nerve above the ankle. Copyright Mayo Clinic.

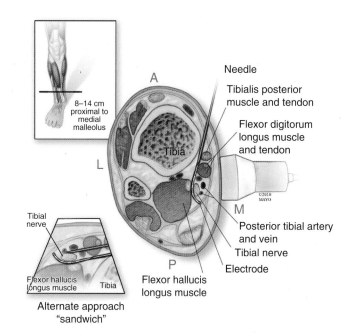

Fig. 18-6 Placement of dual electrodes in progress around the posterior tibial nerve approximately 10 to 14 cm above the malleolus. The needle and electrode are shown "sandwiching" the nerve. Copyright Mayo Clinic.

Conclusion

The novel application of PNS under US scanning may prove to be nothing more than an interesting way to perform a trial of stimulation or the instigator of new research and invention. Future prospective double-blinded studies and development of new electrodes would certainly help to solidify PNS as a viable technique. Safety and migration prevention (reoperation) are of paramount concern with any PNS technique.

References

1. Melzack R, Wall PD: Pain mechanisms: a new theory. *Science* 150:971-979, 1965.
2. Wall PD, Sweet WH: Temporary abolition of pain in man. *Science* 155:108-109, 1967.
3. Nashold BS, et al: Long-term pain control by direct peripheral nerve stimulation. *J Bone Joint Surg Am* 64:1-10, 1982.
4. Strege DW, et al: Chronic peripheral nerve pain treated with direct electrical nerve stimulation. *J Hand Surg (Am)* 19:931, 1994.
5. Hassenbusch SJ, et al: Long-term results of peripheral nerve stimulation for reflex sympathetic dystrophy. *J Neurosurg* 84:415-423, 1996.
6. Stanton-Hicks M, et al: Miscellaneous and experimental therapies. In Wilson PR, Stanton-Hicks M, Harden R, editors: CRPS: *Current diagnosis and therapy, progress in pain research and management*, vol. 32, Seattle, 2005, IASP Press.
7. Huntoon MA, et al: Feasibility of ultrasound guided percutaneous placement of peripheral nerve stimulation electrodes and anchoring during simulated movement. Part Two: Upper extremity. *Reg Anesth Pain Med* 33:558-565, 2008.
8. Huntoon MA, et al: Feasibility of ultrasound guided percutaneous placement of peripheral nerve stimulation electrodes in a cadaver model. Part One: Lower extremity. *Reg Anesth Pain Med* 33:551-557, 2008.
9. Huntoon MA, Burgher AH: Ultrasound-guided permanent implantation of peripheral nerve stimulation (PNS) system for neuropathic pain of the extremities: original cases and outcomes. *Pain Med* 10:1369-1377, 2009.
10. Gan LS, et al: A new means of transcutaneous coupling for neural prostheses. *IEEE Transact Biomed Engin* 54:509-517, 2007.
11. Bittar RG, Teddy PJ: Peripheral neuromodulation for pain. *J Clin Neurosci* 1259-1261, 2009.
12. Davis GA: Commentary: peripheral neuromodulation for pain. *J Clin Neurosci* 16:1262, 2009.
13. Van Calenbergh F, et al: Long-term clinical outcome of peripheral nerve stimulation in patients with chronic peripheral neuropathic pain. *Surg Neurol* 72:330-335, 2009.
14. Eisenberg E, Waisbrod H, Gerbershagen HU: Long- term peripheral nerve stimulation for painful nerve injuries. *Clin J Pain* 20:143-146, 2004.
15. Lavand'homme P, Eisenach JC: Perioperative administration of the alpha-2-adrenoceptor agonist clonidine at the site of nerve injury reduces the development of mechanical hypersensitivity and modulates local cytokine expression. *Pain* 105:247-254, 2003.
16. Agnew WF, et al: Histologic and physiologic evaluation of electrically stimulated peripheral nerve: considerations for the selection parameters. *Ann Biomed Engin* 17:39-60, 1989.
17. Agnew WF, et al: Local anesthetic protects against electrically induced damage in peripheral nerve. *J Biomed Engin* 12:301-308, 1990.
18. Kim JH, et al: Diaphragm-pacing histopathological changes in the phrenic nerve following long-term electrical stimulation. *J Thoracic Cardiovasc Surg* 72:602-608, 1976.
19. Sunderland S: The intraneural topography of the radial, median, and ulnar nerves. *Brain* 68:243-298, 1945.
20. Grinberg Y, et al: Fascicular perineurium thickness, size, and position affect model predictions of neural excitation. *IEEE Transact Neural Syst Rehabil Engin* 16:572-581, 2008.

19 Occipital Neurostimulation

Samer Narouze, Salim M. Hayek, and Timothy R. Deer

CHAPTER OVERVIEW

Chapter Synopsis: Occipital neurostimulation (ONS) provides a minimally invasive, reversible, and effective treatment for a number of intractable headache disorders. The technique is thought to work by inhibiting central nociceptive impulses by stimulation of the peripheral extensions of the trigeminocervical complex, the nerve branches of C2 and C3. A multicenter study showed that the technique shows promise for treatment of chronic headaches. Successful electrode implantation for occipital neurostimulation requires significant consideration of nerve anatomy and technical details of the various available devices. Ideally implantation should avoid unpleasant dysthesias, which can result from superficial placement, and occipital muscle stimulation that causes spasm when electrodes are implanted too deep. As in all forms of neurostimulation, lead migration represents a potential technical failure that can require surgical replacement; incidence is particularly high with ONS.

Important Points:

- Stimulation of the occipital nerve, which originates from the C2 nerve root, is a valuable tool in treating cervicogenic headache, occipital neuritis, chronic migraine, and chronic cluster headache.
- Current prospective randomized studies are pending to access the evidence-based impact of this therapy on migraine.
- In some cases ONS may be combined with stimulation of other cranial nerves to avoid the need for more invasive intracranial procedures.
- The risk of ONS is relatively low compared to spinal cord stimulation or intracranial procedures.
- The most common problems are migration, erosion, and infection. This chapter gives the reader some highlights to reduce complications.

Introduction

Occipital neurostimulation (ONS) or greater occipital nerve (GON) stimulation offers the potential for a minimally invasive, low-risk, and reversible approach to managing intractable headache disorders contrary to neuroablative techniques or other more invasive intracranial procedures.

Indications

ONS has been used successfully in the treatment of occipital neuralgia[1-4] and many primary headache disorders such as migraine,[5] transformed migraine,[4] cluster headache,[5-9] and hemicrania continua.[6,10] Few reports also demonstrated its efficacy in secondary headache disorders, including cervicogenic headache,[11] C2-mediated headaches,[12] posttraumatic,[13] and postsurgical headaches.[14]

Mechanism of Action

The most accepted mechanism of action is that stimulation of the distal branches of C2 and C3, being the peripheral anatomical and functional extension of the trigeminocervical complex, may inhibit central nociceptive impulses.[15] Positron emission tomography (PET) scan studies showed increased regional cerebral blood flow in areas involved in central neuromodulation in chronic migraine patients with occipital nerve electrical stimulation.[16] Additional functional imaging may further define the exact mechanism of

action as these studies become more widely available in multicenter studies.

Efficacy and Safety

Recently the preliminary results of a multicenter prospective randomized single-blind controlled feasibility study that was conducted to examine the safety and efficacy of ONS for treatment of intractable chronic migraine were reported.[17] Patients who responded favorably to occipital nerve block (ONB) were randomized 2:1:1 to adjustable stimulation (AS), preset stimulation (PS), or medical management (MM). Those who did not respond to ONB formed an ancillary group (AG).

Three-month objectives included reduction in headache days/month, decrease in overall pain intensity (0 to 10 scale), and responder rate (>50% drop in headache days/month or >3-point drop in overall pain intensity from baseline). One hundred ten subjects were enrolled from nine centers; 75 were assigned to a treatment group (AS = 33, PS = 17, MM = 17, AG = 8). Sixty-six subjects completed diary data during a 3-month follow-up (AS = 28, PS = 16, MM = 17, AG = 5). At 3 months, percent reduction in headache days/month was 27% (AS), 8.8% (PS) (p = 0.132), 4.4% (MM) (p = 0.058), and 39.9% (AG) (p = 0.566). P values were for comparison to the AS group.

Reduction in overall pain intensity was 1.5 (AS), 0.5 (PS) (p = 0.076), 0.6 (MM) (p = 0.092), and 1.9 (AG) (p = 0.503). Responder rate was 39% (AS), 6% (PS) (p = 0.032), 0% (MM) (p = 0.003), and 40% (AG) (p = 1.000). The authors concluded that ONS may be a promising treatment for intractable chronic migraine and ONB may not be predictive of response to ONS.[17]

Anatomy

The GON arises from the C2 dorsal ramus and curves around the inferior border of the inferior oblique muscle (IOM) to ascend on its superficial surface between the IOM and the semispinalis capitis at the C1 level. Then it penetrates the semispinalis capitis and invariably the splenius muscle to end subcutaneously near the nuchal line by penetrating the trapezius muscle or its aponeurosis.[18-20] There is considerable anatomical variation in the course of the GON. Bovim and colleagues[18] found that the GON pierces the trapezius in nearly half the subjects; however, others have described a much lower likelihood of penetration of the trapezius muscle. The GON was invested in the aponeurosis of the trapezius at its insertion.[19,20]

The GON usually penetrates the semispinalis capitis muscle fibers at a distance between 2 and 5 cm caudad to the occipital protuberance.[18] More cranially it may also penetrate the trapezius muscle fibers or aponeurosis, becoming superficial between 5 and 18 mm below the intermastoid line.[19]

Technique for Occipital Neurostimulation

The procedure can be performed with local anesthetic and conscious sedation, monitored anesthesia care, or general anesthesia (especially in the prone position for better airway control).

The technique was originally reported by Weiner and Reed in 1999.[1] Earlier reports involve placement of the leads subcutaneously at the C1 level. The stimulator lead can be directed medially from a lateral entry point medial and inferior to the mastoid process[1,4,9,12,21,22] or laterally from a midline entry point.[2,7,11,13,23,24]

The authors prefer a lateral point entry in unilateral cases since the patient can be placed in the lateral decubitus position. However, the midline point entry is more appropriate in bilateral cases when the patient is positioned prone.

Level and Depth of Lead Placement

The level and depth of lead placement are crucial for a successful ONS trial. Placing the leads too superficially risks failure of nerve stimulation and lead erosion through the skin or patients experiencing unpleasant burning sensations. On the other hand, leads placed too deep risk stimulating posterior neck muscles and causing unpleasant muscle spasms.[25]

Positioning the stimulator lead subcutaneously at the C1 level places it at a significant distance from the nerve, with the posterior neck muscles (mainly trapezius and semispinalis capitis) intervening. Thus, to stimulate the GON itself, the intervening muscles are likely to be recruited as well (**Fig. 19-1**).

Lead placement adjacent to the nuchal line would be less prone to muscle stimulation because the GON is superficial at this level.[25]

Lead Type

Original reports of the procedure described using quadripolar leads, although recent technical and practice trends favor the use of octipolar leads. There are no comparative studies of quadripolar vs. octipolar lead use in ONS. However, the added electrode contacts in the octipolar leads allow for exponentially more stimulation configuration arrays.[25] Because the lesser occipital nerve runs laterally to the GON at the level of the nuchal line, longer octipolar leads also capture lesser occipital nerve branches, which leads to better coverage (**Fig. 19-2**). Paddle-type leads deliver electric

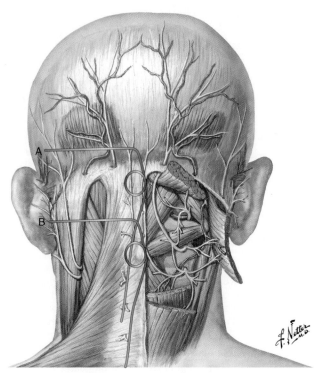

Fig. 19-1 **A**, Occipital neurostimulation lead placed at the nuchal ridge level **B**, Occipital neurostimulation lead placed at C1 level. Netter illustration from www.netterimages.com. ©Elsevier Inc. All rights reserved.

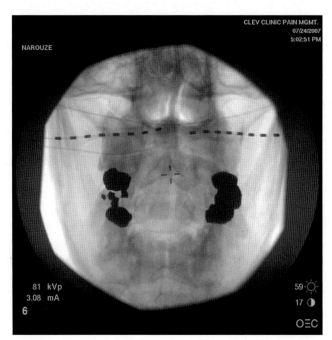

Fig. 19-2 Cylindrical percutaneous occipital neurostimulation lead. Reprinted with permission from Ohio Headache and Pain Institute.

current in one direction only, whereas cylindrical percutaneous leads deliver current circumferentially. Some clinicians prefer the paddle-type leads in redo cases secondary to percutaneous lead migrations because the paddle leads can be easily sutured into the surrounding fascia. The downside of the paddle is that the larger profile may lead to discomfort or erosion. The implanting doctor must weigh the benefits and the risks (**Fig. 19-3**).

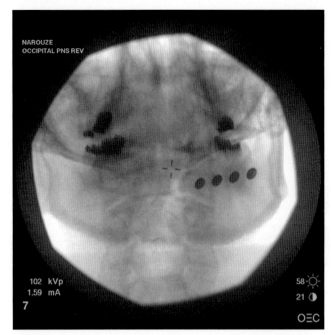

Fig. 19-3 Paddle-type surgical occipital neurostimulation lead. Reprinted with permission from Ohio Headache and Pain Institute.

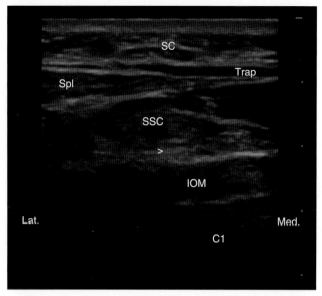

Fig. 19-4 Short axis sonogram at C1 level showing the greater occipital nerve *(arrowhead)*. *IOM,* Inferior oblique muscle, *Spl,* splenius muscle; *SC,* subcutaneous tissue; *SSC,* semispinalis capitis; *Trap,* trapezius muscle; *Med.,* medial; *Lat.,* lateral. Reprinted with permission from Ohio Headache and Pain Institute.

Ultrasound-Guided Occipital Neurostimulation Placement

Traditionally the lead is placed with fluoroscopy; if it is too superficial, one may experience unpleasant dysthesias in the overlying skin area, and if placed deep it may invariably penetrate the occipital muscles, which usually leads to painful muscle spasms on stimulation. Since ultrasound is a great tool in visualizing soft tissue structures, with ultrasound-guided technique the lead can be placed subcutaneously near the nuchal line where the GON is superficial without intervening muscle; or the GON can be recognized, and the lead can be placed intentionally between the inferior oblique and semispinalis muscle (where the nerve runs) at the C1-C2 level (**Fig. 19-4**). In the latter case the GON can be stimulated with minimal settings; this can save the life of the battery. We refer to this latter approach as *occipital PNS*.[26]

Nerve Stimulation-Guided Occipital Neurostimulation Placement

Recently the possibility of using sensory nerve stimulation as a tool to determine depth of lead placement has been recommended and investigated. In 20 patients the mean subcutaneous depth of implant was 11 mm based on sensory nerve stimulation. Although this evaluation was performed prospectively, it is important that this finding be reproduced in a multicenter setting.[27]

Technical Problems and Complications

The major technical problem with ONS is lead migrations. The incidence of lead migration was 24% after 3 months.[17] In another review it was found to be 60% 1 year after implant and 100% 3 years after implant.[5] This led some practitioners to consider the use of self-anchoring leads in ONS with encouraging preliminary results (**Fig. 19-5**). None of 12 patients required a surgical revision for lead migration for a mean follow-up period of 13 months.[28]

The second most common problem is occipital muscle spasms caused by occipital muscle stimulation secondary to improper lead placement as described above.[25]

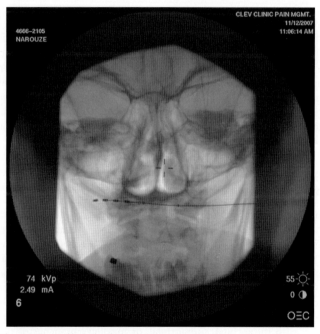

Fig. 19-5 Self-anchoring percutaneous lead. Reprinted with permission from Ohio Headache and Pain Institute.

Other rare complications may include lead fracture or disconnect, lead tip erosion, infection, unpleasant stimulation, and localized pain at implant sites.[29-31]

Mixed Causes of Cephalgia

In some patients stimulation of the ONS only captures a single aspect of a complicated problem. Many patients suffer from pain in the occiput mixed with other neuropathic pain syndromes of the face. Commonly this involves the trigeminal nerve or its nerve

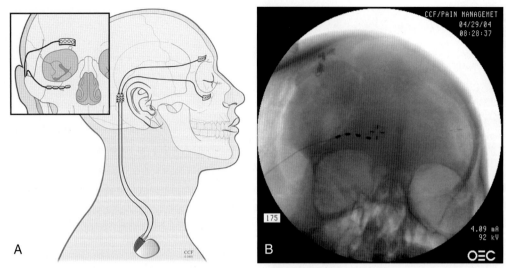

Fig. 19-6 **A**, Schematic diagram illustrating infraorbital and supraorbital peripheral neurostimulator lead placement. Note that the retroauricular anchoring of the leads may be performed with or without extensions. **B**, Radiograph of a supraorbital nerve stimulator lead in a patient with supraorbital neuralgia following frontal craniotomy. ©Cleveland Clinic Foundation.

innervation pathways. In these cases it may be necessary to combine ONS with cranial nerve stimulation of the face. These mixed devices may require repositioning and always require a careful analysis of how the 16 electrode contacts can be used to best cover the area of paresthesia. When a mixed nerve trial is required, it is important that each nerve be assessed in an independent fashion and also combined for an overall impact and decision on the appropriateness of a permanent implant. This combination of two or more peripheral nerve stimulation (PNS) targets may have fewer risks than motor cortex stimulation and may be more acceptable to the patient and insurer. In the event of failure of PNS, motor cortex stimulation should be considered.[32]

Stimulation of the Gasserian Ganglion and Peripheral Nerve Targets

In mixed neuropathic pain of the head and face, some implanters have focused on the gasserian ganglion. These results are often promising in the first few weeks of implant but have been technically challenging and have had mixed long-term results. Additional prospective studies are needed to evaluate the role of this target, as opposed to the branch of the trigeminal nerve, which may be easier to access with a simple percutaneous approach.[33,34] Slavin and colleagues[34] have shown positive outcomes combining ONS stimulation with infraorbital, supraorbital, or maxillary branches of the trigeminal nerve (**Fig. 19-6**). These PNS approaches are low risk and may be attractive when considering the option of significant intracranial procedures.[35] Johnson and Burchiel[36] reported a pilot study involving 10 patients who received subcutaneous infraorbital and/or supraorbital nerve stimulation for trigeminal neuropathic pain. The etiology of the pain was posttraumatic in six of the patients and postherpetic neuralgia in four. Greater than 50% pain relief and significant decrease in analgesic medication use occurred in 70% of patients, with more robust results occurring in the posttraumatic group than in the postherpetic group. Reoperation occurred in 30%, including wound breakdown over the extension in two of the 10 cases. There was a gradual decrease in efficacy of stimulation with time; 80% of patients still experienced ≥50% pain relief 2 years after implant.

Conclusion

The use of subcutaneous peripheral neurostimulation for head and face pain has evolved dramatically over the past decade both in the technique of implant and indications for which these devices are placed. New interest has been developing in areas of ONS for novel indications such as fibromyalgia. The future of this target and that of facial stimulation is certainly intriguing and will be fascinating to watch as more research is performed.

References

1. Weiner RL, Reed KL: Peripheral Neurostimulation for Control of Intractable Occipital Neuralgia. *Neuromodulation* 2:217-221, 1999.
2. Kapural L et al: Occipital nerve electrical stimulation via the midline approach and subcutaneous surgical leads for treatment of severe occipital neuralgia: a pilot study. *Anesth Analg* 101:171-174, 2005.
3. Johnstone CHS, Sundaraj R: Occipital nerve stimulation for the treatment of occipital neuralgia—eight case studies. *Neuromodulation* 9:41-47, 2006.
4. Oh MY et al: Peripheral nerve stimulation for the treatment of occipital neuralgia and transformed migraine using a C1-2-3 subcutaneous paddle style electrode: a technical report. *Neuromodulation* 7:103-112, 2004.
5. Schwedt TJ et al: Occipital nerve stimulation for chronic headache-long-term safety and efficacy. *Cephalalgia* 27:153-157, 2007.
6. Schwedt TJ et al: Occipital nerve stimulation for chronic cluster headache and hemicrania continua: pain relief and persistence of autonomic features. *Cephalalgia* 26:1025-1027, 2006.
7. Burns B, Watkins L, Goadsby PJ: Treatment of medically intractable cluster headache by occipital nerve stimulation: long-term follow-up of eight patients. *Lancet* 369:1099-1106, 2007.
8. Burns B, Watkins L, Goadsby PJ: Treatment of intractable chronic cluster headache by occipital nerve stimulation in 14 patients. *Neurology* 72:341-345, 2009.
9. Magis D et al: Occipital nerve stimulation for drug-resistant chronic cluster headache: a prospective pilot study. *Lancet Neurol* 6:314-321, 2007.
10. Burns B, Watkins L, Goadsby PJ: Treatment of hemicrania continua by occipital nerve stimulation with a BION device: long-term follow-up of a crossover study. *Lancet Neurol* 7:1001-1012, 2008.

11. Rodrigo-Royo MD et al: Peripheral neurostimulation in the management of cervicogenic headache: four case reports. *Neuromodulation* 8:241-248, 2005.

12. Melvin EA, Jr et al: Using peripheral stimulation to reduce the pain of C2-mediated occipital headaches: a preliminary report. *Pain Physician* 10:453-460, 2007.

13. Schwedt TJ et al: Occipital nerve stimulation for chronic headache—long-term safety and efficacy. *Cephalalgia* 27:153-157, 2007.

14. Ghaemi K et al: Occipital nerve stimulation for refractory occipital pain after occipitocervical fusion: expanding indications. *Stereotact Funct Neurosurg* 86:391-393, 2008.

15. Goadsby PJ, Bartsch T, Dodick D: Occipital nerve stimulation for headache: mechanisms and efficacy. *Headache* 48:313-318, 2008.

16. Matharu MS et al: Central neuromodulation in chronic migraine patients with suboccipital stimulation: a PET study. *Brain* 127:120-130, 2004.

17. Saper J et al: Occipital nerve stimulation (ONS) for treatment of intractable migraine headache: 3-month results from the ONSTIM feasibility study (abstract). *Pain Med* 10:225, 2009.

18. Bovim G et al: Topographic variations in the peripheral course of the greater occipital nerve: autopsy study with clinical correlations. *Spine* 16:475-478, 1991.

19. Becser N, Bovim G, Sjaastad O: Extracranial nerves in the posterior part of the head: anatomic variations and their possible clinical significance. *Spine* 23:1435-1441, 1998.

20. Mosser SW et al: The anatomy of the greater occipital nerve: implications for the etiology of migraine headaches. *Plast Reconstr Surg* 113:693-697, 2004.

21. Hammer M, Doleys DM: Perineuromal stimulation in the treatment of occipital neuralgia: a case study. *Neuromodulation* 4:47-51, 2001.

22. Slavin KV, Nersesyan H, Wess C: Peripheral neurostimulation for treatment of intractable occipital neuralgia. *Neurosurgery* 58:112-119, 2006.

23. Johnstone CSH, Sundaraj R: Occipital nerve stimulation for the treatment of occipital neuralgia-eight case studies. *Neuromodulation* 9:41-47, 2006.

24. Popeney CA, Alò KM: Peripheral neurostimulation for the treatment of chronic, disabling transformed migraine. *Headache* 43:369-375, 2003.

25. Hayek SM et al: Occipital neurostimulation-induced muscle spasms: implications for lead placement. *Pain Physician* 12(5):867-876, 2009.

26. Narouze S: Ultrasonography in pain medicine: future directions. *Tech Reg Anesth Pain Manage* 13(3):198-202, 2009.

27. Abejon D, Deer T, Verrils P: Depth determination of subcutaneous stimulation by sensory nerve stimulation. Submitted to *Neuromodulation.*

28. Narouze S et al: Occipital nerve stimulation with self-anchoring leads for the management of refractory chronic migraine headache (abstract). *Pain Med* 10:221, 2009.

29. Trentman TL, Zimmerman RS: Occipital nerve stimulation: technical and surgical aspects of implantation. *Headache* 48:319-327, 2008.

30. Jasper JF, Hayek SM: Implanted occipital nerve stimulators. *Pain Physician* 1:187-200, 2008.

31. Trentman TL et al: Percutaneous occipital stimulator lead tip erosion: report of 2 cases. *Pain Physician* 11:253-256, 2008.

32. Levy R, Deer TR, Henderson J: Intracranial neurostimulation for pain control: a review. *Pain Physician* 13(2):157-165, 2010.

33. Machado A et al: A 12-month prospective study of gasserian ganglion stimulation for trigeminal neuropathic pain. *Stereotact Funct Neurosurg* 85(5):216-224, 2007. Epub May 25, 2007.

34. Slavin KV et al: Trigeminal and occipital peripheral nerve stimulation for craniofacial pain: a single-institution experience and review of the literature. *Neurosurg Focus* 21(6):E5, 2006.

35. Thimineur M, De Ridder D: C2 area neurostimulation: a surgical treatment for fibromyalgia. *Pain Med* 8(8):639-646, 2007.

36. Johnson MD, Burchiel KJ: Peripheral stimulation for treatment of trigeminal postherpetic neuralgia and trigeminal posttraumatic neuropathic pain: a pilot study. *Neurosurgery* 55(1):135-141, 2004.

20 Peripheral Subcutaneous Stimulation for Intractable Pain

Giancarlo Barolat

CHAPTER OVERVIEW

Chapter Synopsis: Peripheral subcutaneous stimulation (PSS) provides a minimally invasive form of neurostimulation for intractable pain. This technique, also called *peripheral nerve field stimulation*, targets the small, arborized fibers in subcutaneous tissue. Originally developed to treat areas difficult to reach with stimulation of the nerve trunk or spinal cord, PSS shows promise in other areas, rendering more central implantation unnecessary. Technical details of device selection should always be considered in advance of implantation. PSS may be optimized with cylindrical rather than paddle leads used in some other applications. Further consideration should be given to the size and site of the painful area to be treated. Large areas of the body can be treated with multiple, widely spaced leads. This chapter provides several technical considerations for optimal implantation. The primary indications for PSS are back pain and headaches that may be neuropathic or nociceptive in origin. The most promising patient candidates can pinpoint areas of their worst pain and the area from which pain originates. Because stimulation is achieved directly at the pain site, precise placement is critical to success. Transcutaneous external nerve stimulation can be considered a less invasive option to PSS and, if effective, should be used in place of PSS. Although PSS is minimally invasive and avoids many risks associated with spinal stimulation, some complications are common to it, including infection and lead migration.

Important Points:
- Map the pain areas very carefully. Highlight the areas of "worse pain."
- Confirm with the patient the mapped pain areas.
- Avoid allodynic areas.
- If the areas of worse pain are very extensive (several square inches), the patient might not be a candidate for the procedure.
- Combine it with intraspinal stimulation if indicated.

Clinical Pearls:
- A 100% pain relief at trial is very worrisome and means strong placebo effect.
- If possible, have the patient or a family member map the pain areas before showing up for surgery.
- Always document the lead position with an intraoperative/postoperative radiograph.
- Always cover with the lead placement either the areas of "worse pain" or the areas where the pain starts (or both, if possible).
- During the first 24 to 48 hours following lead placement, the electrical parameters might not reflect the true characteristics of the stimulation.

Clinical Pitfalls:
- Make sure that the patient is fully awake before starting intraoperative sensory testing.
- Carefully secure the leads, particularly in the cervical area.
- Tip of the lead skin erosion is a common issue in the scalp area.
- When tunneling, avoid hypersensitive areas.
- If the patient is thin, place anchors, connectors, and extensions under the fascia if possible to avoid a later revision.

Introduction

Peripheral subcutaneous stimulation (PSS) is a new and exciting area of neurostimulation. It belongs to the general category of stimulation of the peripheral nervous system. However, instead of stimulating a well-defined nerve trunk, the stimulation is applied to the small terminal branches of one or more peripheral nerves. The target area for the stimulation is the subcutaneous tissue, where the small nervous endings of the nerves arborize in a widespread network.

The technique is known with several different names, such as *subcutaneous stimulation, peripheral nerve field stimulation, regional stimulation,* and *peripheral nerve stimulation.*[1-6] All of these definitions point to the fact that the target is the small peripheral nervous system fibers in the subcutaneous tissue. This is a paradigm switch from previous neurostimulation modalities, in which the stimulation is applied to a well-defined large neural structure (i.e., a large peripheral nerve, the nerve roots, or the spinal cord).

Although the mechanisms of action are unknown, they are most likely similar to the ones described for peripheral nerve stimulation.[7]

This technique has determined a revolutionary change in the paradigm of classical neurostimulation as it has been performed for several decades. In the classical neurostimulation paradigm, the goal is to stimulate some major nervous sensory structures upstream from the painful area to generate paresthesias in that area. With PSS the lead is actually placed within or near the area of the pain (or the area of the projection of the pain). This technique was developed with the goal of stimulating areas that are notoriously difficult or impossible to reach from the spinal cord or major nerve trunk level, including the posterior axial surface of the body from the neck to the lumbar spine. Although originally developed for these difficult situations, PSS is sometimes being used as a first, minimally invasive, neurostimulation procedure if the pain is limited to a relatively small and well-defined area.

Equipment

In the author's experience, PSS is best accomplished with percutaneously placed cylindrical leads and not with paddle leads. The reason lies in the target of the stimulation. When performing dorsal column, nerve root, or large peripheral nerve stimulation, the target is a well-defined neural structure, and the lead(s) is (are) placed on its surface. Therefore the current is unidirectional and best delivered by a paddle lead. With PSS, instead the lead is placed within the target, which is made of all the small sensory nerve endings within the subcutaneous tissues. Therefore the best electrical field is one that is circumferential, like the one delivered by a percutaneously placed cylindrical lead. The type and contact-spacing of the lead depends on the size of the pain area and the number of leads being used. For a very small pain area, a quadripolar lead with 5- to 7-mm intercontact spacing is most likely sufficient. For a large pain area, one or more leads with 9 mm or more intercontact spacing is more appropriate.

Currently there is no implantable equipment developed specifically for this modality. The leads used are the same ones used for intraspinal stimulation. The pulse generators are also borrowed from the spinal cord stimulation (SCS) line of products.

Technique[1]

The principle of PSS is that the lead should be placed within or as near as possible to the painful area. Each electrical contact spreads a circumferential electrical field, which is about 2.5 cm in diameter. Therefore the number, spacing, and distribution of the electrical contacts should be carefully planned according to the size and shape of the painful area. The current can also be driven across leads placed at a distance, thereby increasing the size of the affected electrical field. Larger areas might require several leads placed strategically. I have placed up to four widely spaced percutaneous leads in an effort to cover larger areas of the body.

Almost any area of the body can be reached with this technique. The most commonly addressed areas include lumbar, posterior thoracic, scapular, inguinal, and various regions of the head and face[1-6, 8-17] (**Figs. 20-1 to 20-4**).

A bendable introducer with a blunt obturator is very useful in areas of great curvature such as the forehead, the cervical region, and the knee. A long introducer (6 to 8 inches) can also be useful to avoid placing an incision near painful areas.

The depth of the needle (and therefore the lead) is crucial to the success of the procedure. The lead should be placed in the superficial layer of the subcutaneous tissues. If it is placed in the deep layers of the subcutaneous tissues, no paresthesias will be perceived. If the lead is under the fascia or very close to the muscles, motor contractions will be elicited. If the lead is placed within the dermis, the stimulation will be perceived as extremely painful.

The depth of the needle should satisfy three criteria:

- There should be no indentations in the skin. Indentations mean that the needle is actually in the dermis. If the needle is in the dermis, advancing it is very difficult, and one meets a lot of resistance. If the patient is semiawake, he or she demonstrates a lot of resistance since advancing a needle in the dermis is extremely painful.
- One should be able to visualize a slight "tenting up" caused by the needle in the subcutaneous tissue, and certainly one should be able to readily feel the needle with finger palpation. If the needle cannot be felt, its location is too deep.
- During a percutaneous trial, entry in the subcutaneous tissue is usually characterized by a "pop" feeling caused by the loss of resistance once the needle has penetrated through the epidermis/dermis.

The trial is performed without an incision or with a small nick by inserting the leads in the subcutaneous tissue through the needle provided in the kit or some other inserting device. Even though the procedure is simple, it has to be done with heavy (albeit short) intravenous sedation.

Heavy sedation is highly recommended since inserting a large-bore needle in the subcutaneous tissue parallel to the skin can be extremely painful, particularly since the needle tract cannot be infiltrated with local anesthetic. On insertion of the leads, the trial is undertaken just like a regular SCS trial. One caveat is that sometimes the trauma of the needle insertion causes the tissues to temporarily react abnormally to the stimulation. Impedances can be high, and stimulation might not be perceived fully. A reprogramming session 24 to 48 hours following the lead insertion usually yields much more reliable results.

If the trial is successful in reducing the pain, the whole system is implanted at a second sitting. It is possible to perform a trial with permanent electrodes, but this entails an incision and the use of one or more extension cables.

Implantation of the whole system requires excellent surgical technique and experience. The areas of pain to be addressed must be marked. Possible areas of hypersensitivity or hyperalgesia that must be avoided are then mapped out. The implantable pulse generator (IPG) location must be decided with the above mapping in mind. Sometimes tunneling several electrodes subcutaneously in the posterior thoracic area is not desirable. The same applies to the strategic placement of anchors and connections with extension cables. If not properly placed, these elements alone could lead to later removal of the device. Migration of the leads is the most common complication, and one should make every effort to prevent that occurrence. Anchoring the lead is crucial. Several methods of anchoring are available. One could use the commercially available anchors that come with the lead kit. If more than one anchor per lead is placed, the anchors can be trimmed so as to not be too bulky. Alternatively one could place two or three "drain stitches," with the knots tied semiloosely around the lead so as to not damage it. This is a very effective way of "trapping" the lead without the bulk of an anchor. I always place a loop, which is then secured with a second anchor or another suture. The loop is probably the most significant protection against migration. In some areas such as the posterior cervical region, migrations are much more common.

The implantation of the whole system can be a substantial surgical procedure that cannot be underestimated. Often it requires several incisions and multiple tunneling efforts. A complex PSS procedure could be much more demanding than a simple SCS implant.

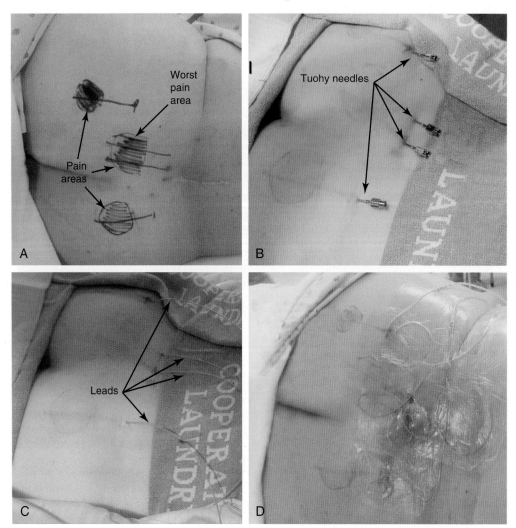

Fig. 20-1 Severe bilateral lumbar pain following several lumbar spine surgical procedures. Test trial patient in right lateral position. **A,** Pain areas. **B,** Tuohy needles placed in pain areas. **C,** Leads placed in pain areas. **D,** Leads attached to extensions and taped with transparent adhesive dressing on left flank.

Indications

Both nociceptive and neuropathic pain can respond positively to this modality.

Criteria for the trial procedure include: (1) severe pain of at least a 6-month duration, (2) failure of conservative treatment, and (3) psychological stability. Both axial and limb painful areas can be targeted (**Figs. 20-5 to 20-7**). In the author's practice the most common indications include intractable axial lumbar pain (whether the patient has received surgical intervention or not), intractable posterior thoracic pain, intractable scapular pain, inguinal pain, thoracic wall pain, shoulder pain, headaches, and atypical facial pain. I have not placed subcutaneous leads in the perineum. I have implanted many patients with severe intractable low back pain whose other alternative was a multilevel spine fusion. When dealing with exclusively axial pain and in the presence of multilevel lumbar spine degenerative disease, a trial with PSS seems to be a reasonable option.

The most important part of the procedure is careful planning. Unlike SCS, in which the lead insertion incision is almost invariably either in the upper lumbar or upper thoracic midline, with PSS the incisions can be numerous and must be strategically placed

according to the pain areas to be covered and the position of the implantable pulse generator (IPG). As a first step, the patient and the implanting physician must agree on which pain areas are to be addressed. Many times, when presented with the question, "where is your pain?" the patient points to very large body areas, often larger than what is reasonable to try to cover with the stimulation. I then usually ask two key questions: (1) Where is the area of your worst pain? (2) Where is the area from which your pain originates? (if there is one). If the patient points to a vague large area and cannot pinpoint the answer to these questions, he or she is not deemed a good candidate for the procedure. Next the areas of pain to be addressed must be outlined in detail. Areas that qualify for criteria 1 and/or 2 are the ones that carry priority in lead placement.

The success of the procedure is directly related to the ability of the patient to guide the implanter to the most crucial pain areas. Experienced implanters often ask the patient to mark the areas of pain before coming to the hospital. Some implanters go as far as asking the patient to assign numerical values to the various pain areas as a reflection of the pain severity.

Strategic placement of the leads can be accomplished either by placing the lead(s) in the center of the painful area or by "bracketing" the area with leads flanking the area. The latter is definitely the

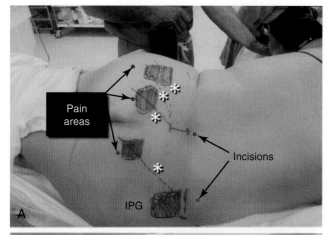

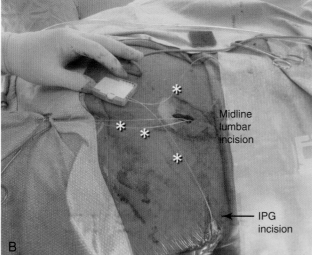

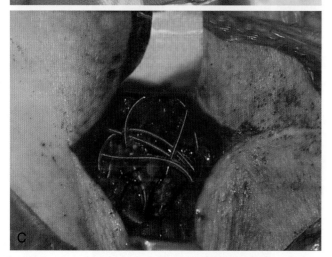

Fig. 20-2 Permanent surgical implant. **A,** Preoperative marking showing pain areas, planned incisions, and planned lead trajectories (*asterisks*). **B,** Three leads placed through midline lumbar incision; one lead placed through IPG incision; three leads tunneled to IPG incision; all leads connected to two bifurcated extensions; two extensions plugged into IPG. Leads being tested intra-operatively (*asterisks*). **C,** Midline lumbar incision. Each of the three leads is anchored with two anchors and a small strain relief loop between the two anchors. *IPG,* Implantable pulse generator.

preferred approach in the case of allodynic areas. Leads placed directly in the allodynic area might be physically bothersome, and the stimulation might be perceived as painful. It is crucial to carefully map the transition zone between the allodynic and nonallodynic area and place the lead exactly in that zone. A centimeter difference could substantially impact the success or failure of the modality.

PSS can also be used in conjunction with intraspinal stimulation and/or large peripheral nerve stimulation.[8] I have several patients in whom both modalities were successfully implemented jointly, either as separate procedures or as part of a single implant procedure. It is not unusual to be able to adequately cover pain in the lower extremities with intraspinal leads, but to rely on leads placed subcutaneously to address pain in the axial low lumbar area. Another common situation for a "mixed" lead placement is in patients who have upper-extremity and scapular pain. In this instance one lead can be placed intraspinally in the cervical area, and another in the scapular area subcutaneously. Both the intraspinal and the subcutaneous leads can be plugged in the same IPG (provided that the total number of contacts does not exceed the capacity of the system). The current can be programmed to flow between the intraspinal and the subcutaneous leads; this might lead to an even broader field of stimulation.

Peripheral Subcutaneous Stimulation and Transcutaneous External Nerve Stimulation

In some respects PSS could be considered the next step in the neurostimulation continuum, after transcutaneous external nerve stimulation (TENS). In fact, many of the indications for PSS are also indications for TENS. The TENS modality(ies) should always be tried before PSS, unless clear contraindications exist: allodynia, pain location not suitable (head, hairy area, perineum). If the TENS treatment is satisfactory, PSS should not be considered.

There are four reasons why TENS might not work:

- The stimulation itself is not effective in reducing the pain.
- The patient might have skin hypersensitivity or allodynia in the pain areas and might not tolerate the electrodes on the skin.
- Some body conditions might not make it possible to use the TENS unit regularly: (a) excessive sweat, (b) hairy areas, and (c) patient might not be able to reach the pain areas and place the electrode pads.
- Even though the TENS helps, the patient might find it awkward to implement it on a daily basis.

If the TENS unit did not work because of the first reason, PSS might still have superior efficacy in relieving pain. If the TENS modality did not work because of reasons two through four, a trial with PSS is definitely indicated; it might be a much more suitable long-term treatment option.

Risk and Complication Avoidance

Because the whole procedure is performed at the level of the subcutaneous tissues, the risk of neurological damage is remote and certainly not in the same category as intraspinal stimulation. The three most common complications are lead migration, skin erosion, and infection. Lead migration can easily occur if the leads are not properly secured as outlined previously. Unlike SCS, in which a small lead migration can be corrected by programming,

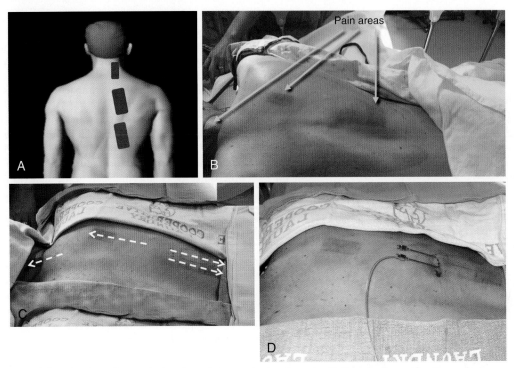

Fig. 20-3 Temporary trial. **A, B,** Posterior cervical and medial scapular border pain. **C,** Four leads: one in the posterior cervical area, one in the upper medial scapular border, and two in the lower thoracic area. **D,** Two Tuohy needles inserted in a caudal direction in the lower pain areas.

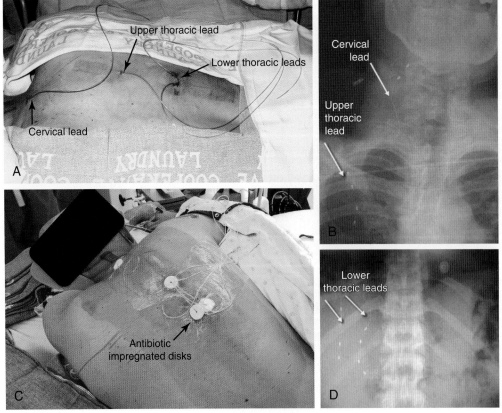

Fig. 20-4 **A, C,** Cervical and thoracic leads. Percutaneous trial with temporary leads. Leads externalized. **B, D,** AP x-rays of the cervical and thoracic spine with the leads in place.

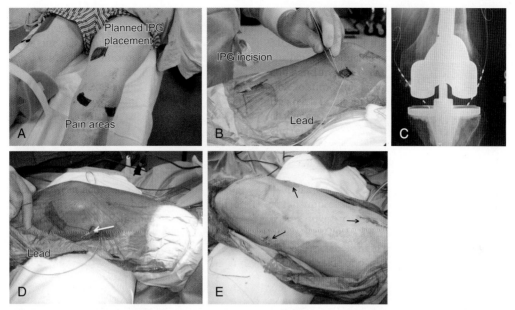

Fig. 20-5   Intractable knee pain. Status post–knee replacement. **A,** Pain areas and planned IPG placement. **B,** Medial lead placement and IPG incision. **C,** Permanent implant. **D,** Lateral lead placement and tunneling tool to IPG *(white arrow).* **E,** Incisions *(black arrows).* *IPG,* Implantable pulse generator.

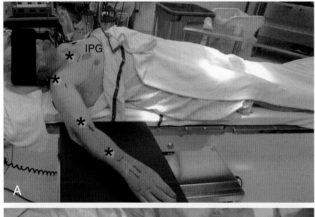

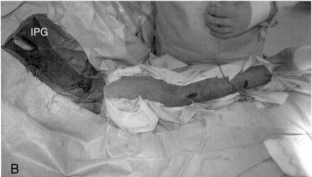

Fig. 20-6   Permanent implant. **A,** Planned incisions *(asterisks).* **B,** IPG shown in incision. *IPG,* Implantable pulse generator.

in PSS, if the lead moves out of the painful area, no reprogramming will be effective in recapturing the pain relief. Skin erosion is possible if the anchors are placed too superficially in the subcutaneous tissue. This is a more frequent issue with leads placed in the scalp area. Skin erosion can also occur at the tip of the lead;

this is also a more frequent problem with scalp stimulation. The risk of infection is not different from other neurostimulation procedures.

Results

Only case reports are available in the literature at the time of writing of this chapter. There are no large series reports or prospective studies. Positive results have been reported in patients with intractable lumbar axial pain, inguinal neuralgia, neuropathic pain, abdominal pain, postherpetic neuralgia, and cervicogenic headaches, to name a few. [3-6, 8-19]

The most comprehensive retrospective study is the one by Verrills and associates.[3] The authors collected data on 13 consecutive patients who had successful trials and were subsequently implanted with Octrode percutaneous leads placed subcutaneously within the major area of pain. Eleven patients met diagnostic criteria for failed back surgery syndrome. A questionnaire assessed outcomes, including pain, analgesic use, and patient satisfaction. The response rate was 93% (13/14; average follow-up time was 7 months). There was a significant decrease in pain levels: an average reduction of 3.77 visual analog scale (VAS) points. Eleven patients (85%) reported successful outcomes and an average pain reduction of 4.18 points, but two reported a poor response. Pain relief was highly correlated with reduced analgesia and patient satisfaction. No complications were reported. Before peripheral nerve stimulation (PNS), the mean VAS was 7.42 ± 1.16 (range 5 to 10). Following PNS, the mean VAS was 3.92 ± 1.72 (range 1 to 6), representing a mean improvement in VAS of 3.77 ± 1.65 (range 1 to 6.5). As a response to PNS, patients were asked to rank their satisfaction with the procedure. One patient considered the outcome to be completely satisfactory. Two patients were very satisfied, and seven were satisfied with the procedure. Two patients were not completely satisfied, and one was not satisfied with PNS.

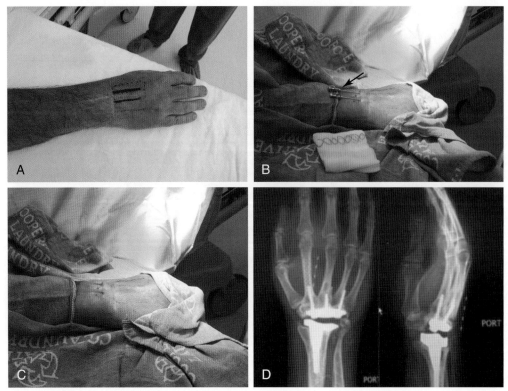

Fig. 20-7 Intractable neuropathic pain following wrist replacement. Temporary test trial. **A,** Planned leads placement. **B,** Tuohy needles for leads placement *(arrow).* **C,** Leads in place for temporary trial. **D,** AP and lateral views of lead in proper position.

The results are promising, but prospective randomized studies are necessary before reaching definitive conclusions for the role of this modality in the management of chronic pain conditions.

Conclusions

Stimulation of the small peripheral nerve fibers in the subcutaneous tissue is promising to become a very important modality in the management of severe pain conditions that have failed more conservative measures. The attractiveness of the modality lies both in its (relative) simplicity and in the fact that one can cover with neurostimulation areas previously deemed almost impossible. A trial is a simple procedure; however, the actual surgical implant is far more complex and tedious and requires substantial intraoperative planning.

The exact role of this modality in the management of refractory pain conditions will have to be defined by large prospective clinical studies.

References

1. Barolat G: Techniques for subcutaneous peripheral nerve field stimulation for intractable pain. In Krames E, Peckham H, Rezai A, editors: *Neuromodulation,* St Louis, 2009, Elsevier, pp 1017-1020.
2. Abejón D, Elliot S: Krames peripheral nerve stimulation or is it peripheral subcutaneous field stimulation; What is in a moniker? *Neuromodulation* 12:1-4, 2009.
3. Verrills P, et al: Peripheral nerve stimulation: a treatment for chronic low back pain and failed back surgery syndrome? *Neuromodulation* 12:68-75, 2009.
4. Al Tamimi M, et al: Successful treatment of chronic neuropathic pain with subcutaneous peripheral nerve stimulation: four case reports. *Neuromodulation* 3:210-214, 2009.
5. Bernstein CA, et al: Spinal cord stimulation in conjunction with peripheral nerve field stimulation for the treatment of low back and leg pain: a case series. *Neuromodulation* 11:116-123, 2008.
6. Krutsch JP, et al: A case report of subcutaneous peripheral nerve stimulation for the treatment of axial back pain associated with postlaminectomy syndrome. *Neuromodulation* 11:112-115, 2008.
7. Ellrich J, Lamp S: Peripheral nerve stimulation inhibits nociceptive processing: an electrophysiological study in healthy volunteers. *Neuromodulation* 8:225-232, 2005.
8. Lipov EG, Joshi JR, Slavin KV: Hybrid neuromodulation technique: use of combined spinal cord stimulation and peripheral nerve stimulation in treatment of chronic pain in back and legs. *Acta Neurochir (Wien)* 150:971, 2008.
9. Mobbs RJ, Nair S, Blum P: Peripheral nerve stimulation for the treatment of chronic pain. *J Clin Neurosci* 14:216-221, 2007.
10. Paicius RM, Bernstein CA, Lempert-Cohen C: Peripheral nerve field stimulation for the treatment of chronic low back pain: preliminary results of long-term follow-up: a case series. *Neuromodulation* 10:279-290, 2007.
11. Paicius RM, Bernstein CA, Lempert-Cohen C: Peripheral nerve field stimulation in chronic abdominal pain. *Pain Physician* 9:261-266, 2006.
12. Rodrigo-Royo MD, et al: Peripheral neurostimulation in the management of cervicogenic headache: four case reports. *Neuromodulation* 8:241-248, 2005.
13. Slavin KV, Nersesyan H, Wess C: Peripheral neurostimulation for treatment of intractable occipital neuralgia. *Neurosurgery* 58:112-119, 2006.
14. Slavin KV: Peripheral nerve stimulation for neuropathic pain. *Neurotherapeutics* 5:100-106, 2008.

15. Stinson LW, et al: Peripheral subcutaneous electrostimulation for control of intractable postoperative inguinal pain: a case report series. *Neuromodulation* 4:99-104, 2001.

16. Yakovlev AE, Peterson A: Peripheral nerve stimulation in treatment of intractable postherpetic neuralgia. *Neuromodulation* 10:373-375, 2007.

17. Lipov E, et al: Use of peripheral subcutaneous field stimulation for the treatment of axial neck pain: a case report. *Neuromodulation* 12:292-295, 2009.

18. Ordia J, Vaisman J: Subcutaneous peripheral nerve stimulation with paddle lead for treatment of low back pain: case report. *Neuromodulation* 12:205-209, 2009.

19. Reverberi C, Bonezzi C, Demartini L: Peripheral subcutaneous neurostimulation in the management of neuropathic pain: five case reports. *Neuromodulation* 12:146-155, 2009.

21 Motor Cortex Stimulation for Relief of Chronic Pain

Claudio Andres Feler

CHAPTER OVERVIEW

Chapter Synopsis: Many types of chronic pain can be improved by electrical stimulation of nerve tissue: in the periphery, at the spinal cord, and even in motor cortex. This chapter describes motor cortex stimulation (MCS) for painful conditions that have not responded to other drug or stimulation therapies. Success with MCS depends on a thorough diagnosis, including parsing chronic pain into nociceptive and neuropathic components whenever possible. Unlike some other stimulation therapies, MCS does not produce paresthesias in patients—a double-edged sword. Although it can make accurate placement of stimulating electrodes more difficult, it does allow for double-blinded studies of efficacy. A review of the literature reveals that MCS has provided positive outcomes for various chronic pain conditions, including facial pain syndromes, neuropathic pain caused by phantom limb, central pain and plexus avulsion, and complex regional pain syndrome (CRPS). The homuncular anatomy of the motor cortex makes treatment of the face and hands relatively simple, whereas leg cortical maps are located deeper in the brain.

Important Points:
- MCS has been available for many years but has recently drawn interest as a viable therapy for the intractable pain patient.
- The Food and Drug Administration (FDA) has not approved MCS as a labeled therapy for the use of humans in the United States. Many neurosurgeons use this therapy in an off-label fashion.
- A proper diagnosis is needed before selecting a patient for MCS.
- Facial and neuropathic pain appear to be the most likely types of disorders to respond to MCS.
- Patients should be treated with spinal cord or peripheral nerve stimulation before MCS if appropriate.
- Attention to detail is important to reduce complications in the patient undergoing MCS.
- More research is needed to determine the best use for this procedure.

Clinical Pearls:
- There is evidence supporting the use of this therapy in those patients who experience neuropathic pain but are anatomically or physiologically unable to obtain paresthetic overlap in their pain areas.
- More conventional stimulation therapies should be attempted first.
- Utility seems to be best in patients with facial distribution pain.

Clinical Pitfalls:
- Anatomical challenges present themselves when trying to stimulate pain in the lower extremity.
- There is no FDA approval for this therapy, making it difficult to provide to many patients.

Introduction

With the advent of modern therapies, a need to determine a proper treatment algorithm is essential to proper use of new advances. Spinal cord stimulation (SCS), peripheral nerve stimulation (PNS) and intrathecal drug delivery (IDD) are options for the patient suffering from severe pain who does not respond to new treatment options.[1,2] Motor cortex stimulation (MCS) is viewed as a new therapy that may play a role in those who do not respond to the treatments noted previously. In fact, MCS is not a new option. The initial report of MCS appeared in the literature 20 years ago and that of deep brain stimulation in the early 1970s, but there is no Food and Drug Administration (FDA) approval for the use of stimulation devices over the cortex of the brain or in the brain to treat pain problems in the United States, making access to these motor cortex and deep brain stimulators for pain difficult.[3,4] This chapter examines the current knowledge base regarding MCS and helps the reader understand critical issues for considering this option for patients.

Establishing Diagnosis

To achieve an optimal selection of a treatment modality, it is necessary to arrive at a correct anatomical and physiological diagnosis. Although chronic pain is often complex from the perspective of centralized messaging, it should usually be possible to deduce a primary and secondary physiological diagnosis by dividing complaints into nociceptive and neuropathic etiologies. This designation is critical and allows for a treatment plan to be crafted for each patient that is relevant to his or her complaint. An example of how this guides therapy selection is a patient with neuropathic leg pain after prior lumbar spine surgery. In such a patient anatomical procedures are not likely to benefit the patient; however, SCS is likely to be very efficacious.

Although the original report by Tsubokawa and associates[4] of MCS for chronic pain considered a group of seven patients who suffered from thalamic pain, this procedure has been used in patients presenting with varied facial pain syndromes in particular, without apparent regard to physiological presentation.[5] In a review of the literature, Nguyen and associates[6] did find results suggestive of modest-to-good improvement of pain in some patients with neuropathic pain. Fontaine, Hamani, and Lozano[7] did an additional review and noted evidence for improvement of patients who experienced neuropathic pain on a variety of causal bases (e.g., phantom limb, central pain and plexus avulsion). Given absence of sensory paresthesias with MCS, two recent studies examined its efficacy using double-blinded stimulation parameters over a 30-day period (Velasco et al, 2009; Lefaucheur et al, 2009). Patients in both studies were then followed long term with active open-label stimulation. One study examined 16 patients with limb or facial neuropathic pain who underwent MCS; 13 were crossed over in a double-blind fashion between active and no stimulation. There were no significant differences between both groups based on visual analog scale (VAS) scores, Brief Pain Inventory (BPI) scores, McGill Pain Questionnaire–Pain Rating Index, Sickness Impact Profile (SIP), or the medication quantification scale. However, in the 12 patients who completed the open-label study, the VAS and SIP scores were significantly reduced compared to baseline. On the other hand, a 2009 study by Velasco and associates trialed five patients with refractory complex regional pain syndrome (CRPS) and implanted four. Clinical signs, VAS, and McGill Pain Scale were monitored while the implanted MCS in each patient was either turned off or on for 30 days between days 30 and 60 and days 60 and 90 following implant in a double-blind fashion. Compared to the off mode, MCS resulted in significant improvement in VAS and McGill Pain Scale and clinical improvements in allodynia, hyperalgesia and sympathetic signs. **Table 21-1** examines studies using MCS for the treatment of pain.

Anatomy

MCS brings with it the anatomy of the cortex itself as a potential challenge, producing possible limitations to the therapy. The face and hand area are over the convexity of the brain and thus are accessible to stimulation without any significant dissection. However, the leg area is in the interhemispheric fissure, which produces technical challenges, both from the point of view of achieving lead placement and retaining the lead in proper position once implanted (**Fig. 21-1**).

Basic Science

Tsubokawa's initial report[5] noted as a rational basis for his series burst suppression in cats that were subjected to MCS. In addition, it was suggested that relevant mechanisms for benefit in these patients included an increase in regional cerebral blood flow and glucose metabolism in both the cortex and the thalamus contralateral to the side of pain. In a later report, Tsubokawa and associates[8] report that patients obtaining benefit from MCS were also found to have pain that was responsive to thiamylal and ketamine infusions but resistant to morphine infusion, again suggesting that patients experiencing relief had neuropathic pain.

Guidelines for Decision Making in Implanting Motor Cortex Stimulation

Consideration of MCS should be given to patients who experience medically refractory neuropathic pain involving areas of the body that are not treatable with more peripherally placed systems

Table 21-1: Summary of Literature Results of Motor Cortex Stimulation for Chronic Neuropathic Pain*

Series	Corresponding Redundant Series*	No. of Patients	FU (mos)	No. of Patients (%)			
				Pain Relief >70%	Pain Relief >50%	Pain Relief >40%	Pain Relief >30%
Tsubokawa et al, 1993	Tsubokawa et al, 1991	11	>24	—	—	6 (54.5)	—
Meyerson et al, 1993	None	10	12.7	2 (20)	5 (50)	—	—
Hosobuchi, 1993	None	6	9-30	—	3 (50)	—	—
Herregodts et al, 1995	None	7	12.7	2 (28.6)	5 (71)	5 (71)	5 (71)
Katayama et al, 1998	Katayama et al, 1994; Yamamoto et al, 1997	31	>24	—	15 (48.3)	—	—
Nguyen et al, 1999	Nguyen et al, 1997 and 2000; Drouot et al, 2002	32	27.3	15 (46.9)	—	23 (71.9)	—
Caroll et al, 2000	Smith et al, 2001; Nandi et al, 2002	10	21-31	3 (30)	4 (40)	—	—
Saitoh et al, 2001	Saitoh et al, 1999 and 2000	15	24.1	—	—	7 (46.7)	—
Sol et al, 2001	Roux et al, 2001	3	27.3	2 (66.7)	2 (66.7)	2 (66.7)	2 (66.7)
Velasco et al, 2002	None	9	12	4 (44.5)	—	6 (66.7)	6 (66.7)
Brown and Pilitsis, 2005	None	10	10	4 (40)	6 (60)	—	—
Nuti et al, 2005	Mertens et al, 1999	31	49	3 (9.7)	7 (22.6)	16 (51.6)	21 (67.7)
Pirotte et al, 2005	None	18	29.7	10 (55.6)	11 (61.6)	11 (61.1)	11 (61.8)
Rasche et al, 2006	Ebel et al, 1996	17	49.7	1 (5.9)	4 (47)	5 (29.4)	8 (47.1)
Velasco et al, 2009	None	5	>36	4 (80)	4 (80)	4 (80)	4 (80)
Lefaucheur et al, 2009	None	16	9-12	5 (31)	8 (50)	9 (56)	10 (62)
Total[†]	—	231	—	53/156 (34)	74/155 (47.7)	94/156 (60.3)	67/99 (67.7)

FU, Follow-up.
*Indicates series published by the same group of authors but not included in our review.
[†]Values are not calculated out of 231 because evaluations were not the same across different studies, and data on pain relief over the defined thresholds were not extractable in all studies.
(Modified from Fontaine D, Hamani C, Lozano A: Efficacy and safety of motor cortex stimulation for chronic neuropathic pain: critical review of the literature. *J Neurosurg* 2009 Feb;110(2):251-6.)

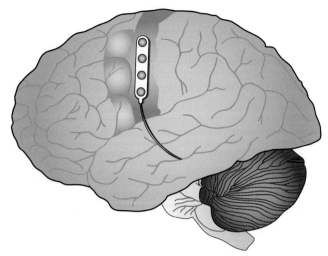

Fig. 21-1 The implanted lead on the brain.

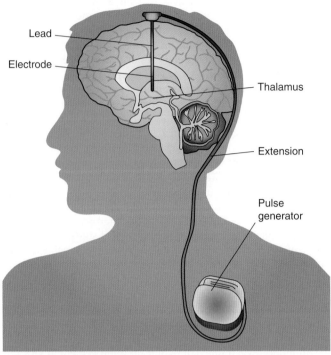

Fig. 21-2 Representation of quadripolar plate electrodes and conventional power supply.

because of topography of pain (e.g., upper face) or inability to obtain overlap of pain with paresthesia caused by the presence of anatomical disruption in the large fiber pathways that results in a need to stimulate a more cranially placed target (e.g., patients with spinal cord injury or wallerian degeneration after a peripheral nerve injury). The implanter must contrast this therapy with deep brain stimulation from the point of view of potential for benefit and both perioperative and postoperative complications.

Indications/Contraindications

Indications for this procedure are medically refractory neuropathic pain syndromes. When appropriate, patients should have failed more commonly used spinal cord or PNS attempts, except patients in whom benefit from such procedures would not be expected to occur (e.g., patients with complete transverse spinal cord injuries).

Patients are contraindicated for this procedure if they have untreated bleeding disorders, localized infection at the surgical site, bacteremia or sepsis, or other intracranial disorders that would make the procedure difficult or impossible or if they are psychologically unstable from severe depression or severe anxiety. The patient should have enough cognitive ability to understand how to use the device.

Equipment

Patients have been implanted most commonly with quadripolar plate electrodes and conventional power supplies (**Fig. 21-2**). Other arrays are usable, and today consideration would be given to more robust electrode arrays to have a better opportunity to improve the patient's pain. New devices are being developed that may have different contours and shapes to better solve the issue of how to best deliver current to this challenging anatomy.

Technique

Before moving forward with MCS the patient should undergo a careful preoperative evaluation. This includes a work-up of the primary pain etiology and a stabilization of concomitant diseases. Issues to consider are infection risks, blood sugar control, clotting function, and nutrition status. Once the patient is considered stable for surgery, intravenous antibiotics are administered, the hair is removed from the surgical site, and the patient is draped and positioned (**Figs. 21-3 to 21-8**). A small craniotomy is performed to

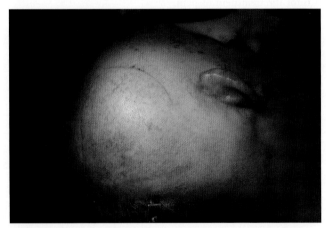

Fig. 21-3 Before the procedure patient's hair is removed from the surgical site.

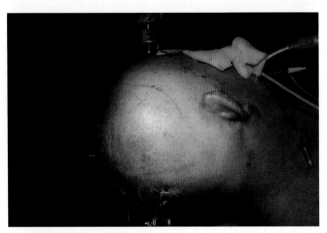

Fig. 21-4 Ensure that patient is positioned correctly.

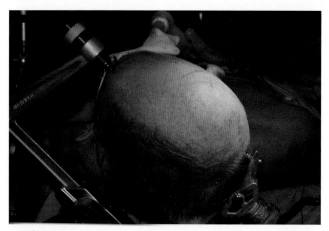

Fig. 21-5 Patient's head must be supported correctly before beginning the procedure.

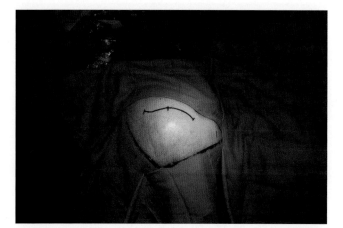

Fig. 21-6 Mark the incision site clearly and apply sterile drapes.

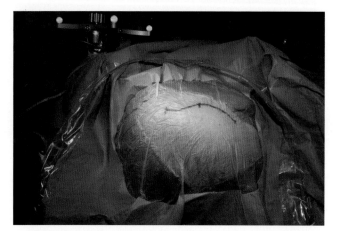

Fig. 21-7 Place a protective film over the incision site.

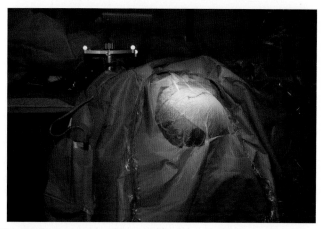

Fig. 21-8 Ensure that blue cord is secure and will not interfere with incision site.

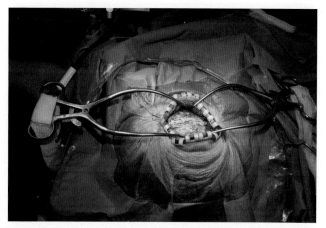

Fig. 21-9 Perform incision and secure layers of skin with surgical tools.

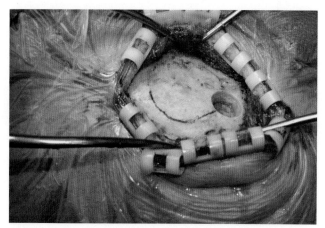

Fig. 21-10 Remove circular section of tissue where lead will be placed.

gain access to the target area of the motor cortex (**Figs. 21-9** to **21-16**). Although operative technique varies somewhat in this procedure, the essential common ground is insertion of a plate electrode over the motor cortex in the area that is somatotopically relevant to the patient's pain (**Figs. 21-17** to **21-27**). This most often involves preoperative imaging with magnetic resonance imaging and intraoperative physiological corroboration using somatosensory data to confirm lead placement over the motor cortex. Leads are most commonly placed epidurally; however, some have used subdural placements for leads, as would be expected in attempts to treat patients with leg pain.

Patient Management/Evaluation

Unlike stimulation at other targets, immediate, direct feedback from patients is not available. The patient does not experience any

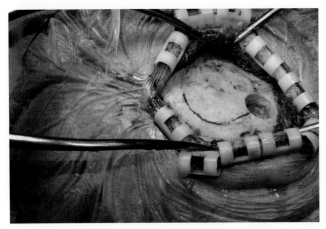

Fig. 21-11 Close-up view of tissue removal.

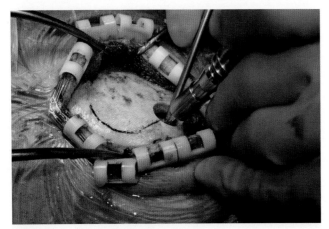

Fig. 21-12 Use surgical tool to remove additional layers of tissue and expose a larger surface area.

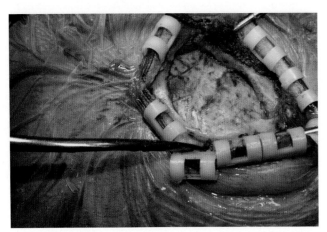

Fig. 21-13 A larger surface area is now exposed.

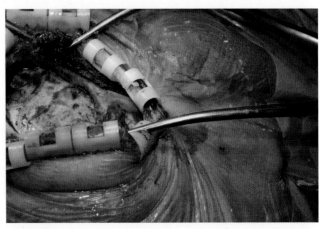

Fig. 21-14 Insert small catheter at one side of the incision site.

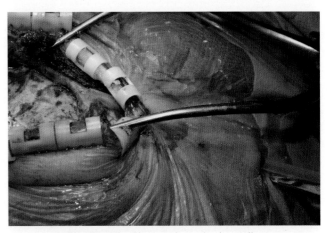

Fig. 21-15 Place catheter horizontally.

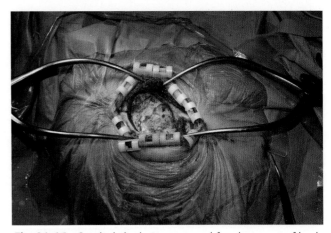

Fig. 21-16 Surgical site is now prepped for placement of lead.

stimulation-induced phenomenon with this method of treatment. The use of specific parameters of stimulation and the frequency of device adjustment/reprogramming are not agreed upon at this time. A protocol for reassessing patients with some reasonable frequency must be agreed on by both the implanter and patient. Assessment of outcome may be based on improvement of VAS and functional measures.

Outcomes Evidence

As noted previously, Nguyen and associates[6] and Fontaine and associates[7] have reviewed the literature and found a variance of positive outcomes from this procedure in the treatment of neuropathic disorders. Notably published reports on this therapy are typically small, poorly controlled, usually retrospective, and have short follow-up. Nonetheless benefit is noted on average in over 50% of patients. These patients report greater than 40% or 50% pain relief, depending on the study measurement. Taking into

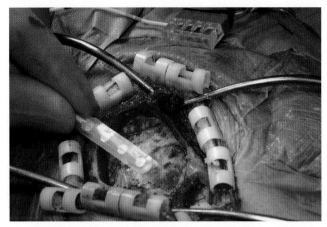

Fig. 21-17 Place lead horizontally in incision site.

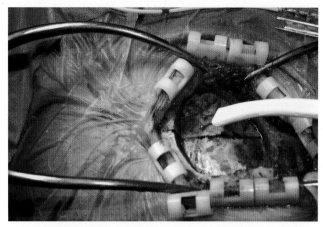

Fig. 21-20 Place probe directly onto tissue.

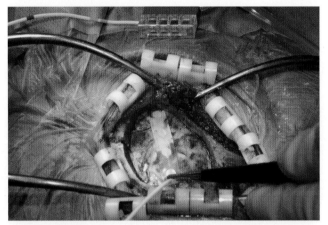

Fig. 21-18 Use surgical tool to apply lead onto tissue.

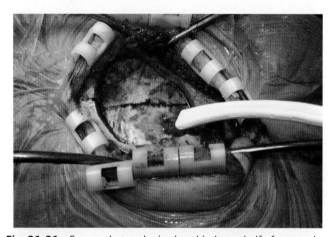

Fig. 21-21 Ensure that probe is placed in lower half of exposed tissue.

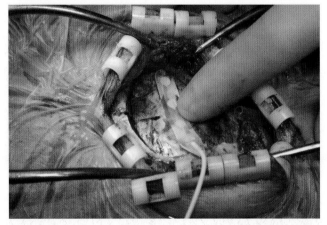

Fig. 21-19 Use index finger to ensure proper placement of lead.

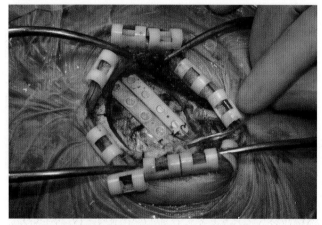

Fig. 21-22 Placement of two leads.

consideration that these patients have no other reasonable available therapy, this is remarkable.[7]

Risk and Complication Avoidance

Common complications of this procedure are infection, which represents ≈5% to 6% incidence; seizures, ≈12%; and hardware dysfunction, ≈5%. Additional, less common complications of extraaxial hemorrhages, motor deficit, and death have been reported. Immediate postoperative deaths from pulmonary embolism and extraaxial hemorrhage have been reported. From the

perspective of hardware malfunction and infections, these rates are average to low.[7] Hardware malfunction/breakage is the most common complication in SCS, expected to occur between 25% and 30% of the time in contemporary practice. The infection rate is similar to that expected with SCS. The mortalities noted occurred from reasons consistent with other intracranial procedures.[7,9]

Conclusions

MCS is a very interesting therapy that has drawn increasing interest for treating severe and intractable pain conditions from pain

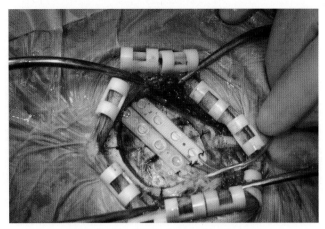

Fig. 21-23 Secure leads with stitches.

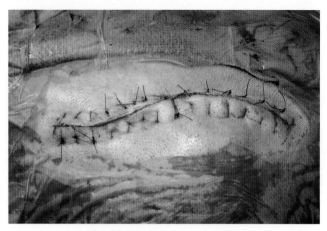

Fig. 21-26 Stitch incision site.

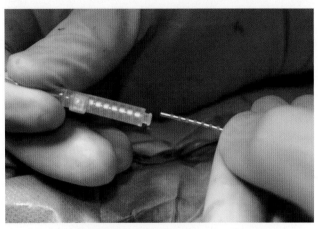

Fig. 21-24 Connect power supply.

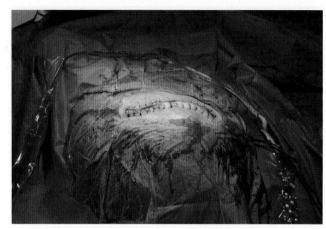

Fig. 21-27 Postprocedure.

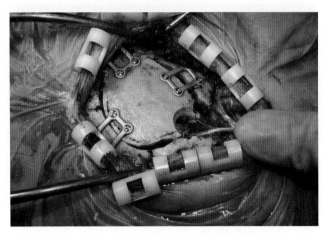

Fig. 21-25 Place screws over removed skin and incision site.

physicians throughout the world. More research and development will be essential in determining the place this procedure plays in the care of the pain patient in future years.

References

1. Krames E et al: rethinking algorithms of pain care: the use of the SAFE principles. *Pain Med* 10(Issue 1):1-5, 2009.

2. Taylor RS et al: The cost effectiveness of spinal cord stimulation in the treatment of pain: a systematic review of the literature. *J Pain Symptom Manage* 27(Issue 4):370-378, 2004.

3. Levy R Deer TR, Henderson J: Intracranial neurostimulation for pain control: a review. *Pain Physician* 13(2):157-165, 2010.

4. Tsubokawa T et al: Treatment of thalamic pain by chronic motor cortex stimulation. *Pacing Clinical Electrophysiol* 14(Issue 1):131-134, 1991.

5. Nguyen JP et al: Motor cortex stimulation in the treatment of central and neuropathic pain. *Arch Med Res* 31(Issue 3):263-265, 2000.

6. Nguyen JP et al: Chronic motor cortex stimulation in the treatment of central and neuropathic pain: correlations between clinical, electrophysiological and anatomical data. *Pain* 82(Issue 3):245-251, 1999.

7. Fontaine D, Hamani C, Lozano A: Efficacy and safety of motor cortex stimulation for chronic neuropathic pain: critical review of the literature. *J Neurosurg* 110(2):251-256, 2009 Feb.

8. Tsubokawa T Katayama Y, Yamamoto T, et al: Chronic motor cortex stimulation in patients with thalamic pain. *J Neurosurg* 78(3):393-401, 1993 Mar.

9. Turner J et al: Spinal cord stimulation for patients with failed back surgery syndrome or complex regional pain syndrome: a systematic review of effectiveness and complications. *Pain* 108(Issue 1):137-147, 2004.

22 Deep Brain Stimulation

Erlick A.C. Pereira and Tipu Z. Aziz

CHAPTER OVERVIEW

Chapter Synopsis: Most applications of electrical stimulation for the treatment of intractable pain are delivered at the spinal cord or in the periphery, but deep brain stimulation (DBS) at central brain structures can also be effective. DBS is indicated for several types of neuropathic pain, including pain after amputation or stroke; plexopathies; and head and face pain, including anesthesia dolorosa. DBS for pain should be undertaken only when all other therapies have failed. The technique is performed at a limited number of centers and would benefit from multicenter studies. Although the spinal cord first- and second-order neuronal hierarchy is well understood, the more central structures involved in pain processing are not, including the targets of DBS for pain, the sensory thalamus and periaqueductal gray. Still-unanswered questions include whether pain processing through these and other brain structures is "top-down" or "bottom-up" and whether endogenous opiates play a role in DBS-induced analgesia. Perhaps it is these unanswered questions that make DBS one of the most fascinating uses of electrical stimulation for intractable pain. Also intriguing is the retention of a somatotopic homunculus in both these centers. This map can provide guidance for electrode implantation; but final placement is determined by an awake, sensing patient who confirms sensations of paresthesias and analgesia with stimulation. These sensations can lend clues as to the complex processing interplay between multiple brain centers that contributes to the overall experience of pain.

Important Points:
- Deep brain stimulation (DBS) is a neurosurgical intervention the efficacy, safety, and utility of which have been robustly demonstrated in the treatment of movement disorders.
- For the treatment of chronic pain refractory to medical therapies, many prospective case series have been reported, but few centers worldwide have published findings from patients treated during the last decade using current standards of neuroimaging and stimulator technology.
- With a clinical experience of DBS of the sensory thalamus and periventricular/periaqueductal gray matter now in over 70 patients treated throughout the last decade, we summarize the historical background, our scientific rationale, patient selection and assessment methods, surgical techniques, and clinical results.
- Several experienced centers continue DBS for chronic pain with considerable success in selected patients, in particular those with pain after amputation; plexopathies; stroke; and head and face pain, including anesthesia dolorosa.
- Other carefully selected patient groups with visceral or genital pain or pain caused by multiple sclerosis, malignancy, and trauma may benefit from DBS; but efficacy in pain after spinal injury might be limited.
- Complications are similar to those of other DBS indications, including small risks of stroke, seizures, hemorrhage, the need for implantable pulse generator revision surgery every 3 to 5 years for nonrechargeable devices, and treatment failure.
- Findings from studies using static and functional neuroimaging modalities and invasive neurophysiological insights from local field potential recording are discussed. Intensive and detailed prospective cohort studies translate into improved patient selection and consistent efficacy, encouraging larger clinical trials.

Clinical Pearls: Although not a new therapy, DBS has metamorphosed considerably over the last decade, concomitant with advances in both stimulator technology and neuroimaging techniques and by corollary improvements in efficacy and reductions in complications. Few centers have published detailed studies of patients treated during the last decade. Our results suggest that DBS gives analgesia most consistently to patients with pain after amputation, either phantom or stump; and cranial and facial pain, including anesthesia dolorosa and plexopathies. Our greater experience of pain after stroke reveals greatest efficacy for stroke patients complaining of burning hyperesthesia.[1,2] Therefore our stroke case series illustrates how important patient selection is to outcome. To improve selection and thus efficacy, objective adjuncts to current pain assessments are desirable. Subjective patient preference for PVG/PAG stimulation over VPL/VPM in stroke together with correlations revealed between cardiovascular effects, analgesic efficacy of DBS and burning hyperesthesia point toward autonomical measures as potential objective markers.[3]

Sustained analgesia by DBS has been shown for myriad indications; our own experience includes multiple sclerosis and genital pain. Each case must be considered individually rather than relying on dogmatic distinctions between neuropathic and nociceptive pain. Consistent with the notion that chronic pain states confer specific central neuropathic changes are results showing poor DBS efficacy for spinal cord–related pain (e.g., from failed back surgery). Predominantly spinal injuries and hence spinal neuropathic changes are unlikely to respond favorably to central brain stimulation. Conversely, causes of chronic pain not traditionally treated by DBS (e.g., visceral pain in which PVG/PAG changes are described using functional neuroimaging)[4,5] have potential for amelioration by DBS worthy of further study.

Investigations both into the mechanisms of DBS and using deep brain recording to elucidate pain processing mechanisms have yielded considerable advances. Future insights will arise from complementary information gathered using new technologies. Diffusion tensor imaging (DTI) using MRI to trace neuronal connections has shown connectivity between PVG/PAG and thalamic structures and may elucidate differential somatotopic connections[6,7]; it also has clinical use to aid targeting in functional neurosurgery.[8] MEG enables whole brain changes to be mapped, with spatial resolution comparable to functional MRI yet temporal resolution of the order of milliseconds, in contrast to functional neuroimaging technique.[9] Our initial investigations have revealed activation of pain-processing neocortical areas during analgesic DBS after filtering out artifactual interference from stimulation.[10,11] Therefore global MEG measurements combined with local deep brain recording holds promise for revealing much about pain processing and DBS-related mechanisms beyond wider neurosurgical applications,[12] toward identifying predictors of efficacy and

Introduction

The pioneer neurosurgeon Lauri Laitinen once commented that "when one sets out to make a historical survey of surgical attempts to relieve the tremor and rigor in Parkinson disease, one cannot help feeling that it would have been a far easier task to list those nervous structures which have not been attacked."[18,19] Neurosurgical attempts to relieve intractable pain mirror his wry observation; all structures from peripheral nerve through dorsal root, spinal cord, midbrain, and thalamus to cingulate cortex have been first lesioned and later electrically stimulated or perfused with analgesics or anesthetics (**Fig. 22-1**). Yet chronic pain continues to present a considerable burden to society, transcending many debilitating medical diseases, including cancer, stroke, trauma, and failed surgery.[20] Its prevalence may be over 20%.[21]

The concept of ameliorating persistent pain by deep brain stimulation (DBS) originates from clinical studies over half a century ago. On the basis of septal self-stimulation experiments in rodents[22] and reports of analgesia in patients receiving septal DBS for psychiatric disorders,[23,24] Heath and Mickle[25] postulated that stimulating the same area that produced pleasure might relieve pain. They successfully reduced a patient's cancer pain over several weeks with intermittent stimulation. The findings were replicated by a case series using improved equipment a decade later.[26]

Further impetus for DBS was provided in the mid-1960s by the theoretical paradigm shift initiated by Melzack and Wall's gate control theory[27] and advances in stimulator technology. The gate control theory was translated first into implantable peripheral nerve stimulators[28] and then into spinal cord stimulation (SCS),[29] developed by Medtronic (Minneapolis, Minn) into a commercially available permanently implantable device.[30,31]

Identification of the periventricular and periaqueductal gray (PVG/PAG) regions as a target for DBS has its origins in animal research. Mayer and associates[32] and Reynolds and others[33] were able to perform major surgery in awake rodents using analgesia induced by PAG stimulation alone. Pain relief by PVG/PAG DBS was first reported in patients by Richardson and Akil[34-36] and then Hosobuchi, Adams, and Linchitz.[37] Evidence supporting ventro-posterolateral and ventroposteromedial (VPL/VPM) thalamic nuclei and adjacent structures as putative targets for DBS came from ablative surgery,[38-41] leading Hosobuchi, Adams, and Rutkin[42] to treat anesthesia dolorosa with VPM thalamic DBS. Several others pioneered thalamic DBS, including Mazars, Merienne, and Cioloca,[43,44] Mazars,[45] Mazars, Roge, and Mazars[46] and Adams and Fields who, along with Hosobuchi,[47-49] also targeted the internal capsule. Observations from inadvertent localization errors and investigations into current spread from the PVG/PAG led others to target more medial thalamic nuclei, including the centromedian-parafascicular complex (Cm-Pf).[50-53]

The rapid diffusion of electrical stimulation treatments for multifarious clinical indications by the mid-1970s led the U.S. Food and Drug Administration (FDA) to sponsor a symposium to evaluate their merits.[54] Only pain treatments were documented to be both safe and effective,[55,56] albeit in an era when the long-term complications of the then recently discovered levodopa on Parkinson disease were yet to be revealed. Crucial primate investigations elucidating basal ganglia functions and presaging a renaissance in DBS for movement disorders had also not yet been undertaken.[19,57]

Despite the consensus, the U.S. Medical Device Amendments of 1976 compelled the FDA to request DBS manufacturers to conduct further studies to show the benefits of DBS for pain, and an additional ruling in 1989 required clinical trials to demonstrate safety and efficacy. Two multicenter trials were conducted, first in 1976 using the Medtronic Model 3380 electrode (196 patients) and then in 1990 with the Model 3387 (50 patients) that superseded it.[58] The two studies were an amalgam of prospective case series from participating neurosurgical centers, neither randomized nor case

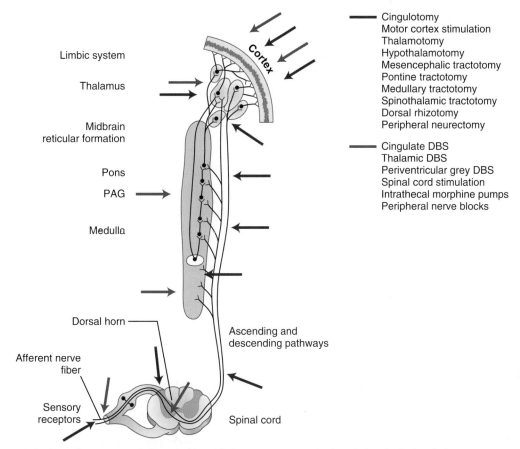

Cingulotomy
Motor cortex stimulation
Thalamotomy
Hypothalamotomy
Mesencephalic tractotomy
Pontine tractotomy
Medullary tractotomy
Spinothalamic tractotomy
Dorsal rhizotomy
Peripheral neurectomy

Cingulate DBS
Thalamic DBS
Periventricular grey DBS
Spinal cord stimulation
Intrathecal morphine pumps
Peripheral nerve blocks

Limbic system

Thalamus

Midbrain
reticular formation

Pons

PAG

Medulla

Dorsal horn

Afferent nerve
fiber

Sensory
receptors

Cortex

Ascending and
descending pathways

Spinal cord

Fig. 22-1   Structures in the pain neuromatrix targeted by ablative neurosurgery *(red)* and electrical stimulation or neuromodulation *(blue)*. *DBS*, Deep brain stimulation; *PAG*, periaqueductal gray.

controlled, and both suffered from poor enrollment and high attrition. Other shortcomings included heterogeneous case mixes with underspecified patient selection criteria and subjective and unblinded assessment of patient outcomes. Confounds arose from inconsistencies in deep brain sites stimulated, numbers of electrodes used per patient, and stimulation parameters chosen. Improvements made to the later Model 3387 trial included limiting deep brain sites stimulated to two per patient and using visual analog scores (VASs) to rate pain intensity for outcome assessment; but its included cases per center were tiny, with a mean of five and median of three patients treated.

Neither trial satisfied study criteria for efficacy of at least half of patients reporting at least 50% pain relief 1 year after surgery. Therefore U.S. FDA approval for analgesic DBS was not sought by the device manufacturer. However, intriguingly, the large numbers of patients lost to follow-up resulted in a steady increase with time in the proportion of patients with at least 50% pain relief; 2 years after implantation they comprised 18 out of the 30 remaining patients (60%) followed up in the Model 3380 trial and 5 out of the 10 in the Model 3387 trial (50%). Nonetheless, the trials resulted in the U.S. FDA giving DBS for pain "off-label" status, thus precluding its approval by medical insurers.[58-60] As a consequence, few clinical investigations into DBS for pain using current technology and techniques have been reported.

In the last decade to our knowledge only five centers, three European and two Canadian, have published case series of more than six patients.[1,61-69] In contrast, both other centrally implantable neurostimulation treatments for pain, SCS and motor cortex stimulation (MCS), have continued to yield research publications,

albeit mostly of uncontrolled case series,[70-75] with small randomized controlled, clinical trials in SCS emerging.[76-78] Over 1300 recipients of DBS for pain have been reported[63,64,68,69,79,80] compared to nearly 400 patients with MCS[73,81] and nearly 4000 with SCS.[74,75]

Our experience is that DBS is superior to MCS for selected refractory pain syndromes.[82] Similarly we find DBS more appropriate than SCS for certain pain etiologies, although little published data exists comparing treatments by the same surgeon in the same group of patients. Two retrospective studies from the same group have compared all three modalities of central neurostimulation, but the results are obfuscated first by different treatments trialed both between and sequentially within patients and second by limited outcome information.[83,84] A recent review has compared the three neurostimulatory therapies but did not include all contemporary DBS case series in its analysis.[85] Over the last decade we have treated over 70 patients with analgesic DBS, regularly publishing results for many implanted and amenable to follow-up.[1,62,65,67,68] Our experience is described, and results reviewed alongside other current studies to clarify the current status of DBS for pain.

Establishing Diagnosis and Indications/Contraindications

Historically, clinical approaches to DBS have sought to categorize patients first by cause of pain and second by dichotomizing the pain into such categories as nociceptive or deafferentation, epicritic or protopathic, peripheral or central. Such distinctions are largely unhelpful to patient selection since a gathering body of human functional neuroimaging and electrophysiological evidence confirms that chronic pain arises concomitant with centrally mediated changes related to neuronal plasticity, regardless of etiology.[86-91] Thus it can be assumed that chronic pain refractory to medical treatment is largely central pain and thus neuropathic. The challenges to patient selection for DBS then become twofold: (1) the confirmation that the patient's pain is neuropathic and neither factitious nor psychogenic, and (2) the selection of those with neuropathic pain who are likely to derive benefit from DBS.

Essential to the patient selection process is assessment by a multidisciplinary team consisting at a minimum of a pain specialist, neuropsychologist, and neurosurgeon. Comprehensive neuropsychological evaluation provides best practice in patient selection for DBS to exclude psychoses, addiction, and medically refractory psychiatric disorders and ensure minimal cognitive impairment.[92-95] Quantitative assessment of the pain and health-related quality of life should be a requirement of the preoperative patient selection process. Our preference is to use both VAS (scale of 0 to 10) to rate pain intensity and the McGill Pain Questionnaire (MPQ) for pain evaluation,[96,97] the latter giving additional qualitative information and including a quality of life assessment. We also assess quality of life using the Short Form 36 (SF-36) and VAS part of the Euroqol five-dimensional assessment tool (EQ-5D).[98-100] The patient records his or her VAS twice daily in a pain diary over a period of 12 days. The 24 VAS scores are reviewed to ensure consistency and clarified with the patient if inconsistent. The EQ-5D, SF-36, and MPQ are administered by the pain specialist before surgery. The MPQ is repeated on a separate occasion independently by the neuropsychologist and scored using the ranked pain rating index. Our experience is that certain items of the MPQ can predict a positive response to DBS. In particular, over 80% of our patients who describe burning pain have found benefit from DBS, regardless of whether VPL/VPM, PVG/PAG or both are stimulated. We have published patient data linking resolution of burning pain with blood pressure reduction and long-term PVG/PAG DBS analgesia implicating cardiovascular changes in this type of pain[3] and found heart rate variability changes consistent with sympathetic suppression and/or parasympathetic augmentation by PVG/PAG DBS[101]; but further multivariate analysis of other MPQ items, other brain targets, and other measurable cardiovascular parameters are required to elucidate further the phenomenon.

The specific etiology of the chronic pain appears less important to efficacy than its symptom history, which may involve hyperalgesia, allodynia, and hyperpathia. The pain must have a definable organic origin with the patient refractory to or poorly tolerant of pharmacological treatments. Surgical treatments may have been attempted (e.g., peripheral neuroablative or decompressive procedures for trigeminal neuralgia); however, we do not consider failure of other neurostimulatory therapies a prerequisite for DBS. Our preference is to trial DBS rather than SCS or MCS in carefully selected patients wherever the etiologies of chronic pain are consistent with neuronal reorganization at multiple levels of the central neuromatrix.

The greater body of clinical studies of SCS,[71,72] coupled with ours and others' lack of success with DBS for spinal injuries,[63,65] favors SCS over DBS as a more appropriate first-line neurostimulatory intervention for spinal cord injury when central reorganization is likely to be mostly at a spinal level. However, our experience of DBS for pain after limb or plexor injury[65,67] encourages us to consider DBS rather than SCS as first-line treatment for complex regional pain syndromes (CRPS). A 100% success rate in 13 implanted patients to date, together with a recent paradigm shift toward central brain reorganization with autonomic dysfunction as the mechanism underlying CRPS,[102-106] supports the treatment

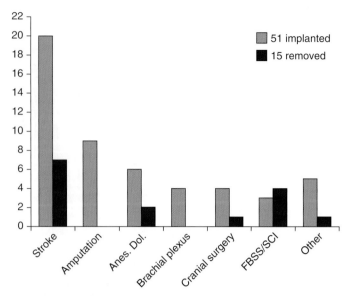

Fig. 22-2 Number of patients proceeding to full implantation by etiology at Oxford 1999 to 2008. *Anes. Dol.*, Anesthesia dolorosa; *FBSS/SCI*, failed back surgery syndrome/spinal cord injury; *Other*, other trauma, malignancy, genital pain, multiple sclerosis.

both for brachial and lumbar plexus injuries and stump pain after amputation and for phantom limb pain.

Other pain etiologies for which we and others have obtained positive outcomes using DBS are stroke[1,2]; facial and head pain, including postherpetic trigeminal neuralgia and anesthesia dolorosa[62,107]; multiple sclerosis[63]; genital pain; and malignancy.[65,68] These are listed for reference by etiology with implantation success rates shown in **Fig. 22-2**; however, we reiterate our position that to select patients for DBS primarily by etiology rather than by findings on history and examination and use of assessment tools is to oversimplify their chronic pain and risk poor outcomes. Rather than using inflexible selection criteria, our preference in patient selection is expert opinion after multidisciplinary assessment demonstrating quantitatively severe pain refractory to medication for at least 1 year, with significantly impaired quality of life and qualitative pain suggestive of neuropathic changes without predominantly spinal involvement. We find little merit in opiate or naloxone administration to determine suitability for DBS, although an historical literature exists.[80] Medical contraindications to DBS include uncorrectable coagulopathy obviating neurosurgery and ventriculomegaly sufficient to preclude direct electrode passage to the surgical target.

Considering cephalalgias, we have also successfully treated cluster headache with DBS of the posterior hypothalamic nuclei and investigated it using multiple translational methods as for chronic pain.[108-110] As we review comprehensively elsewhere,[111] this debilitating condition has responded impressively to DBS in our initial experience and others' and is worthy of multicenter, randomized controlled clinical trials. Further consideration of cluster headache is beyond the scope of this review.

Anatomy

DBS targets are contralateral to the painful side of the body. Currently used sites for DBS can be divided anatomically first into somesthetic regions of the ventrobasal thalamus (VPL/VPM) and second into more medial regions surrounding the third ventricle and aqueduct of Sylvius, including the gray matter (PVG/PAG) and medial thalamic Cm-Pf nuclei. Further anatomical distinction is redundant since accuracy of DBS placement for most practitioners is limited to ±2 mm at best by magnetic resonance imaging (MRI) and computerized tomography (CT) slice thickness.

Moreover, our ultimate adjustment of intracerebral electrode position is directed by awake patient reports of somesthetic localization during intraoperative stimulation. Such subjective information may alter the final electrode site by up to several millimeters from preoperative target coordinates. A guiding principle is the established somatotopic organization of the somesthetic thalamic and PVG/PAG regions. Human microelectrode studies reveal a mediolateral somatotopy in the contralateral ventroposterior thalamus, the head of the homunculus being medial and the feet lateral.[112] Subjective observation of a rostrocaudally inverted sensory homunculus in contralateral PVG/PAG[113] has been confirmed objectively by our human macroelectrode recordings of somatosensory evoked potentials.[114] The PVG/PAG target is found at a point 2 to 3 mm lateral to the third ventricle at the level of the posterior commissure, 10 mm posterior to the midcommissural point. Its pertinent anatomical boundaries in the midbrain include the medial lemniscus laterally, the superior colliculus inferoposteriorly, and the red nucleus inferoanteriorly. Sensory thalamic targets are found 10 to 13 mm posterior to the midcommissural point and from 5 mm below to 2 mm above it. The VPM is targeted for facial pain only and found midway between the lateral wall of the third ventricle and the internal capsule; the arm area of VPL is 2 to 3 mm medial to the internal capsule and the leg area of VPL 1 to 2 mm medial to the internal capsule. The sensory thalamus is bordered by Cm-Pf nuclei medially; the internal capsule laterally; the thalamic fasciculus, zona incerta, and subthalamic nucleus inferiorly; the thalamic nucleus ventralis intermedius anteriorly; and the pulvinar thalamic nucleus posteriorly.

Basic Science

A wealth of electrophysiological, anatomical, and radiological evidence in humans and animals, reviewed elsewhere, establishes both PVG/PAG and ventrobasal thalamus as structures important to pain perception and the pathophysiology of chronic pain syndromes.[9,115-122] The subtleties of hierarchical position and behavioral function of individual brain structures, whether sensory-discriminative, attentional, motivational-affective, or hedonic, are much debated. However, the consensus is toward a pain neuromatrix also involving spinal cord; posterior hypothalamus; amygdala; and neocortical structure, including somatosensory, insular, anterior cingulate, and prefrontal cortex. Whether pain control is top-down or bottom-up in its hierarchy is unresolved and often depends on the experimental paradigm used. Our human electrophysiological studies of neuronal coherence have used somatosensory-evoked potentials and Granger causality predictive modeling to suggest that PVG/PAG exerts ascending modulation on VPM/VPL in a bottom-up model of pain processing,[114] a finding that functional MRI would be unable to confirm because of insufficient temporal resolution.[9,123-125]

Central to the rationale for DBS is the concept of aberrant neuronal firing at the target sites concomitant with the chronic pain. Human and animal electrophysiological experiments show increased thalamic neuronal firing in pain.[126] Comprehensive reviews of electrophysiological studies conclude that the mechanisms of analgesic stimulation are not clearly delineated.[80,127-131] From insights revealed by basal ganglia microelectrode recordings and DBS for movement disorders reviewed elsewhere,[132-134] we postulate that altered rhythmic activity in VPL/VPM and PVG/PAG

neurons is likely to play an important role in the pathophysiology of central pain. At either target our clinical experience is that in general DBS at lower frequencies (≤50 Hz) is analgesic and at higher frequencies (>70 Hz) hyperalgesic,[2,135,136] supporting a dynamic model whereby synchronous oscillations in discrete neuronal populations centrally modulate chronic pain perception. Therefore analgesic DBS may either disrupt pathological high-frequency synchronous oscillations or, more likely, augment pathologically diminished low-frequency synchronous oscillations in the thalamic and reticular components of a reticulothalamocortico-fugal pain neuromatrix. We have shown a positive correlation between analgesic efficacy at either DBS site and the amplitude of slow frequency (<1 Hz) VPL/VPM local field potentials (LFPs),[61,137] allowing for physiologically modulated artifact.[138] We now also have early evidence that patients off DBS have characteristically enhanced low frequency (8 to14 Hz) power spectra of both PVG/PAG and VPL/VPM LFPs when in pain.[139] Further research is required to elucidate if such neuronal signatures could aid patient selection, in particular if combined with technical advances in noninvasive functional neuroimaging and electrophysiological techniques such as single photon emission computed tomography (SPECT) and magnetoencephalography (MEG) to characterize functional neuronal connectivity.[10,11,13]

The PVG/PAG is a structure optimally sited anatomically to integrate interoceptive function, both from adjacent mesencephalic cardiovascular centers and more distal pain processing areas. Its autonomic effects have been well studied in animals,[121,140-143] and changes noted with DBS.[131] We have demonstrated a positive correlation between degree of analgesia in patients receiving PVG/PAG DBS and magnitude of blood pressure reduction[3] and shown that, whereas dorsal PAG stimulation can acutely elevate blood pressure, ventral stimulation reduces it.[144,145] Such findings advance investigations for objective markers of chronic pain and also potential selection of patients who may respond best to PVG/PAG DBS. Indeed our investigations into heart rate variability changes and preliminary findings from ambulatory blood pressure monitoring that such blood pressure changes are sustained may provide objective somatic measures of efficacy that correlate to subjective rating scales.[146,147] Detailed autonomic testing using such equipment as tilt-tables, Portapres, and real-time VAS recording is underway to elucidate such possibilities.

Current thinking is that ventral PVG/PAG DBS engages analgesia commensurate with passive coping behavior, whereas dorsal PVG/PAG DBS may involve "fight or flight" analgesia with associated sympathomimetic effect.[3] However, evidence to substantiate the conjecture that PVG/PAG DBS acts via augmenting endogenous opioid release is contentious. The hypothesis arose from animal experiments revealing stimulation-produced analgesia reversed by naloxone[148,149] and human studies that also showed elevated levels of cerebrospinal fluid enkephalins and endorphins with DBS.[37,150,151] However, the cerebrospinal fluid measures were artifactual,[152,153] and double-blinded investigation in humans has revealed no cross-tolerance between DBS and morphine and similar reversibility between naloxone and saline placebo,[154] confirming others' findings.[52,155] Our preliminary human studies agree that naloxone and placebo effects on DBS are similar, questioning an opioid-dependent mechanism. Furthermore, naloxone and saline seem to have distinct and different effects on the low-frequency power spectra of PVG/PAG and VPL/VPM LFPs, suggesting that both opioids and contextual influences can modulate neuronal responses in the pain neuromatrix independent of DBS, in agreement with the dynamic rate model proposed previously. However, naloxone can potentiate acute withdrawal and psychosis

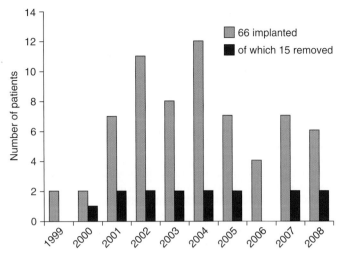

Fig. 22-3 Deep brain stimulation for pain caseload at Oxford during the last decade showing explantation rates. These have remained constant at 23% during the last decade.

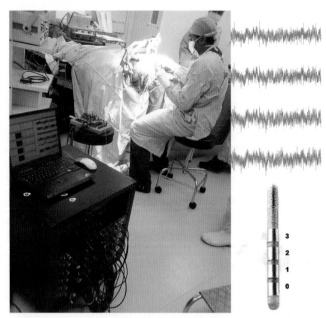

Fig. 22-4 Theater setup. During awake stereotactic surgery a portable recording rig is used for macroelectrode local field potential (LFP) recording if required. LFPs can be recorded from each of the four contacts (*0 to 3*) of the deep brain electrode (*inset right*).

in long-term users of opiate analgesia. Thus we advise against its administration during stereotactic neurosurgical procedures in awake patients.

An obstacle yet to be surmounted in the quest to understand the mechanisms of analgesic stimulation is the lack of adequate animal models of chronic pain.[156,157] In addition to their limited homology in chronic pain paradigms, the smaller brains of rodent and murine models increase targeting inaccuracies, in particular for small brainstem structures such as PVG/PAG. Such experience emphasizes the important opportunities presented by patient-based translational research into DBS to study the mechanisms underlying its efficacious analgesia.

Guidelines

There are no recent North American guidelines for DBS for pain because of its off-label indication in the United States. We have contributed to the European Federation of Neurological Societies' guidelines on neurostimulation therapy for neuropathic pain, which concludes that, because of the few recent case series published, DBS should be limited to specialist centers willing to study and report their outcomes.[158]

Imaging, Equipment, and Technique

Informed written patient consent is obtained after detailed explanations of the risks and potential benefits of the procedure and counseling for its duration of approximately 2 hours under moderate sedation and local anesthesia with the head fixed and cranial stereotaxis applied (**Fig. 22-3**). Our operating theatre setup is shown in **Fig. 22-4**. A week or more before surgery, patients have a T1 weighted MRI scan. For surgery a Cosman-Roberts-Wells (CRW) base ring is applied to the patient's head under local anesthesia. A stereotactic CT scan is then performed, and the MRI scan is volumetrically fused to it using computerized image fusion and stereotactic planning programs to eliminate spatial distortions that arise from magnetic field effects.[159,160] The coordinates for the PVG/PAG and VPL or VPM and entry trajectory are then calculated (**Fig. 22-5**). A frontal trajectory avoiding the lateral ventricles is preferred. DBS targets are described in the previous anatomy section.

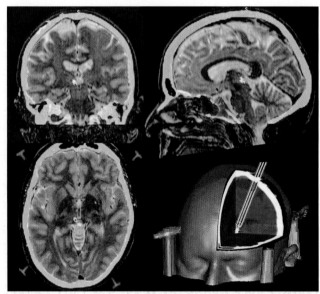

Fig. 22-5 Fused T2 weighted preoperative MRI and postoperative CT images highlighted using heat mapping (axial, coronal, and sagittal clockwise from bottom left) showing left PVG/PAG electrode placement. Three-dimensional reconstruction of electrode trajectory is shown bottom right. *PVG/PAG*, Periventricular and periaqueductal gray.

After a 3-cm parasagittal scalp incision and separate 2.7-mm twist drill craniotomy per electrode, both VPL/VPM and PVG/PAG have been implanted to date with Medtronic Model 3387 quadripolar electrodes. PVG/PAG is implanted first; excellent intraoperative analgesia obviates implantation of a second electrode in VPL/VPM in up to half of patients, in particular those with marked thalamic damage (e.g., following stroke). Thus most of our cohorts have received PVG/PAG or dual-target DBS (**Fig. 22-6**). The minority who have received VPL/VPM DBS alone have either not

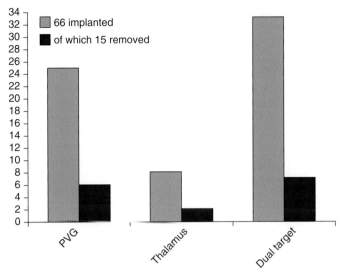

Fig. 22-6 Number of patients proceeding to full implantation by etiology. *PVG/PAG,* Periventricular and periaqueductal gray matter.

experienced efficacy or had side effects with a trial of PVG/PAG DBS. Final electrode position is determined by intraoperative clinical assessment reliant on subjective reporting by the awake patient; microelectrode recording is not routinely used. Bipolar 5- to 30-Hz stimulation is performed initially, pulse width 100 to 450 µs, amplitude 0.1 to 3 V. VPL/VPM stimulation aims to supplant painful sensation by pleasant paresthesia, and PVG/PAG stimulation seeks to induce a sensation of warmth or analgesia in the painful area. Adjustment is primarily somatotopic so as to evoke appropriate topographic responses, but the assessor should be alert to pyramidal signs suggesting capsular involvement with VPL/VPM DBS and with PVG/PAG DBS for oscilliopsia and reports of visual disturbances caused by superior collicular involvement or facial paresthesia arising from medial lemniscus stimulation. Each electrode is fixed to the skull by a miniplate, and its leads externalized parietally via temporary extensions. Immediately after surgery a further stereotactic CT is performed and co-registered as before to confirm electrode position. MRI may be performed after surgery during the week before implantable pulse generator (IPG) insertion for further anatomical target corroboration.

After a week of postoperative clinical assessment, a decision is made whether to permanently implant the electrodes in a second operation under general anesthesia. They are connected to an IPG implanted subcutaneously, usually infraclavicularly or alternatively intraabdominally in subcutaneous fascia. Medtronic Synergy or Kinetra has been used to date. Our surgical technique is detailed further elsewhere.[136,161,162]

Patient Management/Evaluation

All electrodes are externalized for a week of trial stimulation. During this period the patient records VAS scores at least twice daily and is kept blinded to DBS settings. Targets are trialed individually for 1 to 2 days using the stimulator parameters described to determine which settings of quadripolar electrode contact polarities confer maximum analgesia to the optimal somatic region. Monopolar stimulation is also trialed if bipolar settings fail to give pain relief. After this period both electrodes are trialed together for 1 to 2 days. If the patient is satisfied with the degree of pain relief obtained, full implantation of the efficacious electrode(s) is performed, and DBS commenced at the optimized stimulation parameters. In general, we

do not decide between permanent implantation of PVG/PAG, VPL/VPM, or dual-site stimulation on any criteria other than demonstrable efficacy in each individual patient.

Another method favored for evaluating analgesia in single cases and small groups of patients is the N-of-1 trial.[162-164] A randomized, placebo-controlled intrapatient trial is conducted whereby the patient receives pairs of treatment periods during which each intervention, be it DBS on or off or different stimulation targets or parameters, occurs once. The order of treatments is randomized, and the effects of treatment or placebo can be compared between treatment periods. We have demonstrated the validity of N-of-1 trials using the VAS, and their concordance with overall MPQ has been demonstrated for VPL/VPM, PVG/PAG, and dual-target DBS.[165] Blinding and randomization methodologies have also been adopted by others to investigate the efficacy of thalamic DBS.[66] However, the process is labor intensive for the clinician and thus not routinely practicable with limited clinical resources.

Patients ideally leave the hospital the day after IPG implantation and we endeavor to follow their progress with clinic appointments at 1 month, 3 months, 6 months, and annually thereafter. Initially they are given a pain diary to record their VAS and stimulator settings weekly for review at follow-up. In addition to being able to switch the DBS on and off at will, they are usually only given control over its voltage, which is typically limited by the clinician to a maximum efficacious amplitude of up to 6 V.

Outcomes Evidence

Several reviews of DBS for chronic pain have been published, many expert, some commentaries, several systematic.* Our systematic searches have identified a number of primary studies.†

Published case series of at least six patients using current DBS targets are listed in **Table 22-1** and their efficacy summarized. When the same authors reviewed their clinical data more than once, only their latest or largest patient series was considered. Pain relief scores showing 50% or more improvement or verbal ratings of good or excellent after surgery were considered successful outcomes, and patients not permanently implanted included as failed outcomes. However, not all authors reported such failures, leading to overestimation of efficacy in some reports. The literature is also obfuscated by varying and often simplistic or subjective outcome measures with a paucity of double-blind, placebo-controlled studies. To our knowledge only four groups have published studies of at least six patients using current standards of target localization and currently available models of deep brain stimulators in all patients with adequate follow-up and description of outcome.[63,66,68,69] All other primary studies are based on cases first implanted more than a decade ago, some using electrodes now no longer commercially available, and some targeting the internal capsule.

The etiologies and brain targets of our 66 patient-prospective case series are summarized in **Figs. 22-2** and **22-6**. A fifth of all patients had failed other invasive neuromodulatory treatment, including MCS, SCS, and analgesic pump implantation. Fifty-one patients (77%) gained pain relief during the week after procedure and proceeded to full DBS implantation. Mean MPQ-ranked pain indices for the cohort before and after surgery showed significant improvement (p < 0.05) in sensory domains and overall (**Fig. 22-7**). Average improvements in VAS for the cohort of 80% were seen at

---

*See reference numbers 56, 58, 59, 64, 69, 80, 85, 127, 128, 131, 158, and 166-187.
†See reference numbers 15, 34-37, 43, 45, 50, 51, 61-66, 68, 69, 82, 95, 131, 150, 151, 154, 169, and 187-209.

Table 22-1:   Summary of Prospective Case Series of Thalamic and Periventricular Deep Brain Stimulation for Pain

Study Reference	Number of Patients Implanted	Deep Brain Target	% Success: Long-Term (Initially)	Follow-up Time (months): Range (mean)	Evaluation Method Used
43, 45, 188	84 121	PVG/PAG VPL/VPM	0 69	N/A	Verbal report
34-36, 150	30	PVG/PAG	70	1-46 (18)	Self report; NRS
189	7	PVG/PAG	16		Nociceptive stimuli
190	6	PVG/PAG	33	6-42	Verbal report
50	28	PVG/PAG	76	1-33 (14)	N/A
95, 191	24	VPL/VPM	67	1-47 (10)	Verbal report; HRQoL; analgesic use
51, 192	26 20	PVG/PAG VPL/VPM	28	6-54	Three category rating
193	48 12	PVG/PAG VPL/VPM	79	6-42 (36)	VAS
194-196	24	VPL/VPM	63	N/A	Three category rating; activity; analgesic use
197	41	PVG/PAG VPL/VPM	41	N/A	VAS; HRQoL
37, 151, 169 198-202	65 77	PVG/PAG VPL/VPM	77 (82) 58 (68)	14-168	Verbal report; analgesic use
203	141	PVG/PAG VPL/VPM	31 (59)	24-168 (80)	Verbal report
204	89	VPL/VPM	67	N/A	VAS; verbal report; analgesic use
205, 209	36	VPL/VPM	30 (61)	(48)	Nociceptive stimuli
166, 187	25 43 12	VPL/VPM Both Other	14 (overall)	n/a	Verbal report
131, 154, 206, 207	178	PVG/PAG VPL/VPM	50 (80)	12-180 (90)	VAS; analgesic use; HRQoL
15	68	PVG/PAG VPL/VPM	62 (78)	6-180 (78)	VAS, MPQ
64	12	PVG/PAG	n/a	n/a	N/A
130	8 3 45	PVG/PAG VPL/VPM Both	63 33 38	6-66	N/A
66	6	VPL/VPM	83	(42)	NRS, nociceptive and placebo stimuli
63	21	PVG/PAG VPL/VPM	24 (62)	2-108 (24)	VAS, use of DBS
61, 62, 65, 68, 82	47	PVG/PAG VPL/VPM	39 (74)	1-44 (19)	VAS, MPQ, HRQoL

HRQoL, Health-related quality of life; *MPQ,* McGill Pain Questionnaire; *NRS,* numerical rating scale; *PVG/PAG,* periventricular and periaqueductal gray and adjacent mid-line thalamic nuclei; *VAS,* visual analog scale; *VPL/VPM,* ventroposterolateral and ventroposteromedial thalamic nuclei.

3 months after surgery and maintained at 35% to 43% for 4 years thereafter (**Fig. 22-8**). VAS scores frequently did not mirror patients' considerable subjective improvements in function and quality of life, suggesting its limitations as an assessment tool. Other explanations include emergence of a late-tolerance phenomenon or unmasking of other types or regions of pain with restoration of patient activity.

In December 2008 mean efficacious DBS parameters for the entire 51-patient cohort at last clinical follow-up were frequency 18.5 Hz (range 5 to 35 Hz, SD 15 Hz), pulse width 295 μs (range 90-450 μs, SD 93 μs), and amplitude 2.5 V (range 0.5 to 5.2 V, SD 1.2 V). Sixty-seven percent of patients received bipolar stimulation.

Eleven patients (22% of those implanted for at least 1 year) required IPG changes, with a mean time between changes of 25 months in this minority, the mean follow-up of the remaining 78% without IPG changes being 42 months. Mean follow-up of all patients was 55 months (range 1 month to 10 years). Five patients from the cohort died of other causes more than 1 year after their surgery. Four patients developed wound infections, one resolving with antibiotics, one requiring scalp debridement, one IPG site debridement, and one complete system removal. Four patients required DBS lead replacement, two following fall-related fractures and two because of lead tethering; one patient had lead adjustment to improve efficacy. Other complications included visual disturbances

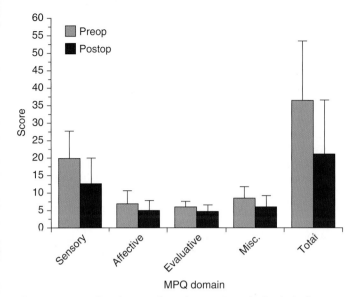

Fig. 22-7 McGill Pain Questionnaire (MPQ) ranked pain indices before and after surgery. Significant improvements (p < 0.05) are seen in the sensory domain and overall. *Misc,* Miscellaneous.

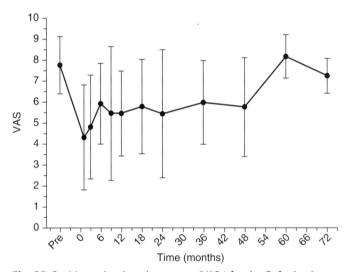

Fig. 22-8 Mean visual analog scores *(VASs)* for the Oxford cohort. Note large error bars suggestive of individual differences and limitations of this subjective rating scale as a long-term outcome assessment. *Pre,* Presurgery.

in three patients with PVG/PAG DBS and one with VPL DBS and dysarthria in one patient with PVG/PAG DBS. Detailed outcomes by etiology from our patient cohort, including quality of life outcomes, are described elsewhere with comprehensive analyses also in progress.[1,62,65,67,68,135,165]

Risk and Complication Avoidance

Specific DBS complications accounted for are stroke (<1%), seizures (<1%), hemorrhage (0.3%), death (0.1%), and the need for IPG revision surgery every 3 to 5 years because of limited battery life and infection (3%); a small proportion of cases required complete removal of the DBS system. Although our overall complication rates are lower than these percentages (e.g., 0.05% hemorrhage; 0.02% death) and IPG changes have been required in a fifth of patients receiving DBS for pain in the last decade, it appears

appropriate to quote figures from prevailing published literature.[161,210,211] Patients are also counseled for the possibility that they may derive no benefit from DBS or not tolerate it well, again necessitating its removal; no specific percentage is quoted since each case is best considered individually, but analysis of our case series suggests that explantation rates caused by poor efficacy have remained constant at 23% during a decade of experience of 66 patients with refining case selection, surgery, and postoperative parameter adjustment (see **Fig. 22-4**).

Conclusion

Our experience of DBS for pain over the last decade has refined our practice in several clinical aspects. It has led us to use it in preference to MCS after back-to-back trials, to continue awake surgery using patient self-reports to refine targeting; to implant PVG/PAG rather than VPM/VPL first for most patients; to actively seek burning hyperesthesia and concomitant autonomic dysfunction as good prognostic indicators for the therapy aiding patient selection; to identify certain etiologies as conferring excellent outcomes; and to refine low-frequency stimulation parameters, including cycling and stimulus breaks to optimize efficacy. We have also developed multiple translational studies using invasive and noninvasive electrophysiology, functional neuroimaging, and autonomic studies aimed not just at understanding brain function and mechanisms of pain perception but at improving selection and efficacy and reducing complications of the procedure. We see several developments coming to fruition over the next 5 years.

Patient selection remains important to success in DBS for pain with objective markers of efficacy lacking preprocedure, in contrast to movement disorders. We predict that breakthroughs will arise either from intensive study of autonomic changes with PVG/PAG DBS, leading to measurable autonomic predictors of efficacy, or from noninvasive modalities such as SPECT and MEG, which may identify patients with altered activity in target brain regions in particular tests. Such findings may lead to DBS targets being chosen on an individual patient basis to optimize success.

Advances in stimulator technology such as the development of rechargeable and demand-driven stimulators may not only obviate the need for IPG replacement and thus improve cost-effectiveness but also enable demand-driven patient controlled analgesia and potentially overcome tolerance or the unmasking of other pain with successful DBS.[212] The characterization by LFP recording in awake patients of neural signatures for pain to which such stimulators could respond forms a firm foundation for research into smart DBS for pain.[139]

LFP recording and diffusion tensor imaging are beginning to objectively characterize objective somatotopy in the PVG/PAG as has previously been described in the thalamus.[112-114] Establishment of deep brain target somatotopy gives objective support to intraoperative electrode position adjustments and can enable the development of intraoperative somatosensory-evoked potential monitoring together with microelectrode or macroelectrode recording to guide electrode positioning, in particular in the anesthetized patient.

There remain groups of patients presently refractory to thalamic or PVG/PAG DBS or whose pain (e.g., whole body pain lacking distinct somatotopy or pain after spinal cord injury) makes them poor candidates for the procedure. We have successfully implanted DBS into the anterior cingulate cortex in such patients with the rationale of reducing the emotional saliency of pain perception while not seeking to alter its nociceptive component. Such work draws on a wealth of literature and our own positive clinical experience of anterior cingulotomy for cancer pain.[213,214] We expect that anterior cingulate DBS will not only become established as a viable novel target in DBS for chronic pain but that its use and related translational investigations will yield many neuropsychological insights into emotion, attention, and executive function.

Further challenges in our DBS for pain service with its international referral patterns are poor recruitment to trials and loss of patients to follow-up. History has demonstrated the potential for unconstrained application of functional neurosurgery in psychiatric disorders; thus patients must be enrolled in formal studies and not lost to clinical follow-up.[215]

An admirable feature of contemporary clinical trials is the a priori standardization of clinical outcomes by collaborative multicenter groups and inclusion of quality of life measures. As DBS for chronic pain illustrates, meta-analyses and systematic reviews become hamstrung in the conclusions that can be drawn from them if the outcome measures of the primary studies analyzed are not standardized.[80,158,162,172] Novel evidence-based methods are being considered and adapted to factor in risks of surgery such as application of a signal-to-noise ratio of treatment effect of DBS compared to expected prognosis of the chronic pain without treatment.[162,216] Treatment effects can be inferred from well-designed case series and nonrandomized cohort studies and justified when a rapid response is seen against a stable or progressively declining disease natural history using such paradigms.

As clinical indications and clinician and patient awareness of DBS continue to increase, costs of both the technology and its implantation will decrease, making the therapy more widely available. Although it is unlikely that DBS will be as widespread and inexpensive as cardiac pacemakers, it may be comparable in cost to SCS within 5 years. A priority is to demonstrate cost-effectiveness by ensuring rigorous and evidence-based studies of DBS for pain and redressing the challenges of past failed trials. A combination of tailored evidence-based methods such as N-of-1 trials and signal-to-noise ratio calculations on intensively studied small cohorts must occur alongside the coordination of multicenter clinical trials with standardized selection, implantation, and outcome data collation protocols. Only then can DBS for pain become reestablished as a widely used therapy rather than one reserved for a select handful of experienced specialist centers willing to carefully study their patients and publish their results.

Key Issues

- DBS for the treatment of chronic pain refractory to drug therapy has been undertaken for half a century, but few centers have reported contemporary findings using current technology. Its use presently remains restricted to experienced, specialist centers willing to publish results, exemplifying the many challenges to demonstrating evidence of efficacy in functional neurosurgery.
- DBS for pain is typically used when all other treatment has failed or is inadequate. This context should be taken into account in evaluating outcomes. Alongside a move to multicenter clinical trials, intrapatient N-of-1 trials and signal-to-noise evidence-based methodology can be applied to DBS for pain to yield robust measures of efficacy from intensively studied case series.

- Our experience over a decade of DBS for pain in 66 patients emphasizes symptomatology rather than etiology in patient selection but reveals positive outcomes after stroke and excellent outcomes for pain after amputation, plexopathies, and head and face pain, including anesthesia dolorosa and postoperative pain.
- PVG/PAG and VPL/VPM remain our targets of choice in DBS for intractable pain, with PVG/PAG assessed first and anterior cingulate cortex DBS considered in refractory or selected cases.
- As with other neuromodulatory therapies, DBS efficacy declines with time when measured by VAS alone, suggesting either a tolerance or unmasking phenomenon likely to be common in neuropathic pain and that may be overcome by stimulation parameter alteration or deramping.
- Translational insights from invasive electrophysiology, MEG, SPECT, DTI, and autonomic testing aim to advance our understanding of DBS for intractable pain and improve patient selection, surgical targeting, and efficacy alongside advances in DBS technology such as the prospect of demand-driven "smart" stimulation.

References

1. Owen SL et al: Deep brain stimulation for the alleviation of post-stroke neuropathic pain. *Pain* 120(1-2):202-206, 2006.
2. Pereira EA et al: Deep brain stimulation for central post-stroke pain-relating outcomes and stimulation parameters in 21 patients. *Acta Neurochir* 150(9):968, 2008.
3. Green AL et al: Stimulating the human midbrain to reveal the link between pain and blood pressure. *Pain* 124(3):349-359. 2006.
4. Dunckley P et al: A comparison of visceral and somatic pain processing in the human brainstem using functional magnetic resonance imaging. *J Neurosci* 25(32):7333-7341, 2005.
5. Chang L: Brain responses to visceral and somatic stimuli in irritable bowel syndrome: a central nervous system disorder? *Gastroenterol Clin North Am* 34(2):271-279, 2005.
6. Owen SL et al: Preoperative DTI and probabilistic tractography in four patients with deep brain stimulation for chronic pain. *J Clin Neurosci* 15(7):801-805, 2008.
7. Sillery E et al: Connectivity of the human periventricular-periaqueductal gray region. *J Neurosurg* 103(6):1030-1034, 2005.
8. Johansen-Berg H, Behrens TE: Just pretty pictures? What diffusion tractography can add in clinical neuroscience. *Curr Opin Neurol* 19(4):379-385, 2006.
9. Kupers R, Kehlet H: Brain imaging of clinical pain states: a critical review and strategies for future studies. *Lancet Neurol* 5(12):1033-1044, 2006.
10. Kringelbach ML et al: Deep brain stimulation for chronic pain investigated with magnetoencephalography. *Neuroreport* 18(3):223-228, 2007.
11. Ray NJ et al: Abnormal thalamocortical dynamics may be altered by deep brain stimulation: using magnetoencephalography to study phantom limb pain. *J Clin Neurosci* 16(1):32-36, 2009.
12. Makela JP et al: Magnetoencephalography in neurosurgery. *Neurosurgery* 59(3):493-511; discussion 493-511, 2006.
13. Pereira EA et al: Regional cerebral perfusion differences between periventricular grey, thalamic and dual target deep brain stimulation for chronic neuropathic pain. *Stereotact Funct Neurosurg* 85(4):175-183, 2007.
14. Kamano S: Author's experience of lateral medullary infarction—thermal perception and muscle allodynia. *Pain* 104(1-2):49-53, 2003.
15. Kumar K, Toth C, Nath R: Deep brain stimulation for intractable pain: a 15-year experience. *Neurosurgery* 40(4):736-746; discussion 746-747, 1997.
16. Romanelli P, Heit G: Patient-controlled deep brain stimulation can overcome analgesic tolerance. *Stereotact Funct Neurosurg* 82(2-3):77-79, 2004.

Disclosure
The authors acknowledge financial support from the UK Medical Research Council, Wellcome Trust, Norman Collisson Foundation, Charles Wolfson Charitable Trust and Oxford Comprehensive Biomedical Research Center.

17. Hariz MI et al: Tolerance and tremor rebound following long-term chronic thalamic stimulation for Parkinsonian and essential tremor. *Stereotact Funct Neurosurg* 72(2-4):208-218, 1999.

18. Laitinen LV: Surgical treatment, past and present, in Parkinson's disease. *Acta Neurol Scand Suppl* 51:43-58, 1972.

19. Pereira EA, Aziz TZ: Surgical insights into Parkinson's disease. *J R Soc Med* 99(5):238-244, 2006.

20. Ashburn MA, Staats PS: Management of chronic pain. *Lancet* 353(9167):1865-1869, 1999.

21. Gureje O et al: Persistent pain and well-being: a World Health Organization Study in Primary Care. *JAMA* 280(2):147-151, 1998.

22. Olds J, Milner P: Positive reinforcement produced by electrical stimulation of septal area and other regions of rat bra. *J Comp Physiol Psychol* 47(6):419-427, 1954.

23. Pool JL et al: *Steroid Hormonal response to stimulation of electrodes implanted in the subfrontal parts of the brain*, Springfield, Ill, 1956, Charles C Thomas.

24. Heath R: *Studies in schizophrenia*, Cambridge, Mass, 1954, Harvard University Press.

25. Heath RG, Mickle WA: *Evaluation of seven years' experience with depth electrode studies in human patients*, New York, 1960, Paul B Hoeber.

26. Gol A: Relief of pain by electrical stimulation of the septal area. *J Neurol Sci* 5(1):115-120, 1967.

27. Melzack R, Wall PD: Pain mechanisms: a new theory. *Science* 150(699):971-979, 1965.

28. Sweet WH, Wepsic JG: Treatment of chronic pain by stimulation of fibers of primary afferent neuron. *Trans Am Neurol Assoc* 93:103-107, 1968.

29. Shealy CN, Mortimer JT, Reswick JB: Electrical inhibition of pain by stimulation of the dorsal columns: preliminary clinical report. *Anesth Analg* 46(4):489-491, 1967.

30. Mullett K: Electrical brain stimulation for the control of chronic pain. *Med Instrum* 12(2):88-91, 1978.

31. Mullett K: State of the art in neurostimulation. *Pacing Clin Electrophysiol* 10(1 Pt 2):162-175, 1987.

32. Mayer DJ et al: Analgesia from electrical stimulation in the brainstem of the rat. *Science* 174(16):1351-1354, 1971.

33. Reynolds DV: Surgery in the rat during electrical analgesia induced by focal brain stimulation. *Science* 164(878):444-445, 1969.

34. Richardson DE, Akil H: Long-term results of periventricular gray self-stimulation. *Neurosurgery* 1(2):199-202, 1977.

35. Richardson DE, Akil H: Pain reduction by electrical brain stimulation in man. Part 1. Acute administration in periaqueductal and periventricular sites. *J Neurosurg* 47(2):178-183. 1977.

36. Richardson DE, Akil H: Pain reduction by electrical brain stimulation in man. Part 2. Chronic self-administration in the periventricular gray matter. *J Neurosurg* 47(2):184-194, 1977.

37. Hosobuchi Y, Adams JE, Linchitz R: Pain relief by electrical stimulation of the central gray matter in humans and its reversal by naloxone. *Science* 197(4299):183-186, 1977.

38. White JC, Sweet WH: *Pain and the neurosurgeon*, Springfield, Ill, 1969, Charles C Thomas.

39. Ervin FR, Brown CE, Mark VH: Striatal influence on facial pain. *Confin Neurol* 27(1):75-90, 1966.

40. Mark VH, Ervin FR: Role of thalamotomy in treatment of chronic severe pain. *Postgrad Med* 37:563-571, 1965.

41. Mark VH, Ervin FR, Hackett TP: Clinical aspects of stereotactic thalamotomy in the human. Part I. The treatment of chronic severe pain. *Arch Neurol* 3:351-367, 1960.

42. Hosobuchi Y, Adams JE, Rutkin B: Chronic thalamic stimulation for the control of facial anesthesia dolorosa. *Arch Neurol* 29(3):158-161, 1973.

43. Mazars G, Merienne L, Cioloca C: Treatment of certain types of pain with implantable thalamic stimulators. *Neurochirurgie* 20(2):117-124, 1974.

44. Mazars G, Merienne L, Ciolocca C: Intermittent analgesic thalamic stimulation: preliminary note. *Rev Neurol (Paris)* 128(4):273-279, 1973.

45. Mazars GJ: Intermittent stimulation of nucleus ventralis posterolateralis for intractable pain. *Surg Neurol* 4(1):93-95, 1975.

46. Mazars G, Roge R, Mazars Y: Results of the stimulation of the spinothalamic fasciculus and their bearing on the physiopathology of pain. *Rev Prat* 103:136-138, 1960.

47. Adams JE, Hosobuchi Y, Fields HL: Stimulation of internal capsule for relief of chronic pain. *J Neurosurg* 41(6):740-744, 1974.

48. Fields HL, Adams JE: Pain after cortical injury relieved by electrical stimulation of the internal capsule. *Brain* 97(1):169-178, 1974.

49. Hosobuchi Y, Adams JE, Rutkin B: Chronic thalamic and internal capsule stimulation for the control of central pain. *Surg Neurol* 4(1):91-92, 1975.

50. Ray CD, Burton CV: Deep brain stimulation for severe, chronic pain. *Acta Neurochir (Wien)* 30(suppl):289-293, 1980.

51. Thoden U et al: Medial thalamic permanent electrodes for pain control in man: an electrophysiological and clinical study. *Electroencephalogr Clin Neurophysiol* 47(5):582-591, 1979.

52. Boivie J, Meyerson BA: A correlative anatomical and clinical study of pain suppression by deep brain stimulation. *Pain* 13(2):113-126, 1982.

53. Andy OJ: Parafascicular-center median nuclei stimulation for intractable pain and dyskinesia (painful-dyskinesia). *Appl Neurophysiol* 43(3-5):133-144, 1980.

54. Gildenberg PL: Symposium on the safety and clinical efficacy of implanted neuroaugmentive devices. *Appl Neurophysiol* 40:69-240, 1977.

55. Gildenberg PL: Neurosurgical statement on neuroaugmentive devices. *Appl Neurophysiol* 40:69-71, 1977.

56. Gildenberg PL: History of electrical neuromodulation for chronic pain. *Pain Med* 7(suppl 1):S7-S13, 2006.

57. Pereira EA, Aziz TZ: Parkinson's disease and primate research: past, present, and future. *Postgrad Med J* 82(967):293-299, 2006.

58. Coffey RJ: Deep brain stimulation for chronic pain: results of two multicenter trials and a structured review. *Pain Med* 2(3):183-192, 2001.

59. Long DM: The current status of electrical stimulation of the nervous system for the relief of chronic pain. *Surg Neurol* 49(2):142-144, 1998.

60. Long DM: Conquering pain. *Neurosurgery* 46(2):257-259, 2000.

61. Nandi D et al: Thalamic field potentials in chronic central pain treated by periventricular gray stimulation—a series of eight cases. *Pain* 101(1-2):97-107, 2003.

62. Green AL et al: Deep brain stimulation for neuropathic cephalalgia. *Cephalalgia* 26(5):561-567, 2006.

63. Hamani C et al: Deep brain stimulation for chronic neuropathic pain: long-term outcome and the incidence of insertional effect. *Pain* 125(1-2):188-196, 2006.

64. Krauss JK et al: Deep brain stimulation of the centre median-parafascicular complex in patients with movement disorders. *J Neurol Neurosurg Psychiatry* 72(4):546-548, 2002.

65. Owen SLF et al: Deep brain stimulation for neuropathic pain. *Neuromodulation* 9(2):100-106, 2006.

66. Marchand S et al: Analgesic and placebo effects of thalamic stimulation. *Pain* 105(3):481-488, 2003.

67. Bittar RG et al: Deep brain stimulation for phantom limb pain. *J Clin Neurosci* 12(4):399-404, 2005.

68. Owen SL et al: Deep brain stimulation for neuropathic pain. *Acta Neurochir Suppl* 97(Pt 2):111-116, 2007.

69. Rasche D et al: Deep brain stimulation for the treatment of various chronic pain syndromes. *Neurosurg Focus* 21(6):E8, 2006.

70. Rasche D et al: Motor cortex stimulation for long-term relief of chronic neuropathic pain: a 10 year experience. *Pain* 121(1-2):43-52, 2006.

71. Taylor RS: Spinal cord stimulation in complex regional pain syndrome and refractory neuropathic back and leg pain/failed back surgery syndrome: results of a systematic review and meta-analysis. *J Pain Symptom Manage* 31(4 Suppl):S13-S19, 2006.

72. Turner JA et al: Spinal cord stimulation for patients with failed back surgery syndrome or complex regional pain syndrome: a systematic

review of effectiveness and complications. *Pain* 108(1-2):137-147, 2004.

73. Brown JA, Barbaro NM: Motor cortex stimulation for central and neuropathic pain: current status. *Pain* 104(3):431-435, 2003.

74. Cameron T: Safety and efficacy of spinal cord stimulation for the treatment of chronic pain: a 20-year literature review. *J Neurosurg* 100(3 suppl Spine):254-267, 2004.

75. Taylor RS, Van Buyten JP, Buchser E: Spinal cord stimulation for chronic back and leg pain and failed back surgery syndrome: a systematic review and analysis of prognostic factor. *Spine* 30(1):152-160, 2005.

76. Kumar K et al: The effects of spinal cord stimulation in neuropathic pain are sustained: a 24-month follow-up of the prospective randomized controlled multicenter trial of the effectiveness of spinal cord stimulation. *Neurosurgery* 63(4):762-770, 2008; discussion 770.

77. Kemler MA et al: Effect of spinal cord stimulation for chronic complex regional pain syndrome type I: five-year final follow-up of patients in a randomized controlled trial. *J Neurosurg* 08(2):292-298, 2008.

78. Manca A et al: Quality of life, resource consumption and costs of spinal cord stimulation versus conventional medical management in neuropathic pain patients with failed back surgery syndrome (PROCESS trial). *Eur J Pain* 12(8):1047-1058, 2008.

79. Gybels J: *Brain stimulation in the management of persistent pain*, ed 4, Philadelphia, London, 2000, Saunders.

80. Levy RM: Deep brain stimulation for the treatment of intractable pain. *Neurosurg Clin North Am* 14(3):389-399, vi, 2003.

81. Smith H et al: Motor cortex stimulation for neuropathic pain. *Neurosurgical focus (electronic resource)* 11(3):E2, 2001.

82. Nandi D et al: Peri-ventricular grey stimulation versus motor cortex stimulation for post stroke neuropathic pain. *J Clin Neurosci* 9(5):557-561, 2002.

83. Katayama YY et al: Motor cortex stimulation for post-stroke pain: comparison of spinal cord and thalamic stimulation. *Stereotact Funct Neurosurg* 77(1-4):183-186, 2001.

84. Katayama Y et al: Motor cortex stimulation for phantom limb pain: comprehensive therapy with spinal cord and thalamic stimulation. *Stereotact Funct Neurosurg* 77(1-4):159-162, 2001.

85. Coffey RJ, Lozano AM: Neurostimulation for chronic noncancer pain: an evaluation of the clinical evidence and recommendations for future trial designs. *J Neurosurg* 105:175-189, 2006.

86. Anderson WS et al: Chapter 21 Plasticity of pain-related neuronal activity in the human thalamus. *Prog Brain Res* 157:353-364, 2006.

87. Melzack R et al: Central neuroplasticity and pathological pain. *Ann N Y Acad Sci* 2001;933:157-174, 2001.

88. Coderre TJ et al: Contribution of central neuroplasticity to pathological pain: review of clinical and experimental evidence. *Pain* 52(3):259-285, 1993.

89. Schweinhardt P, Lee M, Tracey I: Imaging pain in patients: is it meaningful? *Curr Opin Neurol* 19(4):392-400, 2006.

90. Stern J, Jeanmonod D, Sarnthein J: Persistent EEG overactivation in the cortical pain matrix of neurogenic pain patients. *Neuroimage* 31(2):721-731, 2006.

91. Apkarian AV et al: Human brain mechanisms of pain perception and regulation in health and disease. *Eur J Pain* 9(4):463-484, 2005.

92. Saint-Cyr JA, Trepanier LL: Neuropsychologic assessment of patients for movement disorder surgery. *Mov Disord* 15(5):771-783, 2000.

93. Voon V et al: Deep brain stimulation: neuropsychological and neuropsychiatric issues. *Mov Disord* 21(suppl 14):S305-S327, 2006.

94. Lang AE et al: Deep brain stimulation: preoperative issues. *Mov Disord* 21(suppl 14):S171-S196, 2006.

95. Shulman R, Turnbull IM, Diewold P: Psychiatric aspects of thalamic stimulation for neuropathic pain. *Pain* 13(2):127-135, 1982.

96. Carlsson AM: Assessment of chronic pain. I. Aspects of the reliability and validity of the visual analogue scale. *Pain* 16(1):87-101, 1983.

97. Melzack R: The McGill Pain Questionnaire: major properties and scoring methods. *Pain* 1975;1(3):277-299.

98. Ware JE et al: *SF-36 Health survey manual and interpretation guide*, Boston, Mass, 1993, New England Medical Centre, The Health Institute.

99. EuroQol—a new facility for the measurement of health-related quality of life, The EuroQol Group. *Health Policy* 16(3):199-208, 1990.

100. Medical Outcomes Trust: *How to Score the SF-36 Health Survey*, Boston, Mass, 1991, Medical Outcomes Trust.

101. Pereira EA et al: Sustained blood pressure changes with periventricular grey but not posterior hypothalamic deep brain stimulation. *Acta Neurochir* 150(9):933, 2008.

102. Ramachandran VS, Rogers-Ramachandran D: Phantom limbs and neural plasticity. *Arch Neurol* 57(3):317-320, 2000.

103. Janig W, Baron R: Complex regional pain syndrome is a disease of the central nervous system. *Clin Auton Res* 12(3):150-164, 2002.

104. Janig W, Baron R: Complex regional pain syndrome: mystery explained? *Lancet Neurol* 2(11):687-697, 2003.

105. Janig W, Baron R: Is CRPS I a neuropathic pain syndrome? *Pain* 120(3):227-229, 2006.

106. Ramachandran VS: Plasticity and functional recovery in neurology. *Clin Med* 5(4):368-373, 2005.

107. Green AL et al: Post-herpetic trigeminal neuralgia treated with deep brain stimulation. *J Clin Neurosci* 10(4):512-514, 2003.

108. Brittain J-S et al: Local field potentials reveal a distinctive neural signature of cluster headache in the hypothalamus. *Cephalalgia* 29(11):1165-1173, 2009.

109. Owen SL et al: Connectivity of an effective hypothalamic surgical target for cluster headache. *J Clin Neurosci* 14(10):955-960, 2007.

110. Ray NJ et al: Using magnetoencephalography to investigate brain activity during high frequency deep brain stimulation in a cluster headache patient. *Biomed Imag Intervent J* 3(1):25, 2007.

111. Grover PJ et al: Deep brain stimulation for cluster headache. *J Clin Neurosci* 16(7):861-866, 2009.

112. Lenz FA et al: Single-unit analysis of the human ventral thalamic nuclear group: somatosensory responses. *J Neurophysiol* 59(2):299-316, 1988.

113. Bittar RG et al: Somatotopic organization of the human periventricular gray matter. *J Clin Neurosci* 12(3):240-241, 2005.

114. Pereira EAC et al: Stimulating the brain to relive pain: from homunculi to consciousness and deep brain recording to magnetoencephalography. *Neurosurgery* 61(1):221, 2007.

115. Romanelli P, Esposito V: The functional anatomy of neuropathic pain. *Neurosurg Clin North Am* 15(3):257-268, 2004.

116. Peyron R, Laurent B, Garcia-Larrea L: Functional imaging of brain responses to pain: a review and meta-analysis (2000). *Neurophysiol Clin* 30(5):263-288, 2000.

117. Tracey I: Nociceptive processing in the human brain. *Curr Opin Neurobiol* 15(4):478-487, 2005.

118. Sewards TV, Sewards MA: The medial pain system: neural representations of the motivational aspect of pain. *Brain Res Bull* 59(3):163-180, 2002.

119. Gauriau C, Bernard JF: Pain pathways and parabrachial circuits in the rat. *Exp Physiol* 87(2):251-258, 2002.

120. Willis WD, Westlund KN: Neuroanatomy of the pain system and of the pathways that modulate pain. *J Clin Neurophysiol* 14(1):2-31, 1997.

121. Behbehani MM: Functional characteristics of the midbrain periaqueductal gray. *Prog Neurobiol* 46(6):575-605, 1995.

122. Craig AD: Pain mechanisms: labeled lines versus convergence in central processing. *Annu Rev Neurosci* 26:1-30, 2003.

123. Garcia-Larrea L et al: Functional imaging and neurophysiological assessment of spinal and brain therapeutic modulation in humans. *Arch Med Res* 31(3):248-257, 2000.

124. Zambreanu L et al: A role for the brainstem in central sensitisation in humans. Evidence from functional magnetic resonance imaging. *Pain* 114(3):397-407, 2005.

125. Pereira EA et al: Regional cerebral perfusion differences between periventricular grey, thalamic and dual target deep brain stimulation for chronic neuropathic pain. *Stereotact Funct Neurosurg* 85(4):175-183, 2007.

126. Yamashiro K et al: Neurons with spontaneous high-frequency discharges in the central nervous system and chronic pain. *Acta Neurochir Suppl* 87:153-155, 2003.

127. Duncan GH, Bushnell MC, Marchand S: Deep brain stimulation: a review of basic research and clinical studies. *Pain* 45(1):49-59, 1991.

128. Gybels JM, Sweet WH: *Neurosurgical treatment of persistent pain. physiological and pathological mechanisms of human pain*, Basel, 1989, Karger.

129. Weigel R, Krauss JK: Center median-parafascicular complex and pain control. Review from a neurosurgical perspective. *Stereotact Funct Neurosurg* 82(2-3):115-126, 2004.

130. Tronnier VM: *Deep brain stimulation*, Amsterdam London, 2003, Elsevier.

131. Young RF, Rinaldi PC: *Brain stimulation*, New York, 1997, Springer-Verlag.

132. Brown P: Oscillatory nature of human basal ganglia activity: relationship to the pathophysiology of Parkinson's disease. *Movement Disorders* 18(4):357-363, 2003.

133. Engel AK et al: Invasive recordings from the human brain: clinical insights and beyond. *Nat Rev Neurosci* 6(1):35-47, 2005.

134. Hutchison WD et al: Neuronal oscillations in the basal ganglia and movement disorders: evidence from whole animal and human recordings. *J Neurosci* 24(42):9240-9243, 2004.

135. Nandi D, Aziz TZ: Deep brain stimulation in the management of neuropathic pain and multiple sclerosis tremor. *J Clin Neurophysiol* 21(1):31-39, 2004.

136. Bittar RG et al: Deep brain stimulation for movement disorders and pain. *J Clin Neurosci* 12(4):457-463, 2005.

137. Nandi D et al: Thalamic field potentials during deep brain stimulation of periventricular gray in chronic pain. *Pain* 97(1-2):47-51, 2002.

138. Xie K et al: The physiologically modulated electrode potentials at the depth electrode-brain interface in humans. *Neurosci Lett* 402(3):238-243, 2006.

139. Green AL et al: Neural signatures in patients with neuropathic pain. *Neurology* 72(6):569-571, 2009.

140. Rossi F, Maione S, Berrino L: Periaqueductal gray area and cardiovascular function. *Pharmacol Res* 29(1):27-37, 1994.

141. Bandler R et al: Central circuits mediating patterned autonomic activity during active vs. passive emotional coping. *Brain Res Bull* 53(1):95-104, 2000.

142. Carrive P: The periaqueductal gray and defensive behavior: functional representation and neuronal organization. *Behav Brain Res* 58(1-2):27-47, 1993.

143. Bandler R, Carrive P, Zhang SP: Integration of somatic and autonomic reactions within the midbrain periaqueductal grey: viscerotopic, somatotopic and functional organization. *Prog Brain Res* 87:269-305, 1991.

144. Green AL et al: Deep brain stimulation can regulate arterial blood pressure in awake humans. *Neuroreport* 16(16):1741-1745, 2005.

145. Green AL et al: Controlling the heart via the brain: a potential new therapy for orthostatic hypotension. *Neurosurgery* 58(6):1176-1183; discussion 1176-1183, 2006.

146. Pereira EA et al: Sustained reduction of hypertension by deep brain stimulation. *J Clin Neurosci* 17(1):124-127, 2010.

147. Pereira EA et al: Ventral periaqueductal grey stimulation alters heart rate variability in humans with chronic pain. *Exp Neurol* 223(2):574-581, 2010.

148. Akil H, Liebeskind JC: Monoaminergic mechanisms of stimulation-produced analgesia. *Brain Res* 94(2):279-296, 1975.

149. Akil H, Mayer DJ, Liebeskind JC: Antagonism of stimulation-produced analgesia by naloxone, a narcotic antagonist. *Science* 191(4230):961-962, 1976.

150. Akil H et al: Enkephalin-like material elevated in ventricular cerebrospinal fluid of pain patients after analgetic focal stimulation. *Science* 201(4354):463-465, 1978.

151. Hosobuchi Y et al: Stimulation of human periaqueductal gray for pain relief increases immunoreactive beta-endorphin in ventricular fluid. *Science* 203(4377):279-281, 1979.

152. Dionne RA et al: Contrast medium causes the apparent increase in beta-endorphin levels in human cerebrospinal fluid following brain stimulation. *Pain* 20(4):313-321, 1984.

153. Fessler RG et al: Elevated beta-endorphin in cerebrospinal fluid after electrical brain stimulation: artifact of contrast infusion? *Science* 224(4652):1017-1019, 1984.

154. Young RF, Chambi V: Pain relief by electrical stimulation of the periaqueductal and periventricular gray matter: evidence for a non-opioid mechanism. *J Neurosurg* 66(3):364-371, 1987.

155. Meyerson BA: Biochemistry of pain relief with intracerebral stimulation: few facts and many hypotheses. *Acta Neurochir (Wien)* 30(suppl):229-237, 1980.

156. Blackburn-Munro G: Pain-like behaviours in animals—how human are they? *Trends Pharmacol Sci* 25(6):299-305, 2004.

157. Oliveras JL, Besson JM: Stimulation-produced analgesia in animals: behavioural investigations. *Prog Brain Res* 77:141-157, 1988.

158. Cruccu G et al: EFNS guidelines on neurostimulation therapy for neuropathic pain. *Eur J Neurol* 14(9):952-970, 2007.

159. Papanastassiou V et al: Use of the Radionics Image Fusion™ and Stereoplan™ programs for target localization in functional neurosurgery. *J Clin Neurosc* 5(1):28-32, 1998.

160. Orth RC et al: Development of a unique phantom to assess the geometric accuracy of magnetic resonance imaging for stereotactic localization. *Neurosurgery* 45(6):1423-1431, 1999.

161. Joint C et al: Hardware-related problems of deep brain stimulation. *Movement Disorders* 17(suppl 3), 2002.

162. Pereira EA et al: Deep brain stimulation: indications and evidence. *Expert Rev Med Devices* 4(5):591-603, 2007.

163. McLeod RS et al: Single-patient randomised clinical trial. Use in determining optimum treatment for patient with inflammation of Kock continent ileostomy reservoir. *Lancet* 1(8483):726-728, 1986.

164. McQuay H: *N-of-1 Trials*, New York, 1990, Raven Press.

165. Green AL et al: N-of-1 Trials for assessing the efficacy of deep brain stimulation in neuropathic pain. *Neuromodulation* 7(2):76-81, 2004.

166. Kaplitt MG et al: *Deep brain stimulation for chronic pain*, ed 5, Philadelphia, 2004, Saunders.

167. Bendok BR, Levy RM, Onibukon A: Deep Brain Stimulation for the treatment of intractable pain. In Batjer HH, Loftus CM, editors: *Textbook of neurological surgery: principles and practice*, Philadelphia, London, 2003, Lippincott Williams & Wilkins, pp 2673-2681.

168. Meyerson BA: Problems and controversies in PVG and sensory thalamic stimulation as treatment for pain. *Prog Brain Res* 77:175-188, 1988.

169. Adams JE, Hosobuchi Y: Technique and technical problems. *Neurosurgery* 1(2):196-199, 1977.

170. Adams JE, Hosobuchi Y, Linchitz R: The present status of implantable intracranial stimulators for pain. *Clin Neurosurg* 24:347-361, 1977.

171. Burchiel KJ: Deep brain stimulation for chronic pain: the results of two multi-center trials and a structured review. *Pain Med* 2(3):177, 2001.

172. Bittar RG et al: Deep brain stimulation for pain relief: a meta-analysis. *J Clin Neurosci* 12(5):515-519, 2005.

173. Garonzik I et al: Deep brain stimulation for the control of pain. *Epilepsy Behav* 2(suppl 3):3, 2001.

174. Gybels J: Thalamic stimulation in neuropathic pain: 27 years late. *Acta Neurol Belg* 101(1):65-71, 2001.

175. Gybels J et al: Neuromodulation of pain: a consensus statement prepared in Brussels 16-18 January 1998 by the following task force of the European Federation of IASP Chapters (EFIC). *Eur J Pain* 2(3):203-209, 1998.

176. Raslan AM: Deep brain stimulation for chronic pain: can it help? *Pain* 120(1-2):1-2, 2006.

177. Tasker RR, Filho OV: Deep brain stimulation for neuropathic pain. *Stereotactic Functional Neurosurg* 65(1-4):122-124, 1995.

178. Wallace BA, Ashkan K, Benabid A: Deep brain stimulation for the treatment of chronic, intractable pain. *Neurosurg Clin North Am* 15(3):343-357, vii, 2004.

179. Simpson BA: Spinal cord and brain stimulation. In Wall PD, Melzack R, editors: *Textbook of pain,* ed 4, Edinburgh, 1999, Churchill Livingstone, pp 1353-1382.

180. Simpson BA. *Spinal cord and brain stimulation,* ed 5, Edinburgh, 2003, Churchill Livingstone.

181. Siegfried J: Therapeutical neurostimulation—indications reconsidered. *Acta Neurochir* 52(suppl)(Wien):112-117, 1991.

182. North RB, Levy RM: Consensus conference on the neurosurgical management of pain. *Neurosurgery* 34(4):756-760; discussion 760-761, 1994.

183. Osenbach R: Neurostimulation for the treatment of intractable facial pain. *Pain Med* 7(suppl 1):S126-S136, 2006.

184. Hosobuchi Y: The current status of analgesic brain stimulation. *Acta Neurochir* 30(suppl) (Wien):219-227, 1980.

185. Hosobuchi Y: Current issues regarding subcortical electrical stimulation for pain control in humans. *Prog Brain Res* 77:189-192, 1988.

186. Stojanovic MP: Stimulation methods for neuropathic pain control. *Current Pain Headache Rep* 5(2):130-137, 2001.

187. Tasker RR, Vilela Filho O: Deep brain stimulation for neuropathic pain. *Stereotact Funct Neurosurg* 65(1-4):122-124, 1994.

188. Mazars G, Merienne L, Cioloca C: *Comparative study of electrical stimulation of posterior thalamic nuclei, periaqueductal gray, and other midline mesencephalic structures in man,* New York, 1979, Raven Press.

189. Gybels J: Electrical stimulation of the brain for pain control in human. *Verh Dtsch Ges Inn Med* 86:1553-1559, 1980.

190. Schvarcz JR: Chronic self-stimulation of the medial posterior inferior thalamus for the alleviation of deafferentation pain. *Acta Neurochir* 30(suppl)(Wien):295-301, 1980.

191. Turnbull IM, Shulman R, Woodhurst WB: Thalamic stimulation for neuropathic pain. *J Neurosurg* 52(4):486-493, 1980.

192. Dieckmann G, Witzmann A: Initial and long-term results of deep brain stimulation for chronic intractable pain. *Appl Neurophysiol* 45(1-2):167-172, 1982.

193. Plotkin R: Results in 60 cases of deep brain stimulation for chronic intractable pain. *Appl Neurophysiol* 45(1-2):173-178, 1982.

194. Tsubokawa T et al: Thalamic relay nucleus stimulation for relief of intractable pain: clinical results and beta-endorphin immunoreactivity in the cerebrospinal fluid. *Pain* 18(2):115-126, 1984.

195. Tsubokawa T et al: Clinical results and physiological basis of thalamic relay nucleus stimulation for relief of intractable pain with morphine tolerance. *Appl Neurophysiol* 45(1-2):143-155, 1982.

196. Tsubokawa T et al: Deafferentation pain and stimulation of the thalamic sensory relay nucleus: clinical and experimental study. *Appl Neurophysiol* 48(1-6):166-171, 1985.

197. Meyerson BA: Electrostimulation procedures: Effects, presumed rationale, and possible mechanisms. *Adv Pain Res Ther* 5:495-534, 1983.

198. Hosobuchi Y: Chronic brain stimulation for the treatment of intractable pain. *Res Clin Stud Headache* 5:122-126, 1978.

199. Hosobuchi Y: Dorsal periaqueductal gray-matter stimulation in humans. *Pacing Clin Electrophysiol* 10(1 Pt 2):213-216, 1987.

200. Hosobuchi Y: Subcortical electrical stimulation for control of intractable pain in humans: report of 122 cases (1970-1984). *J Neurosurg* 64(4):543-553, 1986.

201. Hosobuchi Y: Combined electrical stimulation of the periaqueductal gray matter and sensory thalamus. *Appl Neurophysiol* 46(1-4):112-115, 1983.

202. Baskin DS et al: Autopsy analysis of the safety, efficacy and cartography of electrical stimulation of the central gray in humans. *Brain Res* 371(2):231-236, 1986.

203. Levy RM, Lamb S, Adams JE: Treatment of chronic pain by deep brain stimulation: long term follow-up and review of the literature. *Neurosurgery* 21(6):885-893, 1987.

204. Siegfried J: Sensory thalamic neurostimulation for chronic pain. *Pacing Clin Electrophysiol* 10(1 Pt 2):209-212, 1987.

205. Gybels J, Kupers R: Deep brain stimulation in the treatment of chronic pain in man: where and why? *Neurophysiol Clin* 20(5):389-398, 1990.

206. Young RF et al: Electrical stimulation of the brain in treatment of chronic pain: experience over 5 years. *J Neurosurg* 62(3):389-396, 1985.

207. Young RF, Brechner T: Electrical stimulation of the brain for relief of intractable pain due to cancer. *Cancer* 57(6):1266-1272, 1986.

208. Katayama Y et al: Deep brain and motor cortex stimulation for post-stroke movement disorders and post-stroke pain. *Acta Neurochir* 87(suppl):121-123, 2003.

209. Gybels J, Kupers R, Nuttin B: Therapeutic stereotactic procedures on the thalamus for pain. *Acta Neurochir (Wien)* 124(1):19-22, 1992.

210. Lyons KE et al: Surgical and hardware complications of subthalamic stimulation: a series of 160 procedures. *Neurology* 63(4):612-616, 2004.

211. Yianni J et al: The costs and benefits of deep brain stimulation surgery for patients with dystonia: an initial exploration. *Neuromodulation* 8(3):155-161, 2005.

212. Toward a demand driven deep-brain stimulator for the treatment of movement disorders: third IEE International Seminar on Medical Applications of Signal Processing, London, UK, 2005.

213. Hassenbusch SJ: Cingulotomy for cancer pain. In Gildenberg P, Tasker R, editors: *Textbook of stereotactic and functional neurosurgery,* New York, 1997, McGraw Hill, pp 1447-1451.

214. Cosgrove GR, Rauch SL: Stereotactic cingulotomy. *Neurosurg Clin North Am* 14(2):225-235, 2003.

215. Pereira EAC: The lobotomist. *J R Soc Med* 98(8):181-182, 2005.

216. Glasziou P et al: When are randomised trials unnecessary? Picking signal from noise. *Br Med J* 334(7589):349-351, 2007.

IV Practice Management

23 Coding and Billing for Neurostimulation

Jeffrey T.B. Peterson

CHAPTER OVERVIEW

Chapter Synopsis: Most physicians want to spend their time treating patients, not dealing with payment issues, but the reality is that coding and billing are an integral part of any medical practice. Electrical stimulation for indications of intractable pain is a widely used and accepted technique with demonstrable benefits to many patients. Proper handling of the documentation associated with payment can protect not only the patient and the clinic but the very practice of electrical stimulation itself. Inappropriate coding or billing can expose the practice to legal liability. This chapter provides some guidance in the proper handling of the process; but, because of regional differences and continual updates to policies, clinicians should regularly refer to relevant guidelines. Medical necessity for the technique needs to be documented, including the patient's disease state, pain characteristics, and failure of other treatments. Providing the most complete documentation of these conditions before treatment increases the likelihood of payment; failure to do so represents the most common cause of nonpayment. The location of the procedure can also affect payment, as can billing by a facility versus by a physician.

Important Points:
- Inappropriate coding and billing practices may expose the practice to financial and legal liability.
- Medical necessity must be properly documented in the note or operative preamble.
- Always refer to national coverage determination (NCD) and local coverage determination (LCD) guidelines for issues specific to the service and practice locale.
- Ensure that billing and documentation are appropriate for the site of service setting.
- Proper authorization is a key component of coding and billing protocol.
- Non-adherence to carrier requirements could lead to denial of authorization.
- Improper documentation may lead to payer audit and payer sanctions.
- Inadequately trained billing personnel can be a compliance and financial risk to the practice.
- Improper modifier usage can result in payer audit.

Introduction

Appropriate documentation and coding for neurostimulation procedures are not only imperative for maintaining a proper record, but, if they are done incorrectly, they can expose the practice to financial and legal liability risk.[1] Because of regionally diverse payer- and carrier-related issues, this chapter presents an overview of coding and billing topics. It is also important to note that regulations pertaining to coding and billing changes are updated routinely; all readers are strongly encouraged to refer to their local carrier policies for the latest information. Although local policies are prone to change, proper documentation as a measure of practice health and stability remains a staple of practice management that demands daily attention.

Proper Documentation and Medical Necessity

Medical necessity should be documented in the office notes or operative preamble. This documentation should include the disease state, pain characteristics, functional limitations, and degree of suffering. Additional documentation should include failed treatments such as physical therapy, medications, injections, and previous surgical efforts. Any current options should be addressed, and a decision to move forward with the device should be noted. The surgical documentation should not only represent justification for necessity, but should contain complete, concise data that support what the practitioner billed and why. An example of this documentation would be, "Before this spinal cord trial the patient underwent medical management with oral medications from different classes (list classes), injections (list injections), physical medicine, and other (list other options). The patient had no acceptable surgical options and wished to move forward. Informed consent was obtained, and the patient was taken to the procedure area."

Spinal Cord Stimulation

The proper current procedural technology (CPT) coding for the trial and permanent stimulator procedures is listed in **Table 23-1**.[2] All patients must meet clinical criteria, and medical necessity should be documented extensively in the patient record. Note that billing for removal of the trial percutaneous leads is not appropriate if no surgical incision and no surgical anchoring were performed in the initial placement. These codes were created specifically for trial leads that were placed using the "cut-down" technique. The global period for the listed surgical codes is 10 days. Wound checks and physical examinations are not typically billable for the first 10 days after placement of the spinal cord stimulation (SCS) system.

Table 23-1: Neurostimulator Current Procedural Technology Codes

63650	Percutaneous implantation of neurostimulator electrode array, epidural
63655	Laminectomy for implantation of neurostimulator electrodes, plate/paddle, epidural
63661	Removal of spinal neurostimulator electrode; percutaneous array, including fluoroscopy when performed
63662	Removal of spinal neurostimulator electrode; plate/paddle, placed via laminotomy or laminectomy, including fluoroscopy when performed
63663	Revision, including replacement when performed, of spinal neurostimulator electrode percutaneous array, including fluoroscopy when performed
63664	Revision, including replacement when performed, of spinal neurostimulator electrode plate/paddle placed via laminotomy or laminectomy, including fluoroscopy when performed
63685	Insertion or replacement of spinal neurostimulator pulse generator or receiver, direct or inductive coupling
63688	Revision or removal of implanted spinal neurostimulator pulse generator or receiver

Analysis-Programming Codes

95971	Electronic analysis of implanted neurostimulator pulse generator system (rate, pulse amplitude and duration, configuration of waveform, battery status, electrode selectability, output modulation, cycling, impedance, and patient compliance measurements[s]); simple spinal cord or peripheral (peripheral nerve, autonomic nerve, neuromuscular) neurostimulator pulse generator/transmitter, with intraoperative or subsequent programming
95972	Electronic analysis of implanted neurostimulator pulse generator system (rate, pulse amplitude and duration, configuration of waveform, battery status, electrode selectability, output modulation, cycling, impedance, and patient compliance measurements[s]); complex spinal cord or peripheral (except cranial nerve) neurostimulator pulse generator/transmitter, with intraoperative or subsequent programming, first hour
+95973	Electronic analysis of implanted neurostimulator pulse generator system (rate, pulse amplitude and duration, configuration of waveform, battery status, electrode selectability, output modulation, cycling, impedance, and patient compliance measurements[s]); complex spinal cord or peripheral (except cranial nerve) neurostimulator pulse generator/transmitter, with intraoperative or subsequent programming, each additional 30 minutes after first hour (list separately in addition to the code for the primary procedure)

If no reprogramming is done, see procedure code 95970.

Modifier Possibilities (But Not Limited to):

58	Staged or related procedure or service by the same physician during the postoperative period: The physician may need to indicate that the performance of a procedure or service during the postoperative period was: (a) planned prospectively at the time of the original procedure (staged); (b) more extensive than the original procedure; or (c) for therapy following a diagnostic surgical procedure.
59	Distinct procedural service: Under certain circumstances the physician may need to indicate that a procedure or service was distinct or independent from other services performed on the same day. Modifier 59 is used to identify procedures/services that are not normally reported together but are appropriate under the circumstances.
51	Multiple procedures: When multiple procedures other than Evaluation and Management services are performed at the same session by the same provider, the primary procedure or services may be reported as listed. The additional procedure(s) may be identified by appending modifier 51 to the additional procedure or services code(s).

Peripheral Nerve Stimulation

The proper CPT coding for the placement of trial and permanent peripheral nerve stimulators is listed in **Table 23-2**.[2] To bill these codes the patient should meet clinical criteria, and medical necessity should be well documented in the record. Please note that it is inappropriate to bill for the removal of the percutaneous electrode leads placed for the trial that are removed in the office setting. The removal codes are intended for leads that have been placed by surgical cut-down and require open surgical removal. Remember that it is appropriate for the physician to bill for the array, not the electrodes. Therefore, if two arrays are tunneled separately to provide stimulation to dual areas, the practitioner can attach either the 51 (multiple procedures) or 59 (distinct procedural service) modifiers, per carrier requirements. The surgical codes listed in the table fall under the 10-day global period. As with SCS, this period applies to wound checks, examinations, and other areas of management regarding the peripheral nerve stimulation system. In some cases insurers do not understand the procedure being performed

with peripheral nerve stimulation. This had led to some denials based on an "experimental therapies" designation. Peripheral nerve stimulation is not experimental; it has been done for many years, and clinical evidence supports its use. It is important for the implanter to educate the medical director of the insurance company about this therapy.

Tools for Billing Compliance

When billing more than one procedure, always refer to the Correct Coding Initiative (CCI) edits updated quarterly on the Centers for Medicare and Medicaid Services (CMS) website. If the code combinations are bundled, it may not be appropriate to bill the codes together; however, the appropriate use of modifiers may allow for the coding combinations selected by the physician. Many Medicare intermediaries have local coverage determination (LCD) guidelines in effect for their various states. The carrier in the local jurisdiction of the practice has those policies available for review. In the absence

Table 23-2: Description of Peripheral Nerve Neurostimulator	
64555	Percutaneous implantation of neurostimulator electrodes; (excludes sacral nerve) peripheral nerve
64575	Incision for implantation of neurostimulator electrodes
64585	Revision or removal of peripheral neurostimulator electrodes
64590	Insertion or replacement of peripheral neurostimulator pulse generator or receiver, direct or inductive coupling
64595	Revision or removal of peripheral neurostimulator pulse generator or receiver

Analysis-Programming Codes

95971	Electronic analysis of implanted neurostimulator pulse generator system (rate, pulse amplitude and duration, configuration of waveform, battery status, electrode selectability, output modulation, cycling, impedance, and patient compliance measurements[s]); simple spinal cord, or peripheral (peripheral nerve, autonomic nerve, neuromuscular) neurostimulator pulse generator/transmitter, with intraoperative or subsequent programming
95972	Electronic analysis of implanted neurostimulator pulse generator system (rate, pulse amplitude and duration, configuration of waveform, battery status, electrode selectability, output modulation, cycling, impedance and patient compliance measurements[s]); complex spinal cord or peripheral (except cranial nerve) neurostimulator pulse generator/transmitter, with intraoperative or subsequent programming, first hour
+95973	Electronic analysis of implanted neurostimulator pulse generator system (rate, pulse amplitude and duration, configuration of waveform, battery status, electrode selectability, output modulation, cycling, impedance, and patient compliance measurements[s]); complex spinal cord or peripheral (except cranial nerve) neurostimulator pulse generator/transmitter, with intraoperative or subsequent programming, each additional 30 minutes after first hour (list separately in addition to the code for the primary procedure)

If no reprogramming is done, see procedure code 95970.

Modifier Possibilities (But Not Limited to):

58	Staged or related procedure or service by the same physician during the postoperative period: The physician may need to indicate that the performance of a procedure or service during the postoperative period was: (a) planned prospectively at the time of the original procedure (staged); (b) more extensive than the original procedure; or (c) for therapy following a diagnostic surgical procedure.
59	Distinct procedural service: Under certain circumstances the physician may need to indicate that a procedure or service was distinct or independent from other services performed on the same day. Modifier 59 is used to identify procedures/services that are not normally reported together but are appropriate under the circumstances.
51	Multiple procedures: When multiple procedures other than E/M services are performed at the same session by the same provider, the primary procedure or services may be reported as listed. The additional procedure(s) may be identified by appending modifier 51 to the additional procedure or services code(s).

of local policy, check the CMS website for national coverage determination (NCD) policy. The NCD for electrical nerve stimulators for back or leg pain includes "surgery" as a required modality that must have been attempted (and failed) before implantation. If the patient was not a surgical candidate, it should be documented that surgery was considered and was not pursued because:

- No surgical lesions existed.
- The patient is contraindicated for surgery.
- The patient does not wish to pursue surgery.

If the clinician's medical record does not indicate to the satisfaction of the insurer why surgery was not selected as a treatment for this patient, the claim may be denied for medical necessity. If the patient's clinical picture does not meet the clinical criteria in a manner of certainty, the patient may be asked to take financial responsibility. Most commercial insurance carriers have an individual policy regarding coverage of the neurostimulation procedure. Check with the individual carrier regarding those requirements before the service. The physician may want to consider generating a letter of predetermination. Document the medical condition of the patient and the procedures believed to be beneficial and why. List patient history, failed therapies and treatments, medications and adverse reactions, and the patient's functional ability in a detailed, comprehensive report. The insurer does not know the patient or his or her condition; thus the more relevant

documentation that can be provided, the better. Keep in mind that a service that has been precertified or preauthorized by an insurance company is still not a guarantee of payment.

Setting

In many circumstances the neurostimulation procedure is not billable at an office location; these services are usually billed in a hospital or ambulatory surgery center facility setting. Some payers do allow the procedures to be performed in the office setting, with a payment differential provided to the physician providing the services. The amount of reimbursement based on the trial or permanent implant stage varies. The implanter and the staff should ensure that the insurance company understands both the setting and the equipment required to achieve the implant.

Facility Billing

Medicare Part B pays the facility fee to certified ambulatory surgical centers (ASCs) for services listed on the Medicare coverage list. Approximately 2400 surgical procedures are paid under "Groupers." If multiple procedures are done at the same setting, expect a reduction of 50% for the additional service. The higher Grouper will be paid at 100%. "Add on" codes are usually reduced 50% as well, although some private payers only pay one facility fee, no matter how many levels the physician treats. The device would be billed separately by the facility or ASC. Hospital facility or Part

A billing typically submits medical claims under revenue codes. As with an ASC, the devices are billed separately. The device codes used by CMS are listed in the Health Care Procedure Coding System (HCPCS), National Level II Medicare Codes book. It is important to remember that not all commercial carriers use this same coding system for the devices as Medicare uses. Checking with each carrier before billing for the devices regarding the codes they accept and pay is necessary. As with all procedure codes, check coding resource books each year for possible changes in either the code or code description.

Remember that facility and physician billing are very different. When a physician submits his claim with a single code for the lead or "array" (63650), the facility can submit the claims per electrode.

Common Errors in Billing

The most common billing errors made for these procedures is lack of supporting documentation to establish medical necessity and failure to predetermine if the insurance will cover the service.[3] Costs are present at the time of implant and also going forward. There is typically a lifetime commitment to follow-up care, which includes analysis, reprogramming, and adjustments. Therefore it is imperative that each aspect of these procedures be addressed.

Authorization

Authorization staff must ask specific questions regarding approval to the patient's insurer. General questioning increases the likelihood of error, including a retroactive denial of service or denial of payment from the carrier. All discussions with the insurer should be carefully documented, including, time, date, and names of representatives with whom the conversation has occurred. It may be helpful for the practice to develop an authorization checklist to ensure that all items have been discussed. On appropriate approval, the patient may then be scheduled for the procedure (**Box 23-1**).

Conclusion

Proper documentation and coding are imperative to proper payment, compliance, and adherence to payer-specific requirements.

> **Box 23-1: Authorization Checklist**
>
> 1. Ensure understanding of the specific insurance plan requirements.
> 2. Provide correct CPT, demographic, and other information required by the plan.
> 3. For work-related injuries, ensure that the primary diagnosis code is covered under the patient's claim.
> 4. Obtain a written authorization or, if verbal, the name of the representative, date, and authorization number.
> 5. Record the authorization number and any expiration date where it can be accessed easily by the scheduling and billing departments.
> 6. Determine if the authorization is also a guarantee of payment under the provisions of the plan. If not, ask for a predetermination of payment in addition to the preauthorization.
> 7. Ensure that patients are scheduled for the procedure before authorization expiration.

CPT, Current procedural technology.

Performing procedures for which the practitioner may not be paid appropriately or not paid at all is a financial and legal risk indicator for the pain practice. A successful practice must focus on excellent patient care as a primary goal, but the factors discussed in this chapter are critical for long-term viability of the practice.

References

1. Jones K, Lebron R, Mangram A: Practice management education during surgical residency. *The American Journal of Surgery* 196(issue 6):878-882, 2008.
2. Abraham M, Beebe M, Dalton J: *AMA Current procedural terminology,* 2010 Professional Edition, ISBN: 978-1-60359-119-5.
3. Manchankanti L, Singh V, Pampati V: Description of documentation in the management of chronic spinal pain. *Pain Physician* 12:E199-E224, 2009.

24 Cost-Effectiveness of Neurostimulation

Rod S. Taylor and Rebecca J. Taylor

CHAPTER OVERVIEW

Chapter Synopsis: Health care is expensive; and the up-front costs of electrical stimulation are significant, particularly when compared to more conventional treatments such as pharmacological interventions. Many insurance payers now require an economic evaluation as evidence of cost-effectiveness before they will commit to covering the costs. This chapter presents such an economic evaluation of neurostimulation (represented by spinal cord stimulation) vs. usual care. One difficulty that analysis presents is that benefits to the patients must be not only quantified but given a monetary value. Elements that may be considered as part of a patient's quality of life include mobility, emotional well-being, and cognitive ability. Ideally the scope of costs and benefits should include those to society overall (e.g., the health service, the patient, social services, and other sectors). Seven studies undertaken as economic evaluations of spinal cord stimulation are considered.

Important Points:

- With increasing pressure on health care budgets, there has been a global trend for health care systems to increasingly require evidence of cost-effectiveness before they will reimburse or cover health care technologies.
- Given the high up-front costs of medical devices and therefore neurostimulation, undertaking a formal economic evaluation is particularly important to demonstrate value for money.
- Economic evaluation is a methodology that involves the comparative analysis of the overall costs and outcomes of using a health technology vs. usual care.
- This chapter illustrates the application of economic evaluation to neurostimulation using the example of spinal cord stimulation.

Introduction

Efficacy and safety have traditionally been the key evidentiary cornerstones for a new health technology to obtain market access. This evidence is a required part of the licensing of a new drug or medical device. However, over the last decade, with increasing pressure on health care budgets there has been a global trend for health care systems to also provide evidence of cost-effectiveness before they will reimburse or cover a new health care technology.[1,2] Indeed, many countries have established agencies such as the National Institute for Health and Clinical Excellence (NICE) in the United Kingdom (UK), with a mandate to undertake economic evaluations of new and emerging treatments and thus determine if they represent good value for money for that health care jurisdiction. Although often focused on drugs, the consequence of economic evaluation for medical devices, and therefore neurostimulation, are even more potentially challenging given their high up-front cost.

The first part of this chapter is an overview of the different types of economic evaluation and guidelines. The second part of this chapter illustrates these methods by reference to the evidence base for the cost-effectiveness of spinal cord stimulation (SCS).

Methods of Economic Evaluation

The term *cost-effectiveness* has become synonymous with health economic evaluation and has been used (and misused) to depict the extent to which interventions measure up to what can be considered to represent value for money. Strictly speaking, however, cost-effectiveness analysis (CEA) is one of a number of techniques of economic evaluation.

Economic evaluation is the "comparative analysis of [two or more] courses of action in terms of their costs and consequences"[3] and is a tool to assist health care policy makers. A decision maker can then decide whether the intervention is worth paying for by comparing its benefits with the benefits foregone (so-called *opportunity cost*), in paying for it. Or, to put it another way, given that budgets are finite, economic evaluation seeks to maximize outcomes for the resources available (so-called *economic efficiency*).

There are four main types of full economic evaluation. Each characterizes costs in the same terms (i.e., in monetary units such as dollars). However, each has a different approach to characterizing health outcomes.

In cost-minimization analysis (CMA), the effectiveness of each of the interventions must have been demonstrated to be equal. Thus the analysis is simply a comparison of costs. The least costly option will be preferred.

In cost-benefit analysis (CBA), both costs and benefits are measured in monetary terms. This has the considerable advantage that the decision to proceed or not is simply a case of measuring whether the value of the benefits exceeds the cost. The disadvantage is that it is difficult (and sometimes objectionable) to effectively put a price on a life. Although often used in areas such as transportation policy, CBA is used infrequently in health care.

Cost-effectiveness analysis (CEA) is concerned with costs and health outcomes and describes health outcomes in naturalistic or disease-specific units. Therefore CEA can tell which strategy maximizes a given objective (e.g., which neurostimulation treatment provides the most pain relief with the lowest cost).

Cost-utility analysis (CUA) is a subgroup of CEA. But, whereas health outcome measures in CEA relate to one aspect of a patient's well-being, health outcome measures in CUA attempt to capture all aspects of well-being in a single composite (utility) value. The quality adjusted life year (QALY) is the typical outcome measure in a CUA. Calculation of QALYs entails first measuring quality of life (utility) on a scale from zero to one (where zero equates to death and one equates to perfect health). The period of time (in years) over which this quality assessment applies is then multiplied by its quality weighting to give the number of QALYs. Given both the comprehensiveness of the QALY and that it allows policy makers to compare value for money across disease areas (e.g., cost-effectiveness of vagal nerve stimulation for refractory epilepsy vs. deep brain stimulation for Parkinson disease or analgesic drug treatments for the management of neuropathic pain syndromes), CUA has been widely regarded as the gold standard by many health economists and policy makers.

Grounded in economic theory, utility measures reflect the preferences of groups of persons for particular treatment outcomes and disease states and combine many different health domains into a single number, weighting the different domains with the values people have for the particular health states. Utilities can be elicited directly, using the standard gamble or time trade-off (TTO) methods, or indirectly, using questionnaire-based measures (such as EuroQol [EQ-5D] or Health Utilities Index [HUI] for which population preference weights have previously been obtained). Indirect preference measurement techniques obtain utilities using questionnaires to elicit individuals' valuations of multiple attributes, or domains, of their quality of life (e.g., mobility, emotional well-being, and cognitive ability); responses are then converted into utility values using preestablished formulas. An example of the utility of a male patient age 65 years with diabetic neuropathic pain based on completion of the EQ-5D is shown in **Box 24-1**. The utility index of 0.228 is contrast to an age-sex matched score of 0.78 for an otherwise healthy member of the UK population.[4]

The result of an economic evaluation is a total cost and total outcome of each of the alternative strategies. However, the results are often presented as an incremental cost-effectiveness ratio (ICER), a summary statistic defined as $\Delta C/\Delta E$, where ΔC is the incremental cost (i.e., the difference in costs) and ΔE is the incremental effectiveness (i.e., the difference in health outcomes) in the comparison of a strategy of interest vs. a baseline, or reference, strategy (**Fig. 24-1**). When one strategy produces greater health outcomes than another but at greater cost, threshold (or trade-off) ratios, or societal willingness-to-pay cut-off points, are used to arrive at a choice among strategies. This threshold may differ among countries (e.g., in the United States it is often quoted as $50,000/QALY,[5] and in the UK it is £20,000 to £30,000/QALY).[6]

Note that cost analysis is an inherently different type of study. It involves the simple assessment of the cost of a health care strategy (e.g., the cost to treat a person with neuropathic pain for 1 year) and in fact is not a true economic evaluation because it does not involve the side-by-side evaluation of competing strategies. For this reason and because health outcomes are left out of consideration, decisions that rely solely on cost analysis can be erroneous: cheap technologies are not necessarily cost-effective.

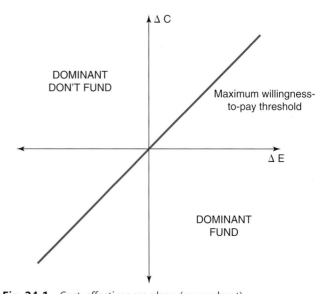

Fig. 24-1 Cost-effectiveness plane (or quadrant). Incremental cost (ΔC) and effectiveness (ΔE) of new health technology vs. an old technology. In the Southeast quadrant the new health technology is more effective and less costly. When this is the case, the new treatment dominates over the old treatment (i.e., the new health technology would be funded and replace the old technology). In the Northwest quadrant the new health technology is less effective and more costly. When this is the case, the old treatment dominates over the old treatment (i.e., the new technology would not be funded, and the old technology would remain). Since new health technologies are often more effective and more expensive than old technologies, the main focus of economic evaluation is the Northeast quadrant. A new technology with an incremental cost-effectiveness ratio (ICER) below the maximum willingness-to-pay (WTP) threshold would be funded, whereas a new technology with an ICER above this threshold would not be funded. In the Southwest quadrant the new technology saves money compared to the old; however, it could be argued that this is at the cost of health. The maximum acceptable ICER is based on the WTP threshold developed for the Northeast quadrant.

Box 24-1: Hypothetical EQ-5D Scoring for a 65-year-old Male with Diabetic Neuropathy

Mobility
I have no problems in walking about. ✓
I have some problems in walking about.
I am confined to bed.

Self-Care
I have no problems with self-care. ✓
I have some problems washing or dressing myself.
I am unable to wash or dress myself.

Usual Activities (e.g., work, study, housework, family or leisure activities)
I have no problems performing my usual activities.
I have some problems performing my usual activities. ✓
I am unable to perform my usual activities.

Pain/Discomfort
I have no pain or discomfort.
I have moderate pain or discomfort.
I have extreme pain or discomfort. ✓

Anxiety/Depression
I am not anxious or depressed.
I am moderately anxious or depressed. ✓
I am extremely anxious or depressed.

EQ-5D index score = 1 − (0.081 + 0 + 0 + 0.036 + 0.386 + 0.071 + 0.269) = 0.228

Guidelines for Conducting Economic Evaluation

A number of international guidelines for conducting economic evaluations have been published, notably Drummond and associates,[3] the U.S. Panel on Cost-Effectiveness in Health and Medicine,[7] and NICE Technology Appraisal Guidance.[8]

A number of steps are needed to carry out an economic evaluation (**Box 24-2**). The first is to define the question. It is critical to define exactly what is being compared with what, who the patients are, and what treatments each group is receiving. For example, is the neurostimulatory device to be applied to patients who are otherwise refractory to drug treatment and is the device regarded as an add-on therapy rather than a specific replacement for a current therapy? The scope is equally important. At whose costs are we looking? At whose outcomes? The ideal scope is that of society, meaning that costs incurred by the health service, patients, social services, voluntary sector and all others are included in the analysis. In practice it is often very difficult to estimate some of these; thus analyses are frequently restricted to a health care perspective.

Cost-Effectiveness of Spinal Cord Stimulation

Over the last 20 years a number publications have included some consideration of the costs of SCS. This economic literature has been the subject to three systematic reviews.[9-11] The literature

Box 24-2: Steps in Conducting an Economic Evaluation
■ Define the question.
■ Define the scope.
■ Specify the method of economic evaluation.
■ Define costs to be estimated.
■ Specify analytical model.
■ Estimate outcomes.
■ Summarize results.
■ Analyze sensitivity.

searches undertaken by these previous reviews across a range of databases (Medline, CINAHL, EMBASE, CDSR, DARE, CENTRAL, NHS EED and HTA) were updated (to March 2010) for the purposes of this article. From these searches, five studies that were full economic evaluations of SCS were identified. Two additional economic evaluations currently in publication were also included. The characteristics of these seven studies are summarized in see **Table 24-1**.[12-18]

The studies were undertaken in a variety of patient groups that included failed back surgery syndrome (FBSS), complex regional pain syndrome (CRPS), refractory angina, and chronic limb ischemia. All studies involved a comparison of costs and outcomes of SCS to usual care, the choice of usual care depending on the medical indication being studied (e.g., analgesia management or spinal reoperation for FBSS and percutaneous myocardial laser revascularization for refractory angina). Studies undertook an analysis of costs and outcomes collected within the trial time horizon (trial-based analysis) or were based on decision analytic modeling to extrapolate beyond the trial data. It is very rare for a single trial to measure all necessary costs and outcomes relevant to decision making; therefore modeling techniques are often used to combine data from different sources (e.g., costs from an observational study and long-term intervention outcomes from a registry) and to project likely future values to arrive at a total cost and consequence from each strategy. Commonly used approaches include decision trees and Markov models.[19] For example, the economic evaluation by Taylor and Taylor[14] used modeling to derive an indirect comparison of SCS vs. medical therapy (from two trials, one comparing SCS vs. reoperation and the other comparing reoperation vs. medical therapy), to convert pain relief into quality of life (utility) and, using observational data on the long-term impact of SCS, to extrapolate 6-month trial data over the patient's lifetime.

The ICERs of these studies generally show that SCS is cost-effective treatment for FBSS and CRPS (i.e., SCS is either less costly and more effective than the comparative therapy, or SCS has an

Table 24-1: Summary of Full Economic Evaluations of Spinal Cord Stimulation

Author (Year) Country	Indication	Type of Economic Evaluation	Comparator	Time Horizon	ICER
Kemler and Furnee (2002)[12] The Netherlands	Complex reflex sympathetic dystrophy	Cost utility analysis Trial and decision analysis model-based	Medical treatment	1 year Patient lifetime	€17,927/QALY SCS dominant
Kemler et al (2010)[13] United Kingdom	Complex regional pain syndrome	Cost utility analysis Decision analysis model-based	Medical treatment	15 years	£4,260/QALY
Taylor & Taylor (2005)[14] United Kingdom	Failed back surgery syndrome	Decision analysis model-based Trial-based	Medical treatment	2 years Patient lifetime	€45,819/QALY SCS dominant
North et al (2007)[15] United States	Failed back surgery syndrome	Cost-effectiveness analysis Cost utility analysis Trial-based	Reoperation	3.1 years	SCS dominant
Taylor et al (2010)[16] United Kingdom	Failed back surgery syndrome	Cost utility analysis Decision analysis model-based	Medical treatment Reoperation	15 years	£5,624/QALY £6,392/QALY
Dyer et al (2008)[17] United Kingdom	Refractory angina pectoris	Cost utility analysis Trial-based	Percutaneous myocardial laser revascularization	2 years	£46,000/QALY
Klomp et al (1999)[18] The Netherlands	Critical limb ischemia	Cost-effectiveness Trial-based	Medical treatment	2 years	€100,000/limb saved

SCS, Spinal cord stimulation.

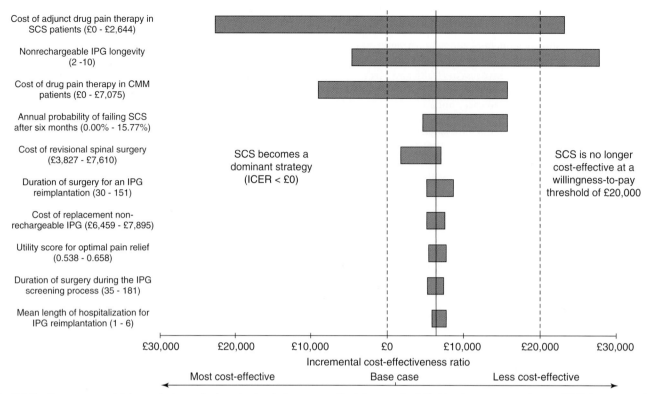

Fig. 24-2 One-way sensitivity analysis—spinal cord stimulation vs. medical therapy for failed back surgery syndrome. *ICER*, Incremental cost-effectiveness ratio; *IPG*, implantable pulse generator; *SCI*, spinal cord stimulation.

ICER of less than a maximal willing threshold of £30,000/QALY). Based on these analyses, NICE in 2009 recommended to the UK National Health Service that SCS be made available routinely to selected patients with FBSS and CRPS[20]:

> "Spinal cord stimulation is recommended as a treatment option for adults with chronic pain of neuropathic origin who: continue to experience chronic pain (measuring at least 50 mm on a 0-100 mm visual analogue scale) for at least 6 months despite appropriate conventional medical management, and who have had a successful trial of stimulation as part of the assessment."

However, the evidence suggested that the cost-effectiveness of SCS for refractory angina and chronic limb ischemia to be less attractive. The ICER for refractory angina is in excess of the £30,000/QALY threshold. The analysis of SCS for critical limb ischemia demonstrates the disadvantage of using CEA: is €100,000/limb saved good value for money? Given this evidence NICE concluded[20]:

> "Spinal cord stimulation is not recommended as a treatment option for adults with complex regional pain syndrome, critical limb ischaemia or refractory angina except in the context of research as part of a clinical trial."

The last stage in an economic evaluation is sensitivity analysis. These "what if" analyses test the robustness of the evaluation and thus the degree of confidence that can be placed in the results. The importance of such analysis is illustrated by the following statement from the Dyer and associates' study assessing the cost-effectiveness of SCS for refractory angina[17]:

> "Exploring the cost-effectiveness of SCS versus PMR [percutaneous myocardial laser revascularization] in the first and second half of the study suggested there was an improvement

over time, which could be indicative of a learning curve effect. For patients recruited during 2000/01, the ICER was estimated at £230,000 per QALY (95% CI: –£2,670,000 to £590,000) whereas for 2002/03, the ICER was estimated at £18,000 per QALY (95% CI: –£21,000 to 51,000). This improvement can largely be explained by better outcomes, in terms of survival and QoL [quality of life], experienced by SCS patients in the second half of the study."

In other words, after a period of clinical learning and familiarity, SCS was a potentially cost-effective therapy (i.e., <£23,000/QALY).

One-way sensitivity analysis has traditionally been used to assess uncertainty in economic evaluations, one variable at a time being changed through a range of values. The resulting set of ICERs is then examined to assess the influence of this variable. **Fig. 24-2** shows the one-way sensitivity analyses for SCS compared to medical therapy for FBSS. For example, although the implantable pulse generator (IPG) longevity was assumed to be 4 years in the base case analysis (shown in fifth row of **Table 24-1**), across a range of plausible range of IPG longevities the cost-effectiveness of SCS could range from being dominant to medical therapy (assuming an IPG longevity as long as 10 years) to be being dominated by medical therapy (assuming an IPG longevity of only 2 years). However, recent methodological advances have motivated the gradual adoption of more sophisticated approaches to measuring and reporting uncertainty in CEA. In probabilistic sensitivity analysis, all model parameters are varied simultaneously over a large number of draws, or simulated trials called *Monte Carlo simulations*.[21] The incremental cost and QALY values arising from 1000 Monte Carlo simulations are shown a cost-effectiveness quadrant in **Fig. 24-3**. That the majority of these simulations lie in the Southeast and lower part of the Northeast quadrants below the £30,000/QALY is evidence that SCS is cost-effective in this case.

COST-EFFECTIVENESS PLANE

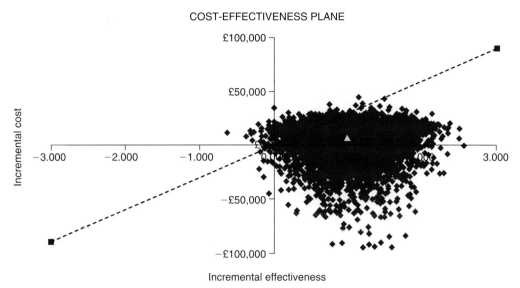

Fig. 24-3 Sample cost-effectiveness quadrant—spinal cord stimulation vs. medical therapy for failed back surgery syndrome.

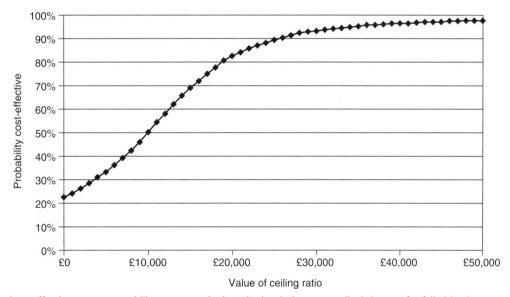

Fig. 24-4 Cost-effectiveness acceptability curve—spinal cord stimulation vs. medical therapy for failed back surgery syndrome.

The cost-effectiveness acceptability curve (CEAC) shows the probability of a health technology being cost-effective over a range of maximum willingness-to-pay thresholds.[22] As shown in **Fig. 24-4**, taking into account all parameter uncertainty, there is a 93% probability that SCS (compared to medical therapy for FBSS) is cost effective at £30,000/QALY.

Summary

Evidence of cost-effectiveness is increasingly required to secure coverage and market access in many countries. For medical devices, including neurostimulation, because of high up-front costs of the technology, demonstrating value for money is particularly important to ensure patient access. Therefore clinicians working in the field of neurostimulation need to be able to understand the methods and interpret and critique the findings of economic evaluations. The purpose of this chapter was to provide an introduction to these issues and, in doing so, provide greater familiarity with a set of research approaches used increasingly to investigate the relationship between costs and the health consequences of health-related policy decisions.

References

1. Taylor RS et al: Inclusion of cost effectiveness in licensing requirements of new drugs: the fourth hurdle. *Br Med J* 23:972-975, 2004.
2. Detsky AS, Laupacis A: Relevance of cost-effectiveness analysis to clinicians and policy makers. *JAMA* 298:221-224, 2007.
3. Drummond MF et al: *Methods for the economic evaluation of health care programmes*, Oxford, 2005, Oxford University Press.
4. Kind P, Hardman G, Macran S: *UK population norms for the EQ-5D*, The University of York Centre for Health Economics, Discussion

Conflict of interest:
RST is a consultant for Medtronic International. The views expressed in this article are entirely those of the authors.

paper 172, November 1999. Accessed March 1, 2010 from http://www.york.ac.uk/inst/che/pdf/DP172.pdf.

5. Neumann PJ, Greenberg D: Is The United States ready For QALYs? *Health Affairs* 28:1366-1371, 2009.

6. Rawlins MD, Culyer AJ: National Institute for Clinical Excellence and its value judgments. *Br Med J* 329:224-227, 2004.

7. Siegel JE et al: Recommendations for reporting cost-effectiveness analyses: Panel on Cost-Effectiveness in Health and Medicine. *JAMA* 276:1339-1341, 1996.

8. NICE: *Guide to the methods of technology appraisal*, London, 2008, National Institute for Health and Clinical Excellence. Accessed September 30, 2009, from http://www.nice.org.uk/media/B52/A7/TAMethodsGuideUpdatedJune2008.pdf.

9. Taylor RS et al: The cost-effectiveness of spinal cord stimulation in the treatment of pain: a systematic review of the literature. *J Pain Symptom Manage* 27:370-378, 2004.

10. Simpson EL et al: Spinal cord stimulation for chronic pain of neuropathic or ischaemic origin: systematic review and economic evaluation. *Health Technol Assess* 13(17):iii, ix-x, 1-154, 2009.

11. Bala MM et al: Systematic review of the (cost-)effectiveness of spinal cord stimulation for people with failed back surgery syndrome. *Clin J Pain* 24:741-756, 2008.

12. Kemler MA, Furnée CA: Economic evaluation of spinal cord stimulation for chronic reflex sympathetic dystrophy. *Neurology* 59:1203-1209, 2002.

13. Kemler MA et al: The cost-effectiveness of spinal cord stimulation for complex regional pain syndrome. *Value in Health* 2010 (in press).

14. Taylor RJ, Taylor RS: Spinal cord stimulation for failed back surgery syndrome: a decision-analytic model and cost-effectiveness analysis. *Int J Technol Assess Health Care* 21:351-358, 2005.

15. North RB et al: Spinal cord stimulation versus reoperation for failed back surgery syndrome: a cost-effectiveness and cost utility analysis based on a randomized controlled trial. *Neurosurgery* 61:361-368, 2007.

16. Taylor RS et al: The cost-effectiveness of spinal cord stimulation in the treatment of failed back surgery syndrome. *Clin J Pain* 26:463-469, 2010.

17. Dyer MT et al: Clinical and cost-effectiveness analysis of an open label, single-centre, randomised trial of spinal cord stimulation (SCS) versus percutaneous myocardial laser revascularisation (PMR) in patients with refractory angina pectoris: The SPiRiT trial. *Trials* 9:40-45, 2008.

18. Klomp HM et al: Spinal cord stimulation is not cost-effective for non-surgical management of critical limb ischaemia. *Eur J Vasc Endovasc Surg* 10:478-485, 1995.

19. Sonnerberg FA, Beck JB: Markov models in medical decision making: a practical guide. *Med Decis Making* 13:322-339, 1993.

20. NICE: *Spinal cord stimulation for chronic pain of neuropathic or ischaemic origin*, London, 2008, National Institute for Health and Clinical Excellence. Accessed September 30, 2009, from http://www.nice.org.uk/Guidance/TA159.

21. Briggs AH: Handling uncertainty in cost-effectiveness models. *Pharmacoeconomics* 17:479-500, 2000.

22. Fenwick E, Claxton K, Sculpher M: Representing uncertainty: the role of cost-effectiveness acceptability curves. *Health Econ* 10:779-787, 2001.

V Future Directions

25 The Future of Neurostimulation

Matthew T. Ranson

CHAPTER OVERVIEW

Chapter Synopsis: Neurostimulation has made significant strides since Shealy first implanted a spinal cord stimulator in 1967. This chapter addresses some of these advances and others that may be on the horizon for neurostimulation. Stimulating electrodes today can be powered by a rechargeable generator, precluding the need to change out batteries every several years to restore power to the device and thereby reducing risks associated with these minor surgeries. Miniaturization of devices has also improved their utility and effectiveness. Devices such as the BION show promise as a single unit with a self-contained power source. Stimulation has also grown from its initial application of spinal cord stimulation (SCS) to peripheral field stimulation and deep brain stimulation among others. Originally thought to be effective only for neuropathic pain, the painful conditions positively affected by neurostimulation have grown tremendously. In some indications, it has been shown that the underlying pathophysiology can be improved as well. Newly tested patterns of stimulation are also emerging, including the so-called "burst" or sub-perception stimulation. Finally, advances in imaging techniques have also improved outcomes in neurostimulation, primarily in placement of devices.

Important Points:

- Neurostimulation is rapidly evolving from spinal cord stimulation to more selective stimulation of peripheral nerves.
- New advances in miniaturization have the potential to increase the application of neuromodulation.
- New forms of stimulation including "burst" and high-frequency stimulation may actually treat the underlying pathophysiology rather than masking neuropathic pain.

Introduction

Neurostimulation has undergone significant advancements since Shealy implanted the first spinal cord column stimulator in 1967.[1] Predictions about the future of neuromodulation have been made previously but often fall short of reality since it is very difficult to comprehend the direction and magnitude of technology that will be available in the future.[2] Today most of the impulse generators that power spinal cord stimulation (SCS) systems approximate the size of cardiac pacemakers and are rechargeable. Many advances have been made in miniaturization, which has afforded physicians both greater flexibility and better outcomes in neurostimulation. Since many of the new technologies currently under development are proprietary, of these new neurostimulation devices are discussed in generalizations. Although at times it is difficult to comment on specific innovations, the body of work and product development in this arena is impressive and ongoing.

Expanding Applications of Neurostimulation

Traditionally neurostimulation has been used in the treatment of chronic pain syndromes such as lumbar and cervical radiculopathy, failed back surgery syndrome, arachnoiditis, complex regional pain syndromes, and other neuropathic syndromes. Today the role of neurostimulation is expanding to include treatment of vascular disease, cardiovascular disease, refractory migraine headaches, chronic pancreatitis, visceral pain, and urological syndromes such as pelvic pain, rectal pain, bladder and fecal incontinence, and erectile dysfunction.[3] In addition, deep brain stimulation has been used effectively to treat central nervous system disorders such as Parkinson disease, and vagal nerve stimulation has been used to treat gastroparesis. Motor cortex stimulation is another exciting area that has shown promise in complex pain patterns of the head and neck.[4]

Advancements in Neurostimulation Electrodes

The development of multicolumn paddle laminotomy lead systems and octrode percutaneous lead systems has revolutionized the treatment of axial low back pain. Many new paddle constructs have three to five columns that allow for selective depolarization of specific spinal structures (**Figs. 25-1 and 25-2**). This allows for more tailored stimulation of the patient based on complex pain patterns. A new generation of percutaneous leads is currently under development that will provide physicians with even greater versatility in the treatment of neuropathic pain syndromes (**Table 25-1**). In addition, percutaneous multilead systems are currently under development that will offer the advantages of a laminotomy lead without the need for an invasive surgical dissection for placement. The use of a percutaneous delivery tool for a paddle construct is now approved in Europe and should be seen in the United States in the near future (**Fig. 25-3**). The improved efficacy and treatment options for SCS coupled with new risks identified for intrathecal drug delivery systems have led to a new interest in using stimulation earlier in the treatment algorithm.[5] SCS has now moved ahead of long-term chronic opioids, reoperation for spinal disorders, and intrathecal drug delivery in patients with neuropathic and mixed pain of the low back and lower limbs.

Microstimulation devices are under development that can be placed directly over damaged peripheral nerves and used to treat neuropathic pain syndromes resulting from pathologies such as cerebral vascular accidents and carpel tunnel syndrome (**Figs. 25-4**

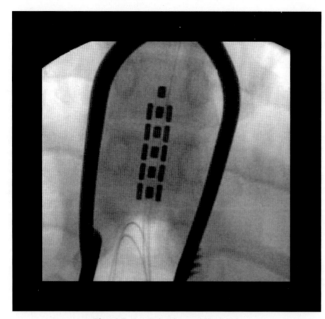

Fig. 25-1 Tripole paddle lead.

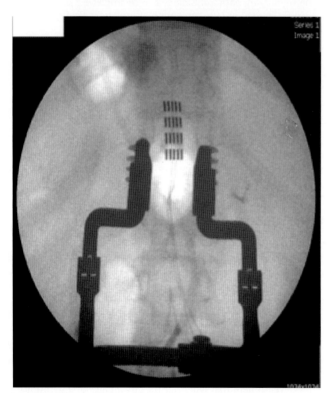

Fig. 25-2 Penta laminotomy lead. Courtesy of Claudio Feler, MD, FACS.

Table 25-1: Comparison of Available and Possible Future Neuromodulation Devices

Available	Now	Future
Percutaneous leads	8 Contacts	64 +
Tripole leads	Surgical laminectomy	Percutaneous tripole
BION	2 Contacts	More ± high frequency
Low frequency	30 Hz-5 kHz	40 kHz +
Wireless generator	Microtransponder	Wireless couple with Bluetooth devices (iPod or cell phone)
Rechargeable generator	10-year life	Infinite recharging capacity
SNRS	Uses quad or octrodes	Intraspinal placement of Microstim devices with wireless capability

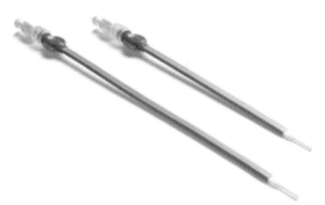

Fig. 25-3 Epiducer.

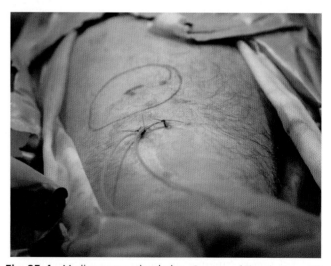

Fig. 25-4 Median nerve stimulation. Courtesy of Timothy Deer, MD.

and 25-5). In addition, microstimulation devices have been used to treat migraine headaches that stem from C2 neuritis. Microstransponder is currently developing a microstimulation device that is a wireless neurostimulation system named *SAINT* (subcutaneous arrangement of implantable neural transponders). The system is purported to eliminate the need for an implantable impulse generator using an external controller that powers the microimplant. Several microstimulation devices (i.e., the BION [Bioness, Valencia, Calif; Boston Scientific, Natick, Mass]) (**Fig. 25-6**) have fully rechargeable lithium ion batteries that obviate the need for an external power source.[6]

Advances in Technique and Targeting of Stimulation

SCS of the posterior spinal column (**Fig. 25-7**), although effective in many chronic pain syndromes, does not provide adequate pain relief from many pain disorders that involve the peripheral nervous

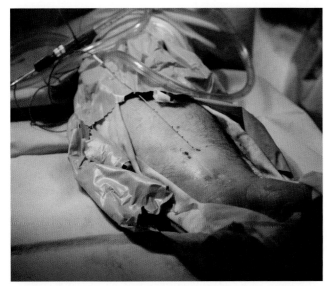

Fig. 25-5 Identification of the median nerve for implantation by nerve stimulation. Courtesy of Timothy Deer, MD.

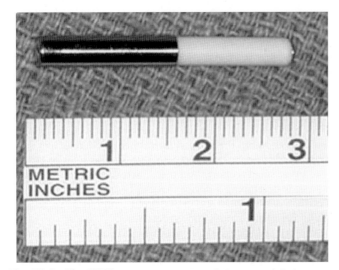

Fig. 25-6 The BION. From Trentmen T et al: Greater occipital nerve stimulation via the Bion microstimulator: implantation technique and stimulation parameters, *Pain Physician* 12:621-628, 2009.

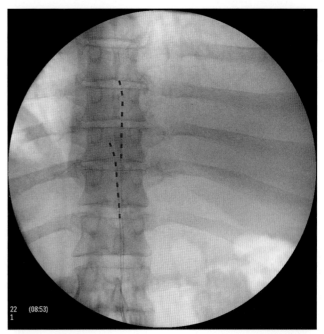

Fig. 25-7 Traditional epidural lead placement x-ray. Courtesy of Timothy Deer, MD.

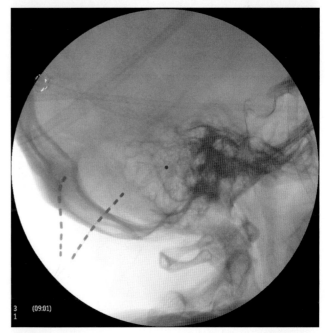

Fig. 25-8 Lateral view of occipital nerve implant. Courtesy of Timothy Deer, MD.

system. Peripheral nerve stimulation (PNS), or the selective targeting of damaged peripheral nerves, has been used successfully in the treatment of painful syndromes refractory to traditional SCS such as intercostal neuralgia and craniofacial pain. In addition, PNS allows for selective targeting of damaged nerves without stimulation of unwanted areas, which can be uncomfortable to many patients. Craniofacial pain has been especially refractory to SCS and is most commonly used to treat occipital and trigeminal nerve lesions (**Figs. 25-8** and 25-9).[7] With advances in microstimulation, it is likely that very selective stimulation will be achieved without many of the complications associated with traditional quadripole and octrode lead placement. Progressive novel uses of stimulation leads in craniofacial nerve lesions have shown great promises but have been complicated by erosion of the leads and anchors. In addition, tunneling of the leads to an area suitable for placement of the impulse generator requires extreme caution because of the proximity of vascular structures, which is not a concern during placement of the new microstimulation devices. New power generators will be available in the future that allow for remote supply

of power to the microstimulation devices by using wireless coil generators.[6] Combinations of peripheral and epidural lead placements with cross-talk between the leads can be used very effectively in the treatment of axial back pain and radiculopathy (**Fig. 25-10**). Alternatively, peripheral lead placement can be used alone for isolated axial back pain refractory to epidural stimulation (**Fig. 25-11**).

Spinal nerve root stimulation (SNRS), or the direct stimulation of the dorsal root, combines the advantages of both peripheral and dorsal column stimulation. As with dorsal column stimulation, SNRS allows for the intraspinal stabilization of the leads with the selectivity of peripheral nerve stimulation.[7] There are two basic approaches to SNRS: (1) the leads are placed laterally over the

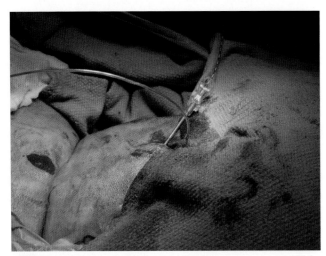

Fig. 25-9 Occipital percutaneous placement. Courtesy of Richard Bowman, MD.

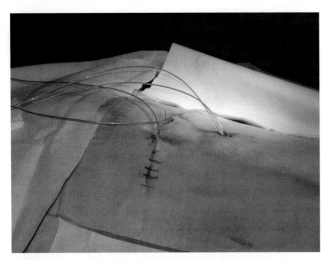

Fig. 25-10 Lumbar and peripheral lead placements. Courtesy of Timothy Deer, MD.

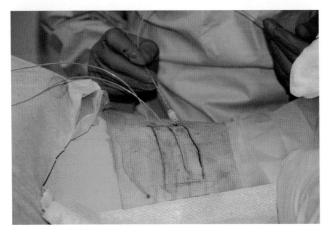

Fig. 25-11 Peripheral nerve leads for pain in the intercostal distribution.

selected dorsal root ganglions, or (2) the leads are placed transforaminally along the desired nerve roots. Some development is occurring in the latter form of SNRS with devices that allow more accurate delivery of transforaminal lead placement.

High-frequency stimulation represents an emerging field of neuromodulation. Neural blockade has been reported using high-frequency alternating currents (HFACs) that resulted in quick onset and reversibility and may represent another treatment alternative in treating pathological peripheral nerve injuries.[7] Neuros is a company that is currently developing a device that stimulates from 5,000 Hz and up to 40,000 Hz compared to traditional SCS systems that stimulate at 30 to 100 Hz.[8] This device will initially be tested in postamputation patients with residual limb pain and, in contrast to SCS, will actually block neural transmission from the severed nerves instead of masking the pain.[9] High-frequency stimulation may ultimately find significant application in many peripheral nerve pain syndromes, including craniofacial pain. Combining the wireless power supply under development by Microtransponder with the high-frequency stimulation provided by Neuros may result in a significant expansion in the application of peripheral neuromodulation.

A microstimulator, the BION (Boston Scientific, Boston Mass) has been used successfully in the treatment of migraine headaches (see **Fig. 25-6**).[10] The device has a cathode on one end and an anode on the other end with a programmable microchip and telemetry capability.[10] Trentman and associates[10] recently reported the results of a clinical trial using the BION in the treatment of refractory migraine headaches. Of the nine patients enrolled in the initial clinical trial, eight completed the follow-up at 1 year and were judged to have fair or better results in reduction of pain and disability, and five out of the eight had greater than 90% reduction in pain.[10] In addition, the successful treatment of hemicrania using the BION device has been reported with success rates of 80% to 90% in a small cohort. Another microstimulation company, Bioness, is developing a device that can be used in the treatment of median neuropathies and in poststroke syndromes that result in painful peripheral neuropathic syndromes.[11]

Another emerging field in neurostimulation is burst stimulation. Traditional dorsal column stimulation results in the perception of paresthesias in the distribution of nerves affected by the neuropathic pain syndrome and often involves recruitment of nerve fibers that are not in the dermatomal distribution of pain. Some failed dorsal column stimulation trials result from either stimulation of unwanted areas or intolerance to the paresthesia that results from traditional dorsal column stimulation. A new technique of burst stimulation has been developed that uses a 40-Hz burst mode with five spikes of 500 Hz per burst.[12] In one clinical trial with a small cohort, burst stimulation resulted in the perception of paresthesias in only 17% of patients, which was stable at 1-year follow-up.[13]

The data on burst stimulation are very limited, and a prospective comparative study would be needed to further evaluate its potential clinical validity.

Advances in Imaging

New methods of imaging and expanded uses of traditional techniques in the placement of both intraspinal and peripheral neurostimulation devices are being developed. Huntoon and Burgher[13] have successfully used ultrasound during placement of standard neurostimulation electrodes targeted to multiple peripheral nerves. The median, ulnar, radial, peroneal, and posterior tibial nerves were all successfully targeted and stimulated with standard electrodes using ultrasonography during the study. The advantages of ultrasound used in peripheral electrode placement include the direct visualization of the nerves and surrounding vascular structures without requiring the skeletonization of the targeted nerve.[13] In addition to ultrasound, several companies are developing stereotactical imaging techniques that will allow for placement of both intraspinal and peripheral neurostimulation devices without the need for continued use of fluoroscopy and the inherent risks of radiation exposure.

Conclusion

New advances in neurostimulation lead technology, the miniaturization of impulse generators, and the development of microstimulation devices are rapidly expanding the application of neurostimulation. The coming health care reform demanding decreased use of resources may increasingly necessitate procedures that can be performed in an outpatient office. Ultrasound-guided peripheral microstimulation implantation directed at peripheral neuropathies may represent a more cost-effective method of treating isolated peripheral nerve injuries compared with traditional dorsal column stimulation. Microstimulation appears to offer the additional advantages of very precise stimulation without the need for tunneling to place an implanted power supply. Burst stimulation, or subperception stimulation, may be more effective than traditional tonic stimulation in the treatment of many chronic neuropathic pain syndromes. Finally, new devices that allow the placement of neurostimulation electrodes without the use of fluoroscopy will significantly reduce the risk to physicians who perform neurostimulation.

References

1. Shealy NC, Mortimer JT, Reswick JB: Electrical inhibition of pain by stimulation of the dorsal columns. *Anes Analg Curr Res* 46(4):489-491, 1967.
2. Deer TR: Current and future trends in spinal cord stimulation for chronic pain. *Curr Pain Headache Rep* 5(6):503-509, 2001.
3. Bernstein AJ, Peters KM: Expanding indications for neuromodulation. *Urol Clin North Am* 32:59-63, 2005.
4. Levy R, Deer TR, Henderson J: Intracranial neurostimulation for pain control: a review. *Pain Physician* 13(2):157-165, 2010.
5. Deer TR: A critical time for practice change in the pain treatment continuum: we need to reconsider the role of pumps in the treatment algorithm. *Pain Med Editorial* 11(7):987-989, 2010.
6. Personal communication. Oct 2009, Bioness Co.
7. Stewart MR, Winfree CJ: Neurostimulation techniques for painful peripheral nerve disorders. *Neurosurg Clin North Am* 20:111-120, 2009.
8. Ackerman DM et al: Effect of bipolar cuff electrode design on block thresholds in high-frequency electrical neural conduction block. *IEEE Trans Biomed Eng* 17(5):469-476, 2009.
9. Stuart M: Device investors look for gains in pain. *Start Up* Feb 1, 2010.
10. Trentman T et al: Greater occipital nerve stimulation via the BION microstimulator: implantation technique and stimulation parameters. *Pain Phys* 12:621-628, 2009.
11. Burns B, Watkins L, Goadsby PJ: Treatment of hemicrania continua by occipital nerve stimulation with a BION device: long-term follow-up of a crossover study. *Lancet Neurol* 7:1001-1012, 2008.
12. De Ridder D et al: Burst spinal cord stimulation: toward paresthesia-free pain suppression. *Neurosurgery* 66:986-990, 2010.
13. Huntoon M, Burgher AH: Ultrasound-guided permanent implantation of peripheral nerve stimulation (PNS) system for neuropathic pain of the extremities: original cases and outcomes. *Pain Med* 10(8):1369-1377, 2009.

Index

Page numbers followed by *f*, *t*, and *b* indicate
figures, tables, and boxes, respectively.